T0344715

CHRONOPHARMACEUTICS

CHRONOPHARMACEUTICS
Science and Technology for Biological Rhythm-Guided Therapy and Prevention of Diseases

Edited by

BI-BOTTI C. YOUAN

University of Missouri–Kansas City

WILEY

A JOHN WILEY & SONS, INC., PUBLICATION

For general information on our other products and services or for technical support, please contact our Customer Care Department within the United States at (800) 762-2974, outside the United States at (317) 572-3993 or fax (317) 572-4002.

Wiley also publishes its books in a variety of electronic formats. Some content that appears in print may not be available in electronic formats. For more information about Wiley products, visit our web site at www.wiley.com.

ISBN: 978-0-471-74343-9

Library of Congress Cataloging-in-Publication Data is available.

Printed in the United States of America

10 9 8 7 6 5 4 3 2 1

CONTENTS

"We must use time creatively."

— Martin Luther King, Jr. (1929–1968)

v

PREFACE

Chronopharmaceutics is an emerging discipline combining the traditional goal of pharmaceutics (sciences of drug delivery systems) with recent knowledge in different disciplines derived from advances in chronobiology. Basically, the advances in chronobiology and related disciplines have led to a plethora of data demonstrating the extent of generality and precision of biological rhythms that may be used intelligently for the development of novel drug delivery systems, as well as drugs, to optimize their efficacy and safety. Furthermore, advances in genomics and nanobiotechnology provide new horizons in disease therapy and prevention. Hence a convergence of pharmaceutics and modern chronobiology is taking place along with the alignment of concomitantly locally and globally monitored environmental and organismic time structures—chronomes. Chronomics is the most ambitious way of optimizing medicines, and thus health care practices so that maximal therapeutic efficacy is achieved with minimal side effects, and is critical in the treatment of cancer and other diseases.

As a new and evolving discipline, chronopharmaceutics has attracted considerable attention from academia and industry. Over the past several years, various courses and workshops in this area have been offered on many campuses worldwide. At the international level, the American Association of Pharmaceutical Scientists, on my initiative, is one of the first to offer a 2004 sunrise school on the topic of "Chronopharmaceutical drug formulation." Frequent requests for a standard textbook from several scholars and publishers on chronopharmaceutics prompted me to propose the current edited book on chronopharmaceutics. At present, there is no comprehensive textbook available on chronopharmaceutics. The various graduate level courses on this interesting topic are being taught by professors who must gather materials from diverse sources. In the search for an ideal controlled release system for a drug, there is no comprehensive book to bridge the gap between current knowledge in pharmaceutics, usually based on physical chemistry, and chronotherapy for effective and safe drug delivery system design, notably for disease prevention using current advances in chronobiology, chronomics, and chronogenetics. This book is intended to increase awareness and initiate discussion in the pharmaceutical and biomedical communities about the importance of rhythms in us and around us in the early design of a delivery system for treatment and more so for the prevention of diseases. Real challenges remain to be solved for ideally controlled drug release and health, for risk elevation, as well as disease monitoring, based on what is known today. To satisfy this urgent need, we have assembled a group of experienced investigator-educators around the world who are on the frontline of chronogenetics, chronopharmacokinetics, chronopharmacodynamics, and chronopharmaceutical drug delivery research to develop a textbook on chronopharmaceutics. This book and specifically the "chronopharmaceutics" topics are intended to be a "hybrid" of both fields ("controlled drug delivery" and "chronotherapy").

This book is intended for undergraduates in their third and fourth year in college and for first and second year graduate students in biomedical and pharmaceutical sciences, first year medical, veterinary, nursing, and dental students and professionals, and researchers in these fields seeking to update their knowledge in a lifelong learning process.

University of Missouri   BI-BOTTI C. YOUAN
Kansas City, Missouri

ACKNOWLEDGMENTS

The idea to start this book on chronopharmaceutics came from Jonathan T. Rose, Editor, Scientific, Technical, and Medical Division, John Wiley & Sons, and caught me by surprise, when we first met at the 2004 meeting of the American Association of Pharmaceutical Scientists (AAPS) in Baltimore. Probably Jonathan had read our first manuscript on the topic, which shortly after publication became one of the 25 hottest papers in the *Journal of Controlled Release* at that time. Shortly after meeting with Jonathan, I developed a book proposal that was kindly reviewed by international experts in the field: Ronald Siegel (Professor and Head, Department of Pharmaceutics, College of Pharmacy, University of Minnesota), Michael M. Smolensky (Professor of Environmental Physiology, The University of Texas, Health Science Center at Houston, School of Public Health), William J. M. Hrushesky (Norman J. Arnold School of Public Health, W. J. B. Dorn Veterans Affairs Medical Center, Columbia, South Carolina), Andrea Gazzaniga (Professor, Istituto di Chimica Farmaceutica e Tossicologica, Faculty of Pharmacy, University of Milan, Italy), and Bjoern Lemmer (Professor, Institute of Pharmacology and Toxicology, University of Heidelberg, Germany). Their expert insights encouraged me to pursue this project at the early stage. I am also extremely thankful to the editorial board for the time and effort they contributed to this endeavor: Robert Langer (Institute Professor, Department of Chemical Engineering, Massachusetts Institute of Technology, Boston, Massachusetts) and Franz Halberg (Professor and Director, Halberg Chronobiology Center, University of Minnesota)—two pioneers in the area of drug delivery and chronotherapy, respectively. I am also indebted to my UMKC colleague and basic circadian rhythm investigator, Jeffrey Price (Associate Professor, School of Biological Sciences, University of Missouri–Kansas City), for the time taken to review and provide constructive comments on my first draft chapter related to chronobiology.

I am grateful to Jonathan T. Rose (John Wiley & Sons), who has always been there to help and support, and perhaps most importantly, to the team of authors from around the world who contributed to this book and assisted in the peer-review process of each chapter. Among reviewers, special thanks are due to Dr. Elena Losi (Dipartimento Farmaceutico, Universita di Parma) and Dr. John Santini Jr. (President, Microchips, Inc., Bedford, Massachusetts), who unfortunately could not contribute to this book due to other commitments.

I would like to sincerely apologize for the delay in the publication of this book due to several life changing events. My first son (Traby) was born on November 12, 2004 and my second son Bobby on August 15, 2006. These changes were also followed by our relocation from Texas (Texas Tech University) to Missouri (University of Missouri–Kansas City), where I began my new position in October 2006 with several new challenges and adaptation issues, as one could imagine. To my wife (Lou Antoinette) and family, I am eternally grateful for always being patient, even on the days when they hardly saw me during the development of this exciting and provocative project.

BI-BOTTI C. YOUAN

CONTRIBUTORS

DANIEL BAR-SHALOM, Department of Pharmaceutics and Analytical Chemistry, Faculty of Pharmaceutical Sciences, University of Copenhagen, Universitetsparken 2, 2100 Copenhagen Ø, Denmark

BERNARD BRUGUEROLLE, Clinical Pharmacology Department, Timone Hospital, 264 Rue Saint Pierre, 13385 Marseille Cedex 5, France

M. CEREA, Dipartimento di Scienze Farmaceutiche "P. Pratesi", Via G. Colombo 71, 20133 Milano, Italy

MICHAEL CIMA, Department of Materials Science and Engineering, Massachusetts Institute of Technology, 77 Massachusetts Avenue, Cambridge, Massachusetts, 02139 USA

GERMAINE CORŃELISSEN, Halberg Chronobiology Center, University of Minnesota, 420 Delaware Street SE, Mayo Mail Code 8609, Minneapolis, Minnesota 55455 USA

KAREN DANIEL, Department of Chemical Engineering, Massachusetts Institute of Technology, 77 Massachusetts Avenue, Cambridge, Massachusetts 02139 USA

FRANCK DELAUNAY, Centre National de la Recherche Scientifigue, University of Nice–Sophia Antipolis, 28 Avenue Valrose–BP 2135, Grand Chateau, 06000 Nice Cedex 2, France

LIANG C. DONG, ALZA Corporation, 1010 Joaquin Road, P.O. Box 7210, Mountain View, California 94039 USA

HONG LINH HO DUC, Department of Materials Science and Engineering, Massachusetts Institute of Technology, 77 Massachusetts Avenue, Cambridge, Massachusetts 02139 USA

A. GAZZANIGA, Dipartimento di Scienze Farmaceutiche "P. Pratesi", Via G. Colombo 71, 20133 Milano, Italy

STEVEN A. GIANNOS, New Product Development, Chrono Therapeutics, Inc., 7 Lehavre Court, Hamilton, New Jersey 08619 USA

FRANZ HALBERG, Halberg Chronobiology Center, University of Minnesota, 420 Delaware Street SE, Mayo Mail Code 8609, Minneapolis, Minnesota 55455 USA

ROBERT LANGER, Department of Chemical Engineering and Division of Biological Engineering, Massachusetts Institute of Technology, 77 Massachusetts Avenue, Cambridge, Massachusetts 02139 USA

A. MARONI, Dipartimento di Scienze Farmaceutiche "P. Pratesi", Via G. Colombo 71, 20133 Milano, Italy

CRYSTAL POLLOCK-DOVE, ALZA Corporation, 1010 Joaquin Road, P.O. Box 7210, Mountain View, California 94039 USA

M. E. SANGALLI, Dipartimento di Scienze Farmaceutiche "P. Pratesi", Via G. Colombo 71, 20133 Milano, Italy

GOPI VENKATESH, Director of Research & Development, Eurand, Inc., 845 Center Drive, Vandalia, Ohio 45377 USA

OTHILD SCHWARTZKOPFF, Halberg Chronobiology Center, University of Minnesota, 420 Delaware Street SE, Mayo Mail Code 8609, Minneapolis, Minnesota 55455 USA

NEENA WASHINGTON, Strathclyde Institute for Biomedical Sciences, The John Arbuthnott Building, University of Strathclyde, 27 Taylor Street, Glasgow GH ONR, Scotland, UK

CLIVE G. WILSON, Strathclyde Institute for Biomedical Sciences, The John Arbuthnott Building, University of Strathclyde, 27 Taylor Street, Glasgow G4 0NR, Scotland, UK

PATRICK S. L. WONG, ALZA Corporation, 1010 Joaquin Road, P.O. Box 7210, Mountain View, California 94039 USA

BI-BOTTI C. YOUAN, Division of Pharmaceutical Sciences, University of Missouri–Kansas City, 5005 Rockhill Road, Room 108E, Kansas City, Missouri 64114 USA

L. ZEMA, Dipartimento di Scienze Farmaceutiche "P. Pratesi", Via G. Colombo 71, 20133 Milano, Italy

ABBREVIATION LIST

ABPM: Ambulatory blood pressure
ACTH: Adenocorticotropic hormone
AD: Alzheimer disease
AIDS: Acquired immune deficiency syndrome
AMS: Accelerator mass spectroscopy
ANOVA: Analysis of variance
ARNT: Aryl hydrocarbon receptor nuclear translocator
ASA: Acetylsalicylic acid (Aspirin)
5-ASA: 5-Aminosalicylic acid
AUC: Area under the curve
AVP: Arginine vasopressin

bHLH: Basic helix-loop-helix, a that characterizes a family of transcription factors
BCNU: bis-Chloronitrosourea (Carmustine)
BHAT: Beta-Blocker Heart Attack Trial
BIOCOS: BIOsphere in the COSmos
Bmal: Brain and muscle aryl hydrocarbon receptor nuclear translocator (ARNT)-like
BZ: Belousov–Zhabotinsky

cAMP: Cyclic adenosine monophosphate
CCGs: Clock-controlled genes
cDNA: Complementary DNA
CGMS: Continuous glucose monitoring system
CHAT: Circadian hyper-amplitude-tension
ChrDDS: Chronopharmaceutical drug delivery systems
CKIε: Casein kinase Iε
CKIδ: Casein kinase Iδ
CLK: Clock
CODAS: Chronotherapeutic oral drug absorption system
COER: Controlled-onset extended-release
CoQ10: Ubiquinone
CREB: cAMP response element-binding

CRM1: see Exportin 1
CRR: Circadian rhythm release
Cry1: Cryptochrome 1
Cry2: Cryptochrome 2
CUSUMs: Cumulative sums
CYC: Cycle

DBP: D-Element-binding protein
D-CHAT: Diastolic circadian hyper-amplitude tension
DHRV: Decreased heart rate variability
DM1: Diabetes mellitus
DNA: Deoxyribonucleic acid
3DP: Three-dimensional printing

EBM: Evidence-based medicine
E-box: sequence which usually lies upstream of a in a region
ECG: Electrocardiogram
EEGs: Electroencephalograms
EPP: Elevated pulse pressure or excessive pulse pressure
ESS: Error sum of squares
EVA: Ethylene-covinyl acetate polymer
EVAc: Ethylene vinyl acetate copolymer
Exportin 1: CRM1 homolog, also known as XPO1, is a human. The protein encoded by this gene mediates leucine-rich nuclear export signal (NES)-dependent protein transport

FAPS: Familial advance sleep phase syndrome
FDA: U.S. Food and Drug Administration
5-FU: 5-Fluorouracil

GERD: Gastroesophageal reflux disorder
GFP: Green fluorescent protein
GH: Gestational hypertension
GIT: Gastrointestinal tract

GPC: Gel permeation chromatography

GPCR: G-Protein coupled receptor

GSK3β: Glycogen synthase kinase 3β

HALO: Hours after light onset

5-HT: 5-Hydroxytryptamine or serotonin

hGH: Human growth hormone

HIV: Human immunodeficiency virus

HLF: Hepatocyte leukemia factor

HPLC: High-performance liquid chromatography

HPMC: Hydroxypropyl methylcellulose

HPMCP: Hypromellose phthalate

IBD: Inflammatory bowel disease

ICD10: International Classification of Diseases, 10th Revision

ICU: Intensive care unit

IL-2: Interleukin-2

IR: Immediate release

IVIVC: In vitro–in vivo correlations

LC: Lipid clinic

LDL: Low-density lipoprotein

LPs: Lipoperoxides

LSC: Liquid scintillation counter

LVMI: Left ventricular mass index

MAP: Mitogen-activated protein

MAP: Mean arterial pressure

M-CSF: Macrophage colony-stimulating factor

MEMS: Microelectromechanical systems

MESOR: Midline estimating statistic of rhythm

MMC: Migrating myoelectric complex

mRNA: Messenger RNA

NA: Noradrenaline

NCEP ATP III: National Cholesterol Education Panel-Adult Treatment Panel III

NES: Nuclear export sequence

NLSs: Nuclear localization signals

NPAS2: Neuronal PAS domain protein 2

ODT: Orally disintegrating tablet

OROS: Osmotic release oral systems

PAI-1: Plasminogen activator inhibitor-1

PAMPS: Poly(2-acrylamido-2-methyl-1-propanesulfonic acid)

PAR bZIP: A family of proteins that are transcription factors; that is, in response to various signals, they combine to other transcription factors to express a gene. The three members of the PAR bZIP family – DBP, HLF and TEF – are involved in the complex world of circadian rhythms: those physiological rhythms which are regulated according to our 24-hour day

PAS: contained in many signalling proteins where they are used as a signal sensor. It was named after three proteins that it occurs in: Per (period circadian protein), Arnt (aryl hydrocarbon receptor nuclear translator protein) and Sim (single-mined protein).

Pdp1ε: PAR domain protein 1ε

Pdxk: Pyridoxal kinase

PE: Pre-eclampsia

PEG: Polyethylene glycol

PEO: Polyethylene oxide

Per: Period

PGA: Polyglycolic acid

PK2: Prokineticin 2

PK/PD: Pharmacokinetic/pharmacodynamic

PLGA: Poly(D,L-lactic-co-glycolic acid)

PLLA: Poly(L-lactic acid)

PORT: Programmable oral release technologies

PP2A: Protein phosphatase

PTH: Parathyroid hormone

QTL: Quantitative trait loci

Rev-erbα: Also known as NR1D1 (nuclear receptor subfamily 1, group D, member 1), is a member of the Rev-ErbA family of nuclear receptors and is a transcriptional repressor. Rev-erbα is highly expressed in the liver, skeletal muscle, adipose tissue and brain, participating in the development and circadian regulation of these tissues

RNA: Ribonucleic acid

RORα: RAR-related orphan receptor alpha (ROR-alpha), also known as NR1F1 (nuclear receptor subfamily 1, group F, member 1), is a nuclear receptor encoded by the *RORA* (RAR-related orphan receptor A)

SCN: Suprachiasmatic nuclei

SEM: Scanning electron microscopy

SiO2: Silicon dioxide

SIF: Simulated intestinal fluid

SIRT1: Silent mating type information regulation 2 homolog, S. cerevisiae stands for sirtuin (silent mating type information regulation 2 homolog) 1 (*S. cerevisiae*). SIRT1 is an enzyme which deacetylates proteins that contribute to cellular regulation (reaction to stressors, longevity)

STN: Subthalamic nucleus

SITT: Small intestinal transit time

SU4885: Metopirone (metyrapone) is a drug used in the diagnosis of adrenal insufficiency and occasionally in the treatment of Cushing's syndrome (hypercortisolism)

SUMO: Small ubiquitin-related modifier protein

TEF: Thyrotroph embryonic factor

TEPP: Time equivalent process parameter

TETP: Time equivalent thickness parameter

Tim: Timeless, timeout

t-PA: Tissue plasminogen activator

TPR: Timed, pulsatile release

TSR: Timed, sustained release

TSS: Total residual sum of squares

UC: Usual care

UGP: Urinary gonadotropin peptide

USP: United States Pharmacopeia

Vri: Vrille

INTRODUCTION: TIME, DIAGNOSTICS, AND THERAPEUTICS—BEYOND CIRCADIAN MARKER RHYTHM-GUIDED TREATMENT

FRANZ HALBERG, GERMAINE CORNÉLISSEN, and OTHILD SCHWARTZKOPFF

> "Surely... [in all of transdisciplinary science, including therapy] the thing to hunt down is a cycle ... and if found, then above all things, and in whatever manner, lay hold of, study it, record it and see what it means."
> — *Sir J. Norman Lockyer (1836–1920)*

The 2-year survival rate of patients with perioral cancers has been doubled by radiation treatment at the peak of the previously monitored tumor temperature. A risk of stroke greater than that associated with hypertension has been detected by taking time structure into account. Aspirin has been found to have drastically different effects with different timing, and agents acting on the central nervous system show different times of maximal toxicity, (Figure 1). While a treatment guided by the circadian tumor temperature rhythm was documented in 1977 (Refs. 532 and 551 in Ref. 1), periodicity in health was experienced and then known as the change from sleeping to waking to the first organisms that sleep or rest, more or less regularly. Periodicity was known in antiquity, probably as fevers of infectious diseases for millennia. For centuries, epilepsy was described to occur in some patients mostly during waking, in others mostly during sleep, or in still others on awakening (if not diffusely during 24 hours—reviewed in Ref. 26 in Ref. 1). It was hence hardly surprising to find circadian rhythms in the human electroencephalogram in disease by 1952 (Ref. 15 in Ref. 1) and in health in 1966 (Ref. 211 in Ref. 1). A history of Minnesota chronobiology is given in Ref. 2542 of Ref. 1. That noise of a fixed intensity to which mice of susceptible strains were exposed can induce convulsions and death at one circadian stage but not at another was reported

Chronopharmaceutics: Science and Technology for Biological Rhythm-Guided Therapy and Prevention of Diseases, edited by Bi-Botti C. Youan
Copyright © 2009 John Wiley & Sons, Inc.

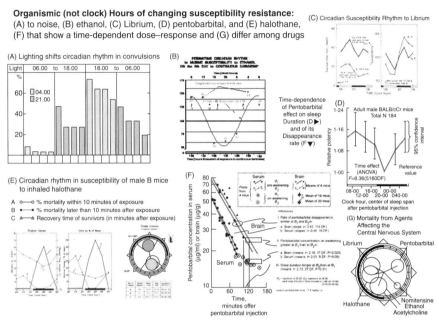

Figure 1. Timing can be as important as dosing, or more so if circadian stage determines the chances of life versus death in response to the same stimuli, as demonstrated for many drugs under the environmental conditions available in a modern laboratory with standardized lighting, environmental temperature and humidity, noise, and odor (while, any associations with magnetic storms that also affect rhythms remain uncontrolled). Part (1A) shows the difference as a function of timing in the response of susceptible mice to noise. On a given lighting scheme (light by day, but not by night), exposure of mice to the ringing of bells at 0800h elicited dashing in very few animals, as seen in the first gray column on the left. Even fewer mice showed clonic or tonic convulsions (the next two columns) and none died (the last column with no entries). By contrast, over 40% of comparable mice of the same susceptible inbred strain exposed to noise in a different stage (at 2100h) dashed, over 20% convulsed, and all of these died from the same stimulus on the same day. The data demonstrate that exposure timing accounted for the difference between life and death in response to the same stimulus. Four days after reversal of the lighting regimen, in addition to an overall elevated susceptibility, there were more rather than fewer deaths at 0800h as compared to exposure at 2100h (Ref. 53 and Ref. 106 in Ref. 1). Part (1B) shows a free-running circadian rhythm in survival after injection every 4 hours of a fixed dose of ethanol to separate groups of comparable mice (Ref. 126 in Ref. 1). Part (1C) (Ref. 137 and 188 in Ref. 1) to (1F) show other circadian toxicity rhythms (Ref. 308 in Ref. 1). A (for us indispensable) point and interval parameter estimation (e.g., by cosinor) is seen in Part (1E) (right) and (1G). For details of the latter, see (Ref. 246 in Ref. 1) [6, 10, 41].

by 1955 (Ref. 53 in Ref. 1) and again in 1958 (Ref. 106 in Ref. 1). The time-varying circadian susceptibility of the nervous system also reveals different phases for the effects of different drugs such as Librium (Ref. 137 in Ref. 1), pentobarbital (Ref. 308 in Ref. 1), nomifensine (Ref. 659 in Ref.1), ethanol (Ref. 110, Ref. 116 and Ref. 126 in Ref. 1), and anesthetics such as halothane (Ref. 188 and Ref. 238 in Ref. 1) and methohexital (Ref. 915 in Ref. 1).

That we are not dealing with a relation to clock-hour [1] was shown not only by the ability to phase-shift rhythms by manipulating the lighting regimen for mice, (Figure 1A) and by changing the sleep–wake schedule for humans (Ref. 107 in Ref. 1), but also by an effect of ethanol that was circadian periodic but free-running with a period close to, but different from, exactly 24 hours in mice kept in continuous darkness, (Figure 1B) (Ref. 126 in Ref. 1). Also in 1958, the effect of ouabain was found to be circadian stage dependent (Ref. 110 and Ref. 119 in Ref. 1). In 1964 (Ref. 188 & Ref. 238 in Ref. 1), the susceptibility resistance cycle to halothane had been extensively documented, to be followed by studies reviewed by Chassard et al. [2]. A circadian rhythm in an experimental oncological therapeutic index appeared in 1973 (Ref. 316 in Ref. 1).

Notwithstanding a mountain of evidence provided from many quarters in this book, indications of timing the use of physical agents [1], drugs [1–7], nutriceuticals [6, 8], or food [4, 9] as yet are missing in their scheduling (e.g., on package inserts or labeling). This undesirable status quo [10] may be due to a central idea in physiology, as also recently noted by Chassard et al. [2] under the title "Timing Is Everything." For too many, nothing in biology makes sense except in the light of homeostasis [11; cf. 12], a concept often used as an excuse to ignore time structures mistakenly assumed to be negligible. A deus ex machina keeps us in a theoretical steady state and, for treatment, leads to what Arthur Jores [13] called "the idiocy of 'three times a day.'" On the left of Figure 2, we resign ourselves, as the aging Claude Bernard [12] did, to assume a relative constancy of the internal environment: homeostasis, which, whether explicit or implied, leads to the treatment of a presumably "true" yet really imaginary steady state, such as a "true" blood pressure or a "true" blood cell count or a "true" hormone level. Alejandro Zaffaroni [14], the original developer of novel drug delivery systems intended for chronotherapy, received his inspiration from his work on steroids, and abandoned "4 tablets a day." Homeostasis can lead to blunders in interpretations of "stress" or "allergy", (Figure 3) and thus to erroneous or incomplete diagnoses and unwarranted treatments. When two groups differ only in the phase of a rhythm (Figure 3) or in its frequency, depending on the time when the groups happen to be compared, one can then encounter large differences in opposite directions, to falsely advocate either (unwarranted) substitution treatment or the removal of (a nonexistent) excess by an inhibitory drug or surgery [15].

Before the era of institutional review boards, endocrine glands were, in good faith but indiscriminately, removed from various kinds of patients simply based on homeostatic ideas underlying research. Alternatively, in this age of computerized data collection and analysis and of programmable pumps, we can do

Figure 2. Let us turn from an imaginary master clock serving an equally imaginary constancy, to an integrative internal–external collateral hierarchy for physiological–environmental coordination. Homeostasis postulates (and laboratory medicine today implements the idea) that physiological processes remain largely within a certain range in health and seeks departures from such "normal values" to diagnose overt disease. Thus, variability within the normal range is often dealt with as if it were narrow, random, and trivial—the body striving for at least a relative "constancy." This status quo (on the left of this figure) should be (but without action by chronomics, as yet is not) improved by learning about a "biological clock" that somehow enables the body to keep track of time. In fact, by removal and replacement experiments, a mechanism was located first in the adrenal and thereafter in the broader pineal–hypothalamic–pituitary–adrenal network [1] and was shown to be responsible for some but not for other circadians that persisted after brain ablation, but all were altered after these procedures. Single cells and even bacteria are genetically coded for a spectrum of rhythmic variation, as are mammalian liver cells. These facts indicate that the concept of a "clock" needs extension, as do biological calendars, when we find biological years longer than a calendar year and recognize, among others, a biological week, an about 0.42 year and a biological decade or two or those in us, and find other new rules in biological variability, such as deterministic chaos and long-known trends, some of which may turn out to be cycles with longer and longer periods. When the giant alga *Acetabularia acetabulum*, a prominent model of a circadian "clock", is placed in continuous light, its spectrum of electrical activity reveals, after signal averaging, the largest amplitude for a component of about 1 week rather than 1 day. When 14 years of studies on this alga are pooled, a cycle slightly but statistically significantly longer than a calendar year, a transyear and an about 10-year cycle, among others, emerge in the data set as a whole and in other data covering decades. The alignment of spectral components and chaos and trends in and around us has also begun (right). Long-term longitudinal, but not yet entire lifetime, monitoring of critical variables complements current linked cross-sectional (hybrid) reference values required for preventive health and environmental care. Changes occurring within the usual value range, as increasingly longer cycles, resolvable as chronomes with a (predictable multifrequency) rhythmic element, allow us to measure the dynamics of everyday life, in order to obtain warnings before the onset of disease, so that prophylactic measures can be introduced in a timely manner. Thus, we find heretofore undetected or largely unquantified, sometimes harmful, environmental effects, all information for timely and timed treatment. The abstract idealized presentation of the sector structure in the interplanetary magnetic field, shown on the top right, consists of three visible arrows, the fourth being covered by a sketch of irregular solar flares, with parameters that are much more variable than originally visualized. Associations between helio- and geomagnetic variability on the one hand and, on the other, of vital signs in health or cardiac arrhythmia, myocardial infarction, stroke and sudden cardiac death are accumulating: they are just the tip of the iceberg, with a highly significant effect of magnetism (recognized by Gilbert in 1600), apparent in the human electrocardiogram in health and disease. In external–internal interactions, a broad spectrum of rhythms (both in the environment and in living matter) organizes deterministic and other chaos and trends. Trends pursued long enough may become low-frequency cycles (e.g., for the detection of any increased risk) so that timely preventive action may be taken (see Figure 6).

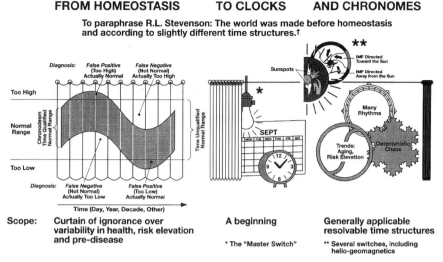

FROM HOMEOSTASIS   TO CLOCKS   AND CHRONOMES

To paraphrase R.L. Stevenson: The world was made before homeostasis and according to slightly different time structures.†

Scope: **Curtain of ignorance over variability in health, risk elevation and pre-disease**   **A beginning**   **Generally applicable resolvable time structures**

* The "Master Switch"   ** Several switches, including helio-geomagnetics

† Inferential statistical methods map chronomes as molecular biology maps genomes; biologic chronomes await resolution of their interactions in us and around us, e.g., with magnetic storms in the interplanetary magnetic field (IMF).

something about recording and analyzing changes in the usual range and about treating accordingly. When asked, the younger Bernard identified as one of his two major discoveries "the extreme variability of the internal environment" [16; cf. 17]. Rhythms and broader time structures, or chronomes [18–22], also consisting of trends when the time series are long enough, and of probabilistic and other chaos when the data are dense enough, are a fact of life, and there are many of them, not only circadians [18–22]. Mapping them all, and eventually correcting their alterations, requires a concerted international effort, a mapping of the chronome project, an endeavor exceeding the scope of mapping genomes. This task can now be implemented to pursue, with prevention in mind, the diagnosis and treatment of conditions such as disorders of variabilities (not only putative "levels") of blood pressure, heart rate, and glycemia [23, 24], among many others, a task not achieved by computing day–night ratios, which latter do not separately assess changes in amplitude and phase and limit one's perspective to only one confounded aspect of circadian systems [25, 26].

Beyond biological clocks and calendars, shown in the middle of Figure 2, chronome elements are shown on the right side of this figure and new and old spectral components are on the bottom right of Figure 4. There, we introduce reciprocal periods in and around us, pertinent to those interested in diseases and threats not only of individuals but also of societies, nations, and ecosystems, and more broadly the environment near and far. We need to recognize and assess these many rhythms in their own right, both in individuals and in populations. For instance, the mapping of circadecadals (Figure 5), has to be considered in seeking indications for hormone replacement therapy [18]. Blunders at many other periods, τ, as in the case of circadians, could be avoided as soon as we knew what to spotcheck with a few strategically placed samples in already mapped rhythms. Unless we sample for a lifetime, and such monitoring is already done for very many thousands of patients with diabetes and should be done in blood pressure disorders, we may as a rule deal with a situation wherein the observation span, T, is much shorter than a decadal and/or many other infradian τ's. We had then better consult maps or prepare them when as yet they are unavailable. There is also a much more important perspective. Some of these periodicities characterize the presumed good and bad: religious motivation, crime and war bear signatures of our cosmos that we can also find in individuals [19–22]. A focus on global diseases is the greatest challenge for industry: by some means we have to shield from or compensate for magnetic effects, as we do already with heating and air conditioning once the still hidden environmental factors underlying mass psychoses are clarified.

Chronome mapping may seem complex and utopian at first, like the building of roads in an unknown terrain or the suggestion to take to the air. But in

---

$\blacktriangleright$

Figure 3. Neglect of timing can lead to inexcusable blunders that were avoided in Minnesota, where they led to chronobiology, and can be avoided everywhere. (A) Eosinophil counts seemingly (but only apparently; see below) lowered by "fasting" and/ or "stress." Effect of a 50% reduction in dietary carbohydrates and fats (with proteins, vitamins, and minerals as in control group) in C_3H mice with a high breast cancer incidence, which is greatly lowered by a diet reduced in calories (not here shown). Is an adrenocortical activation, then assessed by eosinophil depression (as an internal bioassay, in the absence at that time of a chemical assay) *the* answer for treating breast cancer and for prolonging life? It seemed to be an exciting finding at first. Steroids that depress eosinophil cell counts and depress mitoses could be a mechanism through which caloric restriction (and ovariectomy, also done on the calorie-restricted mice) acts in greatly reducing cancer incidence. This seemed to be *the mechanism* to prevent breast cancer, or was this very reasonable and plausible hypothesis a premature extrapolation? (The senior author's chief had taken these results as a statistically significant (and to that extent validated), most promising result to a conference in Paris.) But once the difference in eosinophil count between two groups of mice was found, we attempted to replicate it, because of the importance of its findings to the etiology of cancer, using a larger group of animals, and started earlier in the day. (B) One week later, a follow-up with more animals starting at an earlier clock-hour shows "no difference." By then, a phase difference between the two groups was one explanation for the fact that the large intergroup difference in eosinophil count seen in (A) was not replicated in (B) when more animals were used with an earlier start, as shown in (C). (C) An opposite outcome was observed 1 week later, with a still earlier start: the (without periodicity meaningless) "*stress*" in (A) had become an equally spurious "*allergy*" in (C). Erroneous conclusions concerning therapy result from ignoring in diagnosis a circadian (or other) difference between the timing of rhythms due to differences in their synchronization. This is shown by results from added sampling on the same day, with a validation of a difference in the opposite direction as compared to the difference observed first in (A), as seen in (D) with data and theoretically in (E).

Confusing results, that could wrongly be interpreted as "stress" or "allergy", are accounted for by the action of food (offered mornings) and light as competing synchronizers of circulating eosinophils in C_3H mice with high breast cancer incidence that can be drastically reduced by calorie restriction

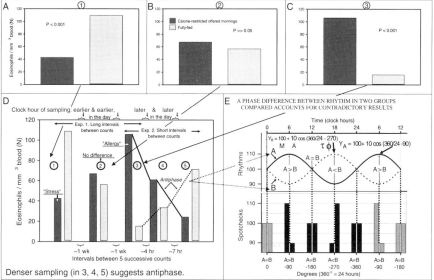

www.JCircadianRhythms.com/content/pdf/1740-3391/1/2.pdf (Halberg F. et al., 2003)

building highways or airplanes to bridge distances, it must be kept in mind that once the roads or the planes are available, they must not be built over and over again for each trip. Users may pay taxes, pay a toll, or buy a ticket. This is what the BIOCOS project is all about, aiming at collecting reference standards that are complex and costly [22]. The new available reference database, used in the interim, will have to be augmented and improved by further work. In science and health care, the introduction of maps about timing means changing a status quo, described by a journal editor in a spontaneous note as "flying blind" [27], and is a raison d'être of any book considering the use of time structures in diagnosis and treatment. To illustrate this need, we refer to the opportunity of dealing with blood pressure and heart rate variabilities [23, 28].

Soon, diagnosis and treatment on repeated yet single blood pressure measurements will be recognized as tunnel vision (which of course is immensely superior to "flying blind" most of the time in the absence of systematically repeated measurements and their chronobiologic interpretation). An about 24-hour profile-based diagnosis and treatment will be identified as bitemporal hemianopsia; albeit much superior to tunnel vision, it is still unsafe in cases of variability disorders (Figure 6), in view of day-to-day variability and rhythms with longer than 24-hour periods, some longer than a year. The circadian and circannual rhythm-based approach (Figure 2 middle), will in time be replaced by continuous chronomically (time structurally) interpreted as-one-goes surveillance with

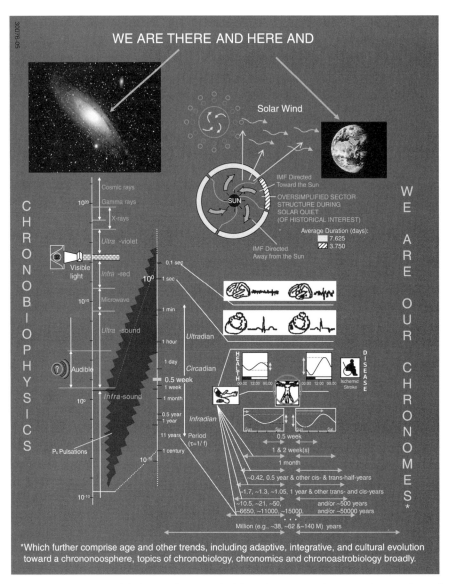

Figure 4. Chronoastrobiology strives to elucidate the past and present integration of organisms into their largely wavy environment. Reciprocal periods in the chronomes of variables in us and around us came about by the eventual genetic coding of the latter in the former. Internal–external interactions await further exploration in health care, notably for stroke prevention in individuals and for the prevention of war, crime, and other diseases of societies and nations. (*See color insert.*)

Contradictory Correlations of Hormonal Metabolites with Age (I, II, IV - 5 of them) or with
Solar Activtiy (V - 5 of them) Stem in part from a Common Years-Long Cycle (III, IV, VI)

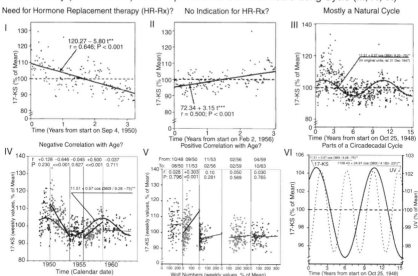

Figure 5. Variabilities along the scale of decades, a confusing source of variation if ignored, can become a new, quantified reference value [18].

sequential testing [29] and parameter tests [30], interpreted in the light of maps, many of them yet to be built and those available yet to be perfected.

Once continuous monitoring is implemented, we can immediately introduce into everyday practice procedures that have become sine qua non in research, including *P*-values and uncertainty estimates in the form of 95% confidence and tolerance or prediction intervals [31, 32]. Today, we can diagnose prehypertension and other increased risks as variability disorders (Figure 6), and can treat them at times of pertinence rather than convenience. We can check the effects of treatment prescribed systematically by sequential tests, in dealing already with prehypertension, with prediabetes and, after more homework is done down the line, with preobesity, eventually to nip a premetabolic syndrome in the bud.

Those who take into account a broader-than-clock-hour and calendar-date-based timing according to time structures can make a big contribution. A bit of attention to the role played by the cosmos (Figure 4) cannot hurt and may help. We can manipulate (treat the amplitude of) a transyear component of blood pressure statistically significantly different from a calendar year, thanks to a contribution by Yoshihiko Watanabe and co-workers [33]. It appears that transyears, at least in sudden cardiac death, are geographic (magnetic) site specific and we have much more to learn [34, 35]. We certainly do not wish to rely only on spotchecks at long intervals and in so doing ignore any variablity disorders and their contributions as vascular variablity syndromes, VVS

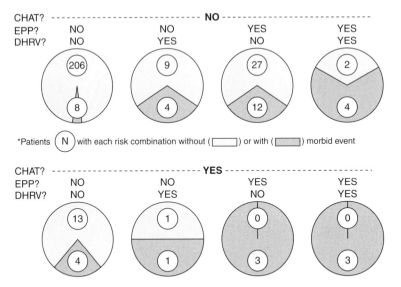

Decreased Heart Rate Variability (DHRV), Circadian Hyper Amplitude Tension (CHAT) and Elevated Pulse Pressure (EPP) are Separate Cardiovascular Disease Risks*

*Patients (N) with each risk combination without (☐) or with (▬) morbid event

*Results from 6-year prospective study on 297 (adding all N's) patients classified by 3 risks (8 circles), supported by findings on total of 2,807 subjects for total of over 160,769 sets of blood pressure and heart rate measurements.   Data from K Otsuka.

Figure 6. Abnormalities in the variability of blood pressure and heart rate, impossible to find in a conventional office visit (the latter aiming at the fiction of a "true" blood pressure), can raise cardiovascular disease risk in the next 6 years from <4% to 100%. As compared to an acceptable variability, the relative vascular disease risk associated with a circadian hyperamplitude tension (CHAT), a decreased circadian heart rate variability (DHRV), and/or an around-the-clock elevated pulse pressure (EPP) is greatly and statistically significantly increased. These silent risks are very great, even in the absence of hypertension. They can often be reversed, notably the risk of CHAT, by a nondrug (relaxation) or drug (specified in timing as well as in kind and dose) approach; and the need for intervention can be found when it occurs by the combination of a closed-loop diagnostic and therapeutic system for chronotheranostics [28]. (See Chapter 11 in this volume.) (*See color insert.*)

(Figure 6). Thirty years ago, hoping that a time structure assessing (chronome-assessing) medicine would eventually come into its own, one of us wrote [5; cf. 4]:

Once the feasibility of manipulating a rhythm's timing and preferably also its amplitude has been demonstrated for a majority of individuals in a population, the procedure may be carried out without individual validation of the specific timing. However, whenever such procedures [for deciding on a timing] are unavailable and individuals differ from each other in terms of the timing of their susceptibility rhythms, sensitivity tests will have to be developed for the given individual by the use of his own markers—say, for bone-marrow depression … in the case of certain chemotherapeutic [and for blood pressure lowering in the case of antihypertensive agents]. These markers will then have to be monitored in close cooperation with the patient and the data thus obtained will have to be analyzed by special techniques. These should allow the identification, inter alia, of individualized acrophases, when the latter correspond to orthophases, while other methods are needed to define the optimal treatment time(s) whenever the acrophase differs from the orthophase.

By 1973, the gains from chronochemotherapy with a sinusoidal pattern, including an improvement of therapeutic index by timing, could be shown in the laboratory. Recently, the optimization of timing nutriceuticals was started with ubiquinone (Q-Gel) [8]. In 1991, Bakken and Heruth [36] cited studies carried out with their then-modern instrumentation that objectively revealed an improved outcome from cyclosporine infused in a circadian sinusoidal pattern versus a constant rate [37; cf. Chapter 11 in this Volume]. A pump (and any treatment more broadly) has to be scheduled by clock-hour. Such scheduling has been a boost to chronotherapy and has worked [38], albeit not invariably [39]. Half a century ago, the manipulability of optimal timing was reviewed [4; cf. 40]. Using circadian and circaseptan rhythms in cancer markers [41, 42], such as CA125 or preferably CA130, to guide treatment, e.g. of ovarian cancer, is a desired individualized alternative to a specification only of clock-hour for all comers [6] and has added years to a cancer patient's survival [43], but as yet is costly and will remain so until its merit further is documented, another challenge for the cooperation of clinicians with industry.

While suggestions made in 1975 and 1991 remain pertinent in 2009, there are now also new diagnostics of disorders of the young Bernard's "extreme variability" for the care, among others, of an above-peer-threshold circadian amplitude of blood pressure and a below-peer-threshold circadian standard deviation of heart rate (Figure 6).

Our editor's thorough review of the background to what he dubs "chronopharmaceutics" rightly raises the question of clinical relevance [44]. Individualized timeliness and timing are obviously needed in support of the promise of chronopharmaceuticals and of corresponding drug delivery systems. In an era of major concerns about the epidemic of obesity and a metabolic syndrome, we learned already that prehypertension [45, 46] and prediabetes [47, 48] may be detected as CHAT. There are also technologies for closing the loop between time structure-based monitoring and analyses for both early diagnosis of elevated risk before actual disease and then timely and timed treatment, with procedures to assess the uncertainties of what is done in individualized practice rather than only in research on groups (See Chapter 11 in this volume). We need not respond only to the values at a given moment, like blood sugar or blood pressure values. When risks higher than those of hypertension are found in variability and when such conditions are documented worldwide [23], as in the case of blood pressure overswinging, there is no safe alternative but to take the broader time structure into account in a budding chronotheranostics (See Chapter 11 in this volume). Figure 7 should convince any reader with high blood pressure that the treatment he or she receives needs to be individualized. We must try not to fly blind [27].

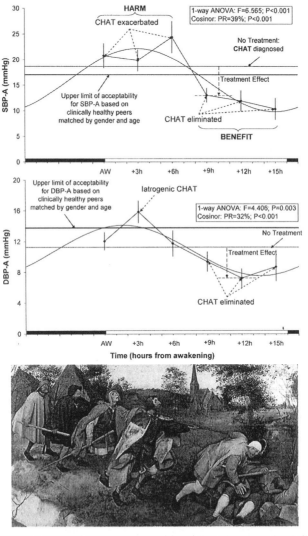

Treatment Beneficial at Certain Other Times (9, 12 or 15 hours after awakening) can EXACERBATE a Pre-existing CHAT in Systolic Blood Pressure (SBP) and INDUCE CHAT in Diastolic Blood Pressure (DBP) when Given at the Wrong Time in Patient Su *

* Su, M, 66y, treated with Losartan (50 mg) and hydrochlorothiazide (12.5 mg). Each point represents 1 week of half-hourly around-the-clock monitoring after ~1 month on a given treatment time.

Figure 7. Monitoring of blood pressure for treatment validation and optimization is not a luxury when, as shown on top and in the middle of this figure, the same currently popular drug Hyzaar can do harm in a patient, Su in the morning, but is beneficial when taken in the same dose by the same person in the evening some weeks later, in each case for ~ 1 month with the blood pressure monitored for the last week, as described in detail by Prof. Watanabe (49). Medication was changed systematically, on a usual routine of living with diurnal activity and nocturnal rest. In the morning the medication raised the circadian amplitude of blood pressure to an extent of exacerbating or inducing a circadian overswing or CHAT, a risk greater than a high blood pressure, whereas at another time it lowered both the circadian amplitude and MESOR, eliminating all abnormality, and thus offered benefit. The painting at the bottom by Pieter Brueghel, "The Parable of the Blind Leading the Blind", is reproduced by kind permission of the Fototeca della Soprintendenza of the BAS PSAE and of the Polo Museale of the City of Naples, in order to emphasize that CHAT is silent to both the caregiver acting on the basis of a conventionally interpreted (chronobiologically uninterpreted) 24-hour blood pressure as well as to the majority of providers treating on the basis of single measurements in their office. © Halberg.

REFERENCES

1. Bibliography of Franz Halberg. Available at http://www.msi.umn.edu/~halberg/.

2. Chassard D, Allaouchiche B, Boselli E. Timing is everything: the pendulum swings on. *Anesthesiology*. 2005; 103: 454–456.

3. Zaffaroni A. New approaches to drug administration. In: *Abstracts, 31st International Congress on Pharmaceutical Science*, September 7–12, 1971, Washington DC, pp. 19–20. Zaffaroni A. Therapeutic implications of controlled drug delivery. In: *Proceedings of the 6th International Congress of Pharmacology*, Forssan Kirjapaine Oy, Helsinki, Finland, 1975; vol. 5, pp. 53–61.

4. Halberg F. Protection by timing treatment according to bodily rhythms: an analogy to protection by scrubbing before surgery. *Chronobiologia*. 1974; 1(suppl. 1): 27–68.

5. Halberg F. When to treat. *Haematologica (Pavia)*. 1975; 60: 1–30.

6. Halberg F, Cornélissen G, Wang ZR, Wan C, Ulmer W, Katinas G, Singh R, Singh RK, Singh R, Gupta BD, Singh RB, Kumar A, Kanabrocki E, Sothern RB, Rao G, Bhatt MLBD, Srivastava M, Rai G, Singh S, Pati AK, Nath P, Halberg Francine, Halberg J, Schwartzkopff O, Bakken E, Shastri VK. Chronomics: circadian and circaseptan timing of radiotherapy, drugs, calories, perhaps nutriceuticals and beyond. *J Exp Ther Oncol*. 2003; 3: 223–260.

7. Carandente A, Halberg F. Drug industry and chronobiology: achievements and prospects. *Ann NY Acad Sci*. 1991; 618: 484–489.

8. Cornélissen G, Halberg F, Schwartzkopff O, Gvozdjakova A, Siegelova J, Fiser B, Dusek J, Mifkova L, Chopra RK, Singh RB. Coenzyme-Q10 effect on blood pressure variability assessed with a chronobiological study design. Abstract. In: *Noninvasive Methods in Cardiology*, Brno, Czech Republic, September 14, 2005; p 10.

9. Halberg F, Haus E, Cornélissen G. From biologic rhythms to chronomes relevant for nutrition. In: Marriott BM, ed. *Not Eating Enough: Overcoming Underconsumption of*

Military Operational Rations. Washington DC: National Academy Press; 1995: 361–372. http://books.nap.edu/books/0309053412/html/361.html#pagetop.

10. Kiser K. Father time. *Minnesota Med.* 2005(Nov); 26–29: 42–43.

11. Cannon WB. The Wisdom of the Body. New York: WW Norton; 1932: 312 pp.

12. Bernard C. *Leçons sur les phénomènes de la vie communs aux animaux et aux végétaux.* Paris: JB Bailliere; 1885.

13. Jores A. 3mal täglich. *Hippokrates (Stutt).* 1939; 10: 1185–1188.

14. Zaffaroni A. Overview and evolution of therapeutic systems. *Ann NY Acad Sci.* 1991; 618: 405–421.

15. Halberg F, Cornelissen G, Katinas G, Syutkina EV, Sothern RB, Zaslavskaya R, Halberg F, Watanabe Y, Schwartzkopff O, Otsuka K, Tarquini R, Perfetto P, Siegelova J. Transdisciplinary unifying implications of circadian findings in the 1950s. *J Circadian Rhythms.* 2003; 1: 2. Available at www.JCircadianRhythms.com/content/pdf/1740-3391/1/2.pdf.

16. Bernard C. De la diversité des animaux soumis à l'expérimentation. De la variabilité des conditions organiques dans lesquelles ils s'offrent à l'expérimentateur. *J Anat Physiol Normales Pathol L'Homme Animaux.* 1865; 2: 497–506.

17. Halberg F. Claude Bernard, referring to an "extreme variability of the internal milieu." In: Grande F, Visscher MB, eds. *Claude Bernard and Experimental Medicine.* Cambridge, MA: Schenkman; 1967: 193–210.

18. Halberg F, Cornélissen G, Watanabe Y, Otsuka K, Fiser B, Siegelova J, Mazankova V, Maggioni C, Sothern RB, Katinas GS, Syutkina EV, Burioka N, Schwartzkopff O. Near 10-year and longer periods modulate circadians: intersecting anti-aging and chronoastrobiological research. *J Gerontol A Biol Sci Med Sci.* 2001; 56: M304–M324.

19. Halberg F, Cornélissen G, Otsuka K, Schwartzkopff O, Halberg J, Bakken EE. Chronomics. *Biomed and Pharmacother.* 2001; 55(suppl 1): 153–190.

20. Halberg F, Cornélissen G, Schack B, Wendt HW, Minne H, Sothern RB, Watanabe Y, Katinas G, Otsuka K, Bakken EE. Blood pressure self-surveillance for health also reflects 1.3-year Richardson solar wind variation: spin-off from chronomics. *Biomed Pharmacother.* 2003; 57(suppl 1): 58s–76s.

21. Halberg F, Cornélissen G, Regal P, Otsuka K, Wang ZR, Katinas GS, Siegelova J, Homolka P, Prikryl P, Chibisov SM, Holley DC, Wendt HW, Bingham C, Palm SL, Sonkowsky RP, Sothern RB, Pales E, Mikulecky M, Tarquini R, Perfetto F, Salti R, Maggioni C, Jozsa R, Konradov AA, Kharlitskaya EV, Revilla M, Wan CM, Herold M, Syutkina EV, Masalov AV, Faraone P, Singh RB, Singh RK, Kumar A, Singh R, Sundaram S, Sarabandi T, Pantaleoni GC, Watanabe Y, Kumagai Y, Gubin D, Uezono K, Olah A, Borer K, Kanabrocki EA, Bathina S, Haus E, Hillman D, Schwartzkopff O, Bakken EE, Zeman M. Chronoastrobiology: proposal, nine conferences, heliogeomagnetics, transyears, near-weeks, near-decades, phylogenetic and ontogenetic memories. *Biomed Pharmacother.* 2004; 58(suppl 1): S150–S187.

22. Halberg F, Cornélissen G, Katinas G, Tvildiani L, Gigolashvili M, Janashia K, Toba T, Revilla M, Regal P, Sothern RB, Wendt HW, Wang ZR, Zeman M, Jozsa R, Singh RB, Mitsutake G, Chibisov SM, Lee J, Holley D, Holte JE, Sonkowsky RP, Schwartzkopff O, Delmore P, Otsuka K, Bakken EE, Czaplicki J, International BIOCOS Group. Part I. Chronobiology's progress: season's appreciations

2004–2005. Time-, frequency-, phase-, variable-, individual-, age- and site-specific chronomics. *J Applied Biomed.* 2006; 4: 1–38.

23. Cornélissen G, Delcourt A, Toussaint G, Otsuka K, Watanabe Y, Siegelova J, Fiser B, Dusek J, Homolka P, Singh RB, Kumar A, Singh RK, Sanchez S, Gonzalez C, Holley D, Sundaram B, Zhao Z, Tomlinson B, Fok B, Zeman M, Dulkova K, Halberg F. Opportunity of detecting pre-hypertension: worldwide data on blood pressure overswinging. *Biomed Pharmacother.* 2005; 59(suppl 1): S152–S157.

24. Sanchez de la Pena S, Gonzalez C, Cornélissen G, Halberg F. Blood pressure (BP), heart rate (HR) and non-insulin-dependent diabetes mellitus (NIDDM) chrono-biology. Abstract S8-06, 3rd Int Congress on Cardiovascular Disease, Taipei, Taiwan, November 26–28, 2004. *Int J Cardiol.* 2004; 97 (suppl 2): S14.

25. Cornélissen G, Otsuka K, Chen C-H, Kumagai Y, Watanabe Y, Halberg F, Siegelova J, Dusek J. Nonlinear relation of the circadian blood pressure amplitude to cardiovascular disease risk. *Scripta Med. (Brno).* 2000; 73: 85–94.

26. Bingham C, Cornélissen G, Chen C-H, Halberg F. Chronobiology works when day–night ratios fail in assessing cardiovascular disease risk from blood pressure profiles. Abstract. In: *III International Conference, Civilization diseases in the spirit of V. I. Vernadsky*, People's Friendship University of Russia, Moscow, October 10–12, 2005, pp. 111–113.

27. Fossel M. Editor's note [to Halberg F, Cornélissen G, Halberg J, Fink H, Chen C-H, Otsuka K, Watanabe Y, Kumagai Y, Syutkina EV, Kawasaki T, Uezono K, Zhao ZY, Schwartzkopff O. Circadian hyper-amplitude-tension, CHAT: a disease risk syndrome of anti-aging medicine. *J Anti-Aging Med* 1998; 1: 239–251]. *J Anti-Aging Med* 1998;1: 239.

28. Cornélissen G, Halberg F, Bakken EE, Singh RB, Otsuka K, Tomlinson B, Delcourt A, Toussaint G, Bathina S, Schwartzkopff O, Wang ZR, Tarquini R, Perfetto F, Pantaleoni GC, Jozsa R, Delmore PA. Nolley E. 100 or 30 years after Janeway or Bartter, Healthwatch helps avoid "flying blind." *Biomed Pharmacother.* 2004; 58(suppl 1): S69–S86.

29. Hawkins DM. Self-starting CUSUM charts for location and scale. *The Statistician.* 1987; 36: 299–315.

30. Bingham C, Arbogast B, Cornélissen-Guillaume G, Lee JK, Halberg F. Inferential statistical methods for estimating and comparing cosinor parameters. *Chronobiologia.* 1982; 9: 397–439.

31. Halberg F, Lee JK, Nelson WL. Time-qualified reference intervals—chronodesms. *Experientia (Basel).* 1978; 34: 713–716.

32. Nelson W, Cornélissen G, Hinkley D, Bingham C, Halberg F. Construction of rhythm-specified reference intervals and regions, with emphasis on "hybrid" data, illustrated for plasma cortisol. *Chronobiologia.* 1983; 10: 179–193.

33. Watanabe Y, Cornélissen G, Watanabe F, Siegelova J, Dusek J, Halberg F. The trans- (~1.3) year in the blood pressure of a 10-year-old boy. Abstract 17. In: *MEFA*, Brno, Czech Republic, November 04–07, 2003; p 22.

34. Halberg F, Cornélissen G, Otsuka K, Fiser B, Mitsutake G, Wendt HW, Johnson P, Gigolashvili M, Breus T, Sonkowsky R, Chibisov SM, Katinas G, Siegelova J, Dusek J, Singh RB, Berri BL, Schwartzkopff O. Incidence of sudden cardiac death, myocardial infarction and far- and near-transyears. *Biomed Pharmacother.* 2005; 59(suppl 1): S239–S261.

35. Halberg F, Johnson EA, Nelson W, Runge W, Sothern R. Autorhythmometry-procedures for physiologic self-measurements and their analysis. *Physiol Teacher*. 1972; 1: 1–11.

36. Bakken EE, Heruth K. Temporal control of drugs: an engineering perspective. *Ann NY Acad Sci*. 1991; 618: 422–427.

37. Cavallini M, Halberg F, Cornélissen G, Enrichens F, Margarit C. Organ transplantation and broader chronotherapy with implantable pump and computer programs for marker rhythm assessment. *J Control Release*. 1986; 3: 3–13.

38. Levi F. From circadian rhythms to cancer chronotherapeutics. *Chronobiol Int*. 2002; 19(1): 1–19.

39. Hrushesky W, Wood P, Levi F, Roemeling Rv, Bjarnason G, Focan C, Meier K, Cornélissen G, Halberg F. A recent illustration of some essentials of circadian chronotherapy study design [letter]. *J Clin Oncol* 2004; 22: 2971–2972.

40. Nagayama H, Cornélissen G, Pandi-Perumal SR, Halberg F. *Time-dependent psychotropic drug effects: hints of pharmacochronomics, broader than circadian time structures*. In: Lader M, Cardinali DP, Pandi-Perumal SP, eds. *Sleep and Sleep Disorders: A Neuropsychopharmacological Approach*. Georgetown, TX: Landes Bioscience; 2005; 34–71.

41. Halberg F, Cornélissen G, Bingham C, Fujii S, Halberg E. From experimental units to unique experiments: chronobiologic pilots complement large trials. *In Vivo*. 1992; 6: 403–428.

42. Halberg F. The week in phylogeny and ontogeny: opportunities for oncology. *In vivo*. 1995; 9: 269–278.

43. Kennedy BJ. A lady and chronobiology. *Chronobiologia*. 1993; 20: 139–144.

44. Youan BBC. Chronopharmacotherapeutics: gimmick or clinically relevant approach to drug delivery? *J Control Release*. 2004; 98: 337–353.

45. Halberg F, Cornélissen G, Halberg J, Schwartzkopff O. Pre-hypertensive and other variabilities also await treatment. *Am J Medicine*, 2007; 120: e19–e20.

46. Cornélissen G, Halberg F, Beaty L, Kumagai Y, Halberg E, Halberg J, Lee J, Schwartzkopff O, Otsuka K. Cugini's syndrome in statu nascendi: Oratio contra morem prevalentem et pro chronobiologica ratione ad pressione sanguinis curandam. *La Clinica Terapeutica*, in press.

47. Sanchez de la Pena S, Gonzalez C, Cornélissen G, Halberg F. Blood pressure (BP), heart rate (HR) and non-insulin-dependent diabetes mellitus (NIDDM) chronobiology. Abstract S8-06, 3rd Int Congress on Cardiovascular Disease, Taipei, Taiwan, 26–28 Nov 2004. *Int J Cardiol*. 2004; 97 (Suppl 2): S14.

48. Gupta AK, Greenway FL, Cornélissen G, Pan W, Halberg F. Prediabetes is associated with abnormal circadian blood pressure variability. *J Human Hypertension*. 2008; 22: 627–633.

49. Watanabe Y, Cornélissen G, Halberg F, Beaty L, Siegelova J, Otsuka K, Bakken EE. Harm vs. benefit from losartan with hydrochlorothiazide at different circadian times in MESOR-hypertension or CHAT. In: Halberg F, Kenner T, Fiser B, Siegelova J, eds. Proceedings, Noninvasive Methods in Cardiology, Brno, Czech Republic, October 4–7, 2008. p. 149–167. Proceedings volume downloadable free of charge from http://web.fnusa.cz/files/kfdr2008/sbornik_2008.pdf.

CHAPTER 1

OVERVIEW OF CHRONOPHARMACEUTICS

BI-BOTTI C. YOUAN

"To every thing there is a season, and a time to every purpose under the heaven."
— *Ecclesiastes 3:1.*

CONTENTS

Chronopharmaceutics: Science and Technology for Biological Rhythm-Guided Therapy and Prevention of Diseases, edited by Bi-Botti C. Youan
Copyright © 2009 John Wiley & Sons, Inc.

1.1   OBJECTIVES

The objectives of this introductory chapter are to (1) introduce this emerging concept of chronopharmaceutics, (2) provide a chronology and comprehensive background literature that support the demand, (3) broadly review diseases for which knowledge gained would be beneficial, (4) classify the chronopharmaceutical drug delivery systems (ChrDDSs) that are on the market or under development, and (5) provide potential resources that may help in future investigation. Chronopharmaceutics may be defined as a branch of pharmaceutics (science and technology of drug dosage forms) devoted to the design and evaluation of drug delivery systems that release a bioactive agent at a rhythm that ideally matches in real time the biological requirement for a given disease therapy or prevention. Ideally, ChrDDSs should embody time-controlled and site-specific drug delivery systems regardless of route of administration. Perhaps the majority of the desirable features for chronopharmaceutics may be found at the interface of chronobiology, chronopharmacology, system biology, and nanomedicine.

1.2   INTRODUCTION TO CHRONOPHARMACEUTICS

The basic concepts of human chronobiology and the rhythm dependence of certain disease states and the pharmacodynamics of medications frequently prescribed for their treatment have been widely reported [1–3]. After we organized the first mini symposium at the 2004 AAPS annual meeting in Baltimore, Maryland, on how to reconcile pharmaceutics with current clinical knowledge, the issue has raised a lot of interest and awareness among pharmaceutical scientists, and several articles have recently focused on chronobiology, drug delivery, and chronotherapeutics from which readers will gain additional insights [3]. It is also now known that the mammalian suprachiasmatic nuclei (SCN) transmit signals to the rest of the brain, organizing circadian rhythms throughout the body. For example, transplants of SCN restored the circadian activity rhythms to animals such as hamsters whose own SCN had been ablated [4].Therefore the concept of *chronotherapy* supported by basic biomedical sciences is not new, as evidenced by the existence of several and peer-reviewed manuscripts and books on the matter (see Table 1.1). However, there is a knowledge gap as far as how novel drug delivery systems can be effectively engineered in order to meet this real medical need and demand. The rationale behind this nonconventional approach to drug design and delivery design is based on the increased awareness about medication safety. The side effect and patience compliance issue with pharmaceuticals is still a major public health problem. For example, in the United States alone, it has been reported that more than 1 million injuries and nearly 100,000 deaths are attributed to medical errors annually [5]. According to the same sources, although few medication errors result in adverse drug events (ADEs), hospitals incur $2200 in additional costs per ADE and $4685 per preventable ADE. Nationally, the cost of ADEs is $2 billion per year, which basically represents the cost to the economy for not solving the problem.

The increasing concern and focus on health care safety has reached the point where, in 1999, the Institute of Medicine (IOM) published a number of reports on how to improve the safety of medical product use. In 1999, the IOM released a landmark report, *To Err is Human*; a second, related report, *Crossing the Quality Chasm*, followed in March 2001. The reports describe a vision for improving health care quality, patient safety, and the safe use of drugs and medical devices. In 2006, the IOM released another report, *The Future of Drug Safety—Promoting and Protecting the Health of the Public* (http://www.iom.edu). Among other suggestions, this IOM report recommended that the U.S. Food and Drug Administration (FDA) identify ways to access other health-related databases and create a public–private partnership to support safety and efficacy studies. The FDA responded to the IOM report with the FDA Amendments Act (FDAAA) of 2007, calling for active postmarket safety surveillance and analysis. As planned, the Sentinel Initiative will fulfill many of the requirements of FDAAA while fulfilling needs of the FDA not contemplated by the law's requirements. In June 2008, the U.S. Department of Health and Human Services (DHHS) announced efforts between the FDA and the Centers for Medicare & Medicaid Services (CMS) to enhance patient safety as well as the quality of medical care patients receive. These collective efforts included the CMS regulations and the Sentinel Initiative. The CMS regulations now enable federal agencies, states, and academic researchers to use Medicare prescription drug claims data for public health research and analysis; *The Sentinel Initiative: National Strategy for Monitoring Medical Product Safety* describes a new program that includes the creation of an electronic system for assessing information to detect potential postmarket adverse events.

The foregoing observations suggest that a chronopharmaceutical approach may provide safer and more effective drug product. Although it is now established that the effectiveness and toxicity of many drugs vary depending on dosing time associated with the circadian rhythm, many drugs are still administered without regard to the time of day. Recently, a few high profile works suggested the possibility to engineer rhythms [6–8]. Based on these recent advances, perhaps an early integration of the current advances in chrono-biology and engineering in the discovery, research and development, clinical testing, and marketing phase of these drugs would lead to a significant decrease in medication error and an increase in patient treatment outcome. But this ideal objective may not be successful without the continuous education of the health care professional and researcher about new developments in this field.

1.3   DEFINITION AND CONCEPT OF CHRONOPHARMACEUTICS

Chronobiology is the study of biological rhythms and their mechanisms. Biological rhythms are defined by a number of characteristics [1]. The term "circadian" was coined by Franz Halberg from the Latin *circa*, meaning about, and *dies*, meaning day [9]. Oscillations of shorter duration are termed "ultradian" (more than one cycle per 24 hours). Oscillations that are longer than 24 hours are "infradian" (less than one cycle per 24 hours). Ultradian, circadian, and infradian rhythms coexist at all levels of biologic organization [1, 10]. *Pharmaceutics* is an area of biomedical and pharmaceutical sciences that deals with the design and evaluation of pharmaceutical dosage forms (or drug delivery systems) to assure their safety, effectiveness, quality, and reliability. Based on the previous definitions, *chronopharmaceutics* is a branch of pharmaceutics (science and technology of drug dosage forms) devoted to the design and evaluation of drug delivery systems that release a bioactive agent at a rhythm that ideally matches in real time the biological requirement of a given disease therapy or prevention. Ideally, chronopharmaceutical drug delivery systems (ChrDDSs) should embody time-controlled and site-specific drug delivery systems [11] regardless of the route of administration. We have discussed the advantages of ideal systems elsewhere [12]. To our knowledge, such ideal ChrDDSs are not yet available on the market. Perhaps the majority of the desirable features for chronopharmaceutics may be found at the interface of chronobiology, chronopharmacology, system biology, and nanomedicine.

1.4   CHRONOLOGY OF CHRONOTHERAPY AND RELATED CONCEPTS: FOUNDATION FOR CHRONOPHARMACEUTICS

Table 1.1 shows a comprehensive list of findings that provide a strong basis for future chronopharmaceutical research. Readers are invited to refer to specific references for more details. It is beyond the scope of this Chapter to comment on each of the references. However, it is important to underline the contributions from researchers such as Julien-Joseph Virey [13], Pittendrigh and Aschoff [1, 10, 14], Benzer [15], Hall [16], Young [17], Rosbash and Takahashi [18], Francis Halberg [19], and Robert Langer [20], whose works have greatly impacted the emergence of chronopharmaceutics and chronotherapy. For example, Julien-Joseph Virey (1775–1846) held the position of

Table 1.1. Milestones in Chronobiology, Chronotherapy, and Relevant Sciences and Technologies

Date	Key Concepts and Findings Contributing to Feasibility and Need of Chronopharmaceutics	Author(s)
7th Century BCE	Importance of rhythms ("Recognize what sort of rhythm governs man"); description of solar eclipse of April 6, 648 BCE ("Zeus, father of the Olympians, made night from mid-day, hiding the light of the shining Sun")	Archilochus of Paros [22–24]
~324 BCE	Daily periodic movements of leaflets: sleep of plants found by Androsthenes of Thasos	Theophrastus; cf. Bretzl [25]
1729, 1731	Sleep movements of the sensitive plant continue in continuous darkness: de Mairan did not wish to cross disciplinary barriers; his professional focus ruled out magnetism with respect to the aurora borealis	de Mairan [26, 27]
1797	Importance of 24-hour period	Hufeland [28]
1814	Thesis on periodicity in health and disease	Virey [29]
1832	Free-running in botany	De Candolle [30]
1922	Sunspot effects on mild and severe clinical symptoms	Vallot, Sardou, and Faure [31]
1934	"Life on earth is an echo of the sun"	Chizhevsky [32–35]
1934, 1935	Solar emission and human mortality	Düll and Düll [36, 37]
1939	"Exceptionally substantial and durable self-winding and self-regulating physiological clock"	Johnson [38]
1939	"The idiocy of '3 times a day'"	Jores [39]
1950	Genetics, not stress, hint at built-in 24-h periodicity in hematology: sampling each animal only once, mice from inbred stocks show great differences in extent of within-day change of blood cell counts	Halberg and Visscher [40]
1951	Removal of the adrenal glands by surgery abolished circadian eosinophil rhythm gauging built-in adrenocortical cycle	Halberg, Visscher, Flink, Berge, and Bock [41]
1952	24-h periodicity in electroencephalographic pathology	Halberg, Engel, Halberg, and Gully [42]
1952	Importance of circadian adrenal cycle which persists on a diet reduced in calories that eliminates the gonadal cycle	Halberg and Visscher [43]
1952–1953	2800-fold decrease in needed dosage of steroid by replacing an approach eliminating a rhythm (1952) with one testing in a specified circadian stage (1953)	Halberg [44, 45]

(Continued)

Table 1.1. Continued

Date	Key Concepts and Findings Contributing to Feasibility and Need of Chronopharmaceutics	Author(s)
1953	Concept: neuroendocrine and cellular cycle built-in and preparing for everyday activity rather than a mere response to everyday "stress"	Halberg [45]
1953	Multiple synchronizers: with ad libitum feeding, lighting schedule dominating and phase-shifting while on a diet reduced in calories, feeding time overrides lighting	Halberg, Visscher, and Bittner [46]
1954	Circadian desynchronization after loss of eyes by surgery or genetics (anophthalmic ZRD mice)	Halberg [19]; Halberg, Visscher, and Bittner [47]
1955	Convulsions or death versus survival as a function of circadian stage in response of sensitive mice to noise	Halberg, Bittner, Gully, Albrecht and Brackney [48]
1955	Circadian susceptibility rhythm to an endotoxin (*Brucella*)	Halberg, Spink, Albrecht and Gully [49]
1956	Therapy from the viewpoint of biological rhythms	Menzel [50]
1957	Contrary to earlier reports a circadian peripheral mitotic rhythm can be shifted by manipulating lighting, albeit more slowly than a shift in liver glycogen rhythm	Halberg, Bittner, and Smith [51]
1958	Audiogenic abnormality spectra, 24-hour periodicity, and lighting	Halberg, Jacobson, Wadsworth, and Bittner [52]
1958	Circadian rhythm in RNA and DNA formation as well as mitoses and in circulating corticosterone of mice	Halberg, Barnum, Silber, and Bittner [53]
1958	24-hour rhythms in blood eosinophils and *Wucheria bancrofti* microfilariae before and after delta 1-9 alpha-fluorocortisol	Engel, Halberg, Dassanayake, and De Silva [54]
1959	Definition of the concept of circadian rhythm	Halberg [55]
1959	Circadian susceptibility rhythm to a drug (ouabain)	Halberg, Haus, and Stephens [56]
1959	Formulation of interaction of cellular, endocrine and neural, notably hypothalamic mechanisms of periodicity Concepts of interacting (1) CNS, (2) endocrine and (3) peripheral internal timers with environment as external but open system synchronizer	Halberg, Halberg, Barnum, and Bittner [57]
1960	Right time differing for first maps of body as a whole, organs, and tissues; hours of changing resistance differ for different agents, first LD_{50} rhythm in response to whole-body irradiation	Halberg [58]

(*Continued*)

Table 1.1. Continued

Date	Key Concepts and Findings Contributing to Feasibility and Need of Chronopharmaceutics	Author(s)
1960	Persistence of a susceptibility rhythm (to ethanol) in continuous darkness	Halberg [59]
1960	Gradual circadian system development in infancy	Hellbrügge [60]
1960	Subtle factors	Brown [61]
1961	Susceptibility to Librium	Marte and Halberg [62]
1961	Circadian mapping of EEG and cortisol in human health	Halberg et al. [63]
1961	Circadian rhythm in a prokaryote (*E. coli*)	Halberg and Conner [64]
1962	Reserpine effect upon core temperature rhythm spectrum	Halberg, Adkins, Marte, and Jones [65]
1962	Spontaneous in vivo rhythm versus circadian rhythm in the in vitro response of mouse adrenal to adrenocorticotropic hormone	Ungar and Halberg [66]
1963	SU4885 as a function of circadian stage life or death from an adrenal cortical modulator	Ertel, Ungar, and Halberg [67]; Ertel, Halberg, and Ungar [68]
1963	Circadian susceptibility rhythm to acetylcholine	Jones, Haus, and Halberg [69]; Halberg [70]
1963	Circadian adrenal cycle in C mice kept without food and water for a day and a half	Galicich, Halberg, and French [71]
1965	Circadian rhythms in man	Aschoff [14]
1965	Mapping spectrum of rhythm in 17-ketosteroid circaseptan desynchronization	Halberg, Engeli, Hamburger, and Hillman [72]
1966	Circadian rhythms: variation in sensitivity of isolated rat artria to acetylcholine	Spoor and Jackson [73]
1967	Cosinor method	Halberg, Tong ,and Johnson [74]
1967	Circadian rhythm of the central temperature of subject given free rein for 6 months	Colin, Houdas, Boutelier, Timbal, and Siffre [75]
1967	Circadian pattern of plasma 17-hydroxycorticosterol: alteration by anticholinergic agents	Krieger and Krieger [76]
1968	Anesthesia: fluothane	Matthews, Marte, and Halberg [77]
1968	Template-directed synthesis with adenosine-5'-phosphorimidazolide	Weimann, Lohrmann, Orgel, Schneider-Bernloehr, and Sulston [78]
1968	Daily circadian rhythm in rats to D-amphetamine sulfate: effect of blinding and continuous illumination on the rhythm	Scheving, Vedral, and Pauly [79]
1969	Ultradians in narcolepsy	Passouant, Halberg, Genicot, Popoviciu, and Baldy-Moulinier [80]

(*Continued*)

Table 1.1. Continued

Date	Key Concepts and Findings Contributing to Feasibility and Need of Chronopharmaceutics	Author(s)
1969	Coining of "chronobiology" (Current Contents "Citation Classic")	Halberg [81]
1970–1979	Ara-C: chronotherapy in the laboratory; test case at NIH and FDA	Cardoso, Scheving, and Halberg [82]; Hauset et al. [83]; Halberg et al. [84]; Scheving, Burns, Pauly, Halberg, and Haus [85]; Halberg et al. [86]
1970	Education: chronobiologic literacy	Halberg [87]
1970	The biology of circadian rhythms from human to microorganism	Hastings [88]
1970	Circadian rhythm of gastric acid secretion in humans	Moore and Englert [89]
1971	Occupational health	Halberg [90]
1971	Dose response evaluation of circadian rhythm to ouabain	Nelson, Kupferberg, and Halberg [91]
1972	Circadian corticosteroid periodicity: critical period for abolition by neonatal injection of corticosteroid	Krieger [92]
1972	Autorhythmometry by self-measurement and single cosinor analysis	Halberg, Johnson, Nelson, Runge, and Sothern [93]
1972–1973	Chronobiology of the life sequence; laboratory techniques and rhythmometry	Smolensky, Halberg, and Sargent [94]; Halberg [95]
1973	Chronobiotic (Quiadon®)	Simpson et al. [96]
1973	When to eat can make the difference between life and death	Nelson, Cadotte, and Halberg [97]
1973	Circannual rhythmic ovarian recrudescence in catfish	Sundararaj, Vasal, and Halberg [98]
1973	Chronotherapeutic index	Rosene, Lee, Kühl, Halberg, and Grage [99]
1974	Circadian oscillations in rodents: a systematic increase of their frequency with age	Pittendrigh and Daan [100]
1974	Tracing developments up to the cosinor	Aschoff [101]
1975	Chronotypic action of theophylline and of pentobarbital as circadian zeitgebers in the rat	Ehret, Potter, and Dobra [102]
1976	Differential circadian rhythms in pineal and hypothalamic 5-HT induced by artificial photoperiods or melatonin	Yates and Herbert [103]
1976	Melatonin: effects on the circadian locomotor rhythm of sparrows	Turek, McMillan, Menaker [104]
1976	Polymers for the sustained release of proteins and other macromolecules	Langer and Folkman [105]
1977	Doubling of 2-year survival rate by timing radiation therapy	Halberg [106]
1977	Estradiol shortens the period of hamster circadian rhythms	Morin, Fitzgerald, and Zucker [107]

(Continued)

Table 1.1. Continued

Date	Key Concepts and Findings Contributing to Feasibility and Need of Chronopharmaceutics	Author(s)
1978	Serotonin shifts the phase of the circadian rhythm in the *Aplysia* eye	Corrent, McAdoo, and Eskin [108]
1979	Transplantation of a circadian pacemaker in *Drosophila*	Handler and Konopka [109]
1980	Human sleep: its duration and organization depend on its circadian phase	Czeisler, Weitzman, Moore-Ede, Zimmerman, and Knauer [110]
1980	Nocturnal asthma and changes in circulating epinephrine, histamine, and cortisol	Barnes, FitzGerald, Brown, and Dollery [111]
1981	Biologic rhythms, hormones, and aging	Halberg, Nelson, and Haus [112]
1982	Rotating shift work schedules that disrupt sleep are improved by applying circadian principles	Czeisler, Moore-Ede, Coleman [113]
1982	Regulation of circadian rhythmicity	Takahashi and Zatz [114]
1983	Free-running activity rhythms in the rat: entrainment by melatonin	Redman, Armstrong, Ng [115]
1983	Adenylate cyclase activation shifts the phase of a circadian pacemaker	Eskin and Takahashi [116]
1983	Chronobiologic abnormality in luteinizing hormone secretion in teenage girls with the polycystic-ovary syndrome	Zumoff et al. [117]
1983	Role for acetylcholine in mediating effects of light on reproduction	Earnest and Turek [118]
1983	Light and propranolol suppress the nocturnal elevation of serotonin in the cerebrospinal fluid of rhesus monkeys	Garrick, Tamarkin, Taylor, Markey, and Murphy [119]
1984	Avian pancreatic polypeptide phase shifts hamster circadian rhythms when microinjected into the suprachiasmatic region	Albers, Ferris, Leeman, Goldman [120]
1984	Spectral sensitivity of a novel photoreceptive system mediating entrainment of mammalian circadian rhythms	Takahashi, DeCoursey, Bauman, and Menaker [121]
1985	Circadian timing of cancer chemotherapy	Hrushesky [122]
1985	Multiple circadian oscillators regulate the timing of behavioral and endocrine rhythms in female golden hamsters	Swann and Turek [123]
1985	Circadian variation in the frequency of onset of acute myocardial infarction	Muller et al. [124]
1986	Benzodiazepine used in the treatment of insomnia phase-shifts the mammalian circadian clock	Turek and Losee-Olson [125]
1986	Bright light resets the human circadian pacemaker independent of the timing of the sleep–wake cycle	Czeisler et al. [126]

(Continued)

Table 1.1. Continued

Date	Key Concepts and Findings Contributing to Feasibility and Need of Chronopharmaceutics	Author(s)
1987	Concurrent morning increase in platelet aggregability and the risk of myocardial infarction and sudden cardiac death	Tofler et al. [127]
1988	Creatine accelerates the circadian clock in a unicellular alga	Roenneberg, Nakamura, and Hastings [128]
1989	Chronobiologic pilot study with special reference to cancer research	Cornélissen, and Halberg [129]
1988	The circadian rhythm of LH release can be shifted by injections of a benzodiazepine in female golden hamsters	Turek and Losee-Olson [130]
1990	Cancer chronotherapy: a drug delivery challenge	Hrushesky [131]
1990	Exposure to bright light and darkness to treat physiologic maladaptation to night work	Czeisler et al. [132]
1991	When should the immune clock be reset? From circadian pharmacodynamics to temporally optimized drug delivery	Levi, Canon, Dipalma, Florentin, and Misset [133]
1992	From experimental units to unique experiments: chronobiologic pilots complement large trials.	Halberg, Cornélissen, Bingham, Fujii, and Halberg [134]
1992	Circadian clock genes are ticking	Takahashi [135]
1993	Timing increases safety and efficacy of antihypertensive medication	Zaslavskaya [136]
1994	Introduction to chronobiology	Halberg and Cornélissen [137]
1994	Forward and reverse genetic approaches to behavior in the mouse	Takahashi, Pinto, and Vitaterna [138]
1994	Mutagenesis and mapping of a mouse gene, *clock*, essential for circadian behavior	Vitaterna et al. [139]
1995	Clinical chronopharmacology: the importance of time in drug treatment	Lemmer [140]
1995	Resolution from a meeting of the International Society for Research on Civilization Diseases and the Environment: timing antihypertensive treatment	Halberg and Cornélissen [141]
1995	Positional cloning and sequence analysis of the *Drosophila clock* gene, timeless	Myers, Wager-Smith, Wesley, Young, and Sehgal [142]
1995	Rhythmic expression of timeless: a basis for promoting circadian cycles in period gene autoregulation	Sehgal et al. [143]
1995	Isolation of timeless by PER protein interaction: defective interaction between timeless protein and long-period mutant PERL	Gekakis et al. [144]
1995	Ultrasound-mediated transdermal protein delivery	Mitragotri, Blankschtein, and Langer [145]

(Continued)

Table 1.1. Continued

Date	Key Concepts and Findings Contributing to Feasibility and Need of Chronopharmaceutics	Author(s)
1996	A diffusible coupling signal from the transplanted suprachiasmatic nucleus controlling circadian locomotor rhythms	Silver, LeSauter, Tresco, and Lehman [4]
1996	Light-induced degradation of TIMELESS and entrainment of the *Drosophila* circadian clock	Myers, Wager-Smith, Rothenfluh-Hilfiker, and Young [146]
1997	Individual assessment of antihypertensive response by self-starting cumulative sums	Cornelissen, Halberg, Hawkins, Otsuka, and Henke [147]
1997	Positional cloning of the mouse circadian clock gene	King et al. [148]
1997	Functional identification of the mouse circadian *clock* gene by transgenic BAC rescue	Antoch et al. [149]
1997	RIGUI, a putative mammalian ortholog of the *Drosophila period* gene	Sun et al. [150]
1997	Circadian oscillation of a mammalian homologue of the *Drosophila period* gene	Tei et al. [151]
1997	Two period homologs: circadian expression and photic regulation in the suprachiasmatic nuclei	Shearman, Zylka, Weaver, Kolakowski, and Reppert [152]
1997	A differential response of two putative mammalian circadian regulators, mper1 and mper2, to light	Albrecht, Sun, Eichele, and Lee [153]
1997	cDNA cloning and tissue-specific expression of a novel basic helix–loop–helix/PAS protein (BMAL1) and identification of alternatively spliced variants with alternative translation initiation site usage	Ikeda and Nomura [154]
1998	A serum shock induces circadian gene expression in mammalian tissue culture cells	Balsalobre, Damiola, and Schibler [155]
1998	Circadian rhythms: new cogwheels in the clockworks	Schibler [156]
1998	New mammalian period gene predominantly expressed in the suprachiasmatic nucleus	Takumi et al. [157]
1998	Light-independent oscillatory gene *mPer3* in mouse SCN and OVLT	Takumi et al. [158]
1998	Role of the CLOCK protein in the mammalian circadian mechanism	Gekakis et al. [159]
1998	Three period homologs in mammals: differential light responses in the suprachiasmatic circadian clock and oscillating transcripts outside of brain	Zylka, Shearman, Weaver, Reppert [160]

(Continued)

Table 1.1. Continued

Date	Key Concepts and Findings Contributing to Feasibility and Need of Chronopharmaceutics	Author(s)
1998	Molecular analysis of mammalian *timeless*	Zylka et al. [161]
1998	Identification of the mammalian homologs of the *Drosophila* timeless gene, *Timeless1*	Koike et al. [162]
1998	Mammalian circadian autoregulatory loop: a *timeless* ortholog and *mPer1* interact and negatively regulate *CLOCK-BMAL1*-induced transcription	Sangoram et al. [163]
1999	Familial advanced sleep-phase syndrome: a short-period circadian rhythm variant in humans	Jones et al. [164]
1999	Oscillation and light induction of timeless mRNA in the mammalian circadian clock	Tischkau et al. [165]
1999	Narcolepsy genes wake up the sleep field	Takahashi [166]
1999	Mammalian ortholog of *Drosophila timeless*, highly expressed in SCN and retina, forms a complex with mPER1	Takumi et al. [167]
1999	Light-independent role of CRY1 and CRY2 in the mammalian circadian clock	Griffin, Staknis, Weitz [168]
1999	Mammalian Cry1 and Cry2 are essential for maintenance of circadian rhythms	van der Horst et al. [169]
1999	Photic induction of mPer1 and mPer2 in cry-deficient mice lacking a biological clock	Okamura et al. [170]
1999	Familial advanced sleep-phase syndrome: a short-period circadian rhythm variant in humans	Jones et al. [164]
1999	Controlled release microchip	Santini, Cima, and Langer [171]
2000	Resetting central and peripheral circadian oscillators in transgenic rats	Yamazaki et al. [172]
2000	Therapeutic implications of circadian rhythms in cancer patients	Levi [173]
2000	Positional syntenic cloning and functional characterization of the mammalian circadian mutation tau	Lowrey et al. [174]
2000	Mop3 (also known as BMAL1) is an essential component of the master circadian pacemaker in mammals	Bunger et al. [175]
2000	Resetting of circadian time in peripheral tissues by glucocorticoid signaling	Balsalobre et al. [176]
2001	New role for cryptochrome in a *Drosophila* circadian oscillator	Krishnan et al. [177]
2001	Night shift work, light at night, and risk of breast cancer	Davis, Mirick, and Stevens [178]
2001	hPer2 phosphorylation site mutation in familial advanced sleep phase syndrome	Toh et al. [179]

(Continued)

Table 1.1. Continued

Date	Key Concepts and Findings Contributing to Feasibility and Need of Chronopharmaceutics	Author(s)
2001	Changing the dosing schedule minimizes the disruptive effects of interferon on clock function	Ohdo, Koyanagi, Suyama, Higuchi, and Aramaki [180]
2001	Molecular mechanisms of the biological clock in cultured fibroblasts	Yagita, Tamanini, van Der Horst, and Okamura [181]
2001	Night shift work, light at night, and risk of breast cancer	Davis, Mirick, and Stevens [178]
2001	Circadian rhythms. Chronobiology—reducing time	Schibler, Ripperger, Brown [182]
2002	Coordinated transcription of key pathways in the mouse by the circadian clock	Panda et al. [183]
2002	Increase in nocturnal blood pressure and progression to microalbuminuria in type 1 diabetes	Lurbe et al. [184]
2002	Circadian rhythms from flies to human	Panda, Hogenesch, and Kay [185]
2002	Extensive and divergent circadian gene expression in liver and heart	Storch et al. [186]
2002	Transcription factor response element for gene expression during circadian night: role of the Rev-ErbA/ROR	Ueda et al. [187]
2002	Circadian gene *Period2* plays an important role in tumor suppression and DNA damage response in vivo	Fu, Pelicano, Liu, Huang, and Lee [188]
2002	Circadian rhythms: the cancer connection	Rosbash and Takahashi [18]
2002	Web of circadian pacemakers	Schibler and Sassone-Corsi [189]
2003	Circadian rhythms. Liver regeneration clocks on	Schibler [190]
2003	Synchronization of cellular clocks in the suprachiasmatic nucleus	Yamaguchi et al. [191]
2003	Control mechanism of the circadian clock for timing of cell division in vivo	Matsuo et al. [192]
2003	Rhythmic histone acetylation underlies transcription in the mammalian circadian clock	Etchegaray, Lee, Wade, and Reppert [193]
2003	Orphan nuclear receptor REV-ERBα controls circadian transcription within the positive limb of the mammalian circadian oscillator	Preitner et al. [194]
2003	Circadian clock: pacemaker and tumor suppressor	Fu and Lee [195]
2003	Individualized time series-based assessment of melatonin effects on blood pressure: model for pediatricians	Zaslavskaya et al. [196]
2003	Clockwork web: circadian timing in brain and periphery, in health and disease	Hastings Reddy and Maywood [197]

(*Continued*)

Table 1.1. Continued

Date	Key Concepts and Findings Contributing to Feasibility and Need of Chronopharmaceutics	Author(s)
2004	Autonomous molecular computer for logical control of gene expression	Benenson, Gil, Ben-Dor, Adar, and Shapiro [198]
2004	Reciprocal regulation of heme biosynthesis and the circadian clock in mammals	Kaasik and Lee [199]
2005	Obesity and metabolic syndrome in circadian clock mutant mice	Turek et al. [200]
2005	Circadian sensitivity to the chemotherapeutic agent cyclophosphamide depends on the functional status of the CLOCK/ BMAL1 transactivation complex	Gorbacheva et al. [201]
2005	Functional consequences of CKIdelta mutation causing familial advanced sleep syndrome	Xu et al. [202]
2006	Jetlag resets the *Drosophila* circadian clock by promoting light-induced degradation of TIMELESS	Koh, Zheng, and Sehgal [203]
2006	Ancestors of the extended cosinor in what became chronobiology, chronomics, chronobioethics, and chronoastrobiology	Schwartzkopff et al. [204]
2006	Circadian timing in health and disease	Maywood, O'Neill, Wong, Reddy, and Hastings [205]
2006	Shift work and pathological conditions	Van Mark, Spallek, Kessel, and Brinkmann [206]
2006	Hypothalamic H1 receptor: a novel therapeutic target for disrupting diurnal feeding rhythm and obesity	Masaki and Yoshimatsu [207]
2006	*Clock* genes: influencing and being influenced by psychoactive drugs	Manev and Uz [208]
2006	Protein arrays: growing pains	Eisenstein [209]
2007	Psychiatric research. Is internal timing key to mental health?	Bhattacharjee [210]
2007	Modeling of a human circadian mutation yields insights into clock regulation by PER2	Xu et al. [211]
2007	Neural–immune interactions in disorders of sleep–wakefulness organization	Bentivoglio and Kristensson [212]
2007	Sense of time: how molecular clocks organize metabolism	Kohsaka and Bass [213]
2007	Circadian sleep disorder reveals a complex clock	Mignot and Takahashi [214]
2007	Modeling of human circadian mutation yield insights into clock regulation	Xu et al. [211]
2007	Engineering complex dynamical structures: sequential patterns and desynchronization	Kiss, Rusin, Kori, and Hudson [6]

(*Continued*)

Table 1.1. Continued

Date	Key Concepts and Findings Contributing to Feasibility and Need of Chronopharmaceutics	Author(s)
2007	Automated reverse engineering of nonlinear dynamical systems	Bongard and Lipson [7]
2008	Complementary and alternative medicine for sleep disturbances in older adults	Gooneratne [215]
2008	Evaluation of sleep disturbances in older adults	Misra and Malow [216]
2008	The meter of metabolism	Green, Takahashi, and Bass [217]
2008	SIRT1 is a circadian deacetylase for core clock components	Belden and Dunlap [218]
2008	SIRT1 regulates circadian *clock* gene expression through PER2 deacetylation	Asher et al. [219]
2008	Differential rescue of light- and food-entrainable circadian rhythms	Fuller, Lu, and Saper [220]
2008	cAMP-dependent signaling as a core component of the mammalian circadian pacemaker	O'Neil, Maywood, Chesham, Takahashi, and Hastings [221]
2008	Integrating circadian timekeeping with cellular physiology	Harrisingh and Nitabach [222]
2008	Hematopoietic stem cell release is regulated by circadian oscillations	Mendez-Ferrer, Lucas, Battista, and Frenette [223]

Pharmacist-in-Chief at the Val-de-Grace, a military hospital. Virey deserves credit for establishing the field of chronobiology based on his insights and writings [13]. Franz Halberg (1906–present) is a scientist and the founder of modern chronobiology. He first began his experiments in the 1940s and later founded the Halberg Chronobiology Laboratories at the University of Minnesota [19]. Robert S. Langer (1948–present) is an Institute Professor at the Massachusetts Institute of Technology. He is a distinguished and highly regarded researcher in biotechnology, especially in the fields of drug delivery systems and tissue engineering. Langer's contributions to medicine and the emerging fields of biotechnology are highly recognized and respected around the world. He is considered a pioneer of many new technologies, including transdermal delivery systems, which allow the administration of drugs or extraction of analytes from the body through the skin without needles or other invasive methods [20].

The future of ChrDDSs is promising if more creative work can be done based on these pioneering and seminal works. In the era of nanoscience and nanotechnology, it is reasonable to predict that a "hybrid" approach integrating basic knowledge of biomedical engineering, chronobiology, and related fields will be needed in order to optimize the chronopharmaceutics or chronomedicine or nanomedicine of the future [21].

1.5 BIOLOGICAL RHYTHMS, HEALTH, AND DISEASES

Hasting et al. [197] have provided some aspects of the circadian timing in the brain and periphery, in relation to health and disease. This section is a brief and broad overview to underscore the importance of the concept on virtually all major health issues.

1.5.1 Biological Rhythms and Sleep Disorders

The importance of biological rhythms on sleep disorders may be discussed in terms of shift work and disorders of the sleep–wake cycle. With increasing economic and social demands, we are rapidly evolving into a 24-hour society. In any urban economy, about 20% of the population is required to work outside the regular 0800–1700h working day and this figure is likely to increase. Although the increase in shift work has led to greater flexibility in work schedules, the negative effects of shift work and chronic sleep loss on health and productivity are now being appreciated [224]. Some professions such as the military and health care professions (nurse, physicians, pharmacists, airline pilots, and crew members in submarines) and patients with particular health problems (e.g., blindness) may be more subject to sleep disorders than others. Wagner [225] reviewed several disorders of the circadian sleep–wake cycle, including delayed sleep phase syndrome, advanced sleep phase syndrome, non-24-hour sleep–wake syndrome, irregular sleep–wake pattern, time zone change (jet lag) syndrome, and shift work sleep disorder. The hypothalamus is now recognized as a key center for sleep regulation, with hypothalamic neurotransmitter systems providing the framework for therapeutic advances. An increased awareness of the close interaction between sleep and homeostatic systems is also emerging. Progress has occurred in the understanding of narcolepsy—molecular techniques have identified the lateral hypothalamic hypocretin (orexin) neuropeptide system as key to the disorder [226]. The contribution of genetic components to the pathology of sleep disorders is increasingly recognized as important [227].

It is well known that the brain area with the highest concentration in noradrenergic nerve terminals and noradrenaline (NA) have a circadian rhythm in their content of NA [228]. Moreover, it has been shown that human sleep, its duration, and organization depend on its circadian phase [110]. A breakthrough chronopharmaceutical formulation against insomnia that plagues many people would be one that addresses the entire oscillatory cycle of the human sleeping process.

In search of treatment and cure for sleep disorders in humans, melatonin (with its chronobiotic properties) has been able to phase shift strongly endogenous rhythms, such as core temperature and its own endogenous rhythm, together with the sleep–wake cycle. When suitably timed, most studies indicate that fast release preparations are able to hasten adaptation to phase shift in both field and simulation studies of jet lag and shift work [229].

It was suggested that prior knowledge of the subject's type of circadian rhythm, and timing of treatment in relation to the individual's circadian phase, may improve the efficacy of melatonin [230]. Other drugs (see Table 1.1) such as theophylline and pentobarbital, in addition to having a number of already established pharmacological properties, have been further identified as chronobiotics; or drugs that may be used to alter the biological time structure by rephasing a circadian rhythm [102]. These chronobiotic effects (either desirable or undesirable) may raise the new concept of side effects of some existing drugs. Besides the use of chronobiotics, illumination has been used as an alternative approach to treat sleep disorders. For example, the peak of sensitivity of the human circadian pacemaker to light was blue-shifted relative to the three-cone visual photopic system [231]. The blue shift is likely to arise from novel photoreceptor proteins—melanopsins [232, 233] and cryptochromes [234].

These findings also suggest special precautions may be warranted (as is now done for pregnant women, children, the elderly, and patients with kidney and liver failures) when formulating and administering drug treatment to patients exhibiting biological rhythm disorders.

1.5.2 Biological Rhythms and Respiratory Diseases

The chronobiology of asthma has been extensively reviewed elsewhere [235, 236]. Basically, the symptoms of allergic asthmatic patients typically worsen during the night, especially during the early morning hours. The exacerbation of asthma during the night represents the changing status of biological functioning due to circadian rhythms in bronchial patency; airways hyperreactivity to acetylcholine, histamine, and house dust; and plasma cortisol, epinephrine, histamine, and cyclic AMP, among others [237]. For example, a study in France with 765 subjects suffering from allergic rhinitis validated the existence of an annual change and peak time of disease severity being January to April. In addition, the elevated severity of symptoms in the morning experienced by 60–70% of patients was recommended as a guide to individually optimize dosing time(s) of medications, such as antihistamines [238, 239].

These observations provide a strong rationale for the chronotherapy of respiratory diseases. For example, the effects of antihistamine and anti-inflammatory medicines may be enhanced by timing them to the day–night temporal pattern in symptom manifestation and intensity to achieve optimization of their beneficial effects with control of toxicity, that is, as a chronotherapy [240].

1.5.3 Biological Rhythms and Cancer

The toxicity and/or efficacy of several anticancer agents has been shown in various experimental systems to be dependent on the circadian timing of their bolus administration or the circadian shaping of their continuous infusion [131]. Moreover, it was suggested that the timing of cancer chemotherapy at the time of maximal resistance of the hematopoietic system to a certain drug may improve the often dose-limiting toxicity of the agent. However, this approach may be difficult to apply because of the large individual differences in the timing of the rhythms, and because of the interaction of circadian, circaseptan, and circannual rhythms [241]. Therefore improved chronopharmaceutical systems may be required to solve these challenges.

Recently, the chronogenetic contributions underscored the importance of biological rhythms in chemotherapy based on the connection between cancer and circadian rhythms [18]. One of the cellular processes that are regulated by circadian rhythm is cell proliferation, which often shows asynchrony between normal and malignant tissues. This asynchrony highlights the importance of the circadian clock in tumor suppression in vivo and is one of the theoretical foundations for cancer chronotherapy which might lead to new therapeutic targets [195]. For example, it has been shown that CLOCK genes dictate sensitivity to the anticancer drug cyclophosphamide [242]. It was shown that both time-of-day and allelic-dependent variations in response to chemotherapy correlated with the functional status of the circadian $CLOCK/BMAL1$ trans-activation complex, suggesting that this complex affected the lethality of chemotherapeutic agents by modulating the survival of the target cells [201]. Collectively, these observations suggest that ChrDDSs may decrease adverse drug events and increase patient treatment outcome in future cancer management.

1.5.4   Biological Rhythms and Cardiovascular Diseases

One of the pioneer works in this field was related to platelet aggregability. In fact, the time of day of onset of platelet aggregability, nonfatal myocardial infarction, and sudden cardiac death had prominent circadian rhythms with a primary peak in the morning and a secondary peak in the evening [243]. The blood pressure and heart rate in normotensives and essential (primary) hypertensive patients display highest values during daytime followed by a nightly drop and an early morning rise. In about 70% of forms of secondary hypertension, however, this rhythmic pattern is abolished or even reversed, exhibiting nightly peaks in blood pressure [239]. It was also suggested that predictable changes in responsiveness of the hematopoietic and immune system provide an opportunity to improve the effects of growth factors and cytokines and decrease their undesirable side effects [241]. Moreover, a relatively recent study of the differences in the pharmacokinetic patterns of metoprolol between a pulsatile drug delivery system using a pulsatile capsule, an immediate release tablet, and a controlled release tablet suggested that pulsatile drug delivery offers a promising way for chronopharmacotherapy [244]. Based on these observations, several chronotherapeutic agents for hypertension and angina pectoris, controlled onset, extended release had been developed and are being marketed [245, 246]. These observations call for a circadian time-specified drug dosage form design and delivery treatment for heart disease as well. Chapter 10 provides more insight into the chronopharmacodynamics of cardiovascular diseases.

1.5.5 Biological Rhythms and Neurodegenerative Diseases

Circadian timing in the brain and periphery and its implications in health and disease have been reported by Hastings et al. [197]. Important brain diseases that may benefit from chronopharmaceutical systems include anxiety, insomnia, epilepsy, and Alzheimer and Parkinson diseases. The circadian variability in hemorrhagic stroke has also been reported [247]. Chronobiology makes possible the discovery of new regulation processes regarding the central mechanisms of epilepsy [248, 249]. For example, the electroencephalogram (EEG) in an animal model for generalized absence epilepsy showed that a circadian pattern emerged for the number of spike-wave discharges [250]. Recent studies have implicated dysfunction of the circadian pacemaker in the etiology of these disturbances in dementia. For example, Alzheimer disease (AD) patients showed increased nocturnal activity and a significant phase delay in their rhythms of core-body temperature and activity compared with patients with frontotemporal degeneration and controls [251]. AD also causes disturbances of circadian rhythms, and sundowning (the occurrence or exacerbation of behavioral symptoms of AD in the afternoon and evening) is related to a phase delay of body temperature caused by AD [252]. The subthalamic nucleus (STN) has a key role in the pathophysiology of Parkinson disease and is the primary target for high-frequency deep brain stimulation. Multiple rhythms are consistent with the hypothesis of multiple oscillating systems, each possibly correlating with specific aspects of human STN function and dysfunction [253]. The altered expression of *clock* genes, as evidenced in transgenic mice, had a profound influence on the behavioral effects of psychoactive drugs. It is envisioned that research focusing on *clock* genes expressed in the brain might lead to the discovery of novel drug–target pathways [208]. Besides drugs, although rhythm and music are not entirely synonymous terms, rhythm constitutes one of the most essential structural and organizational elements of music. These facts suggest that the interaction between auditory rhythm and physical [254] and/biological response could be effectively harnessed for specific therapeutic purposes in the rehabilitation of persons with movement disorders or for alternative treatment of anxiety and neurodegenerative disorders.

1.5.6 Biological Rhythms and Metabolic Disorders

Metabolic status varies predictably on a daily and seasonal basis in order to adapt to the cyclical environment. The hypothalamic circadian pacemaker of the suprachiasmatic nuclei (SCN) coordinates these metabolic cycles.

Disturbances of this coordination, as occur in long-term shift work, have a major impact on health [205], including metabolic disorders such as obesity, diabetes, and hypercholesterolemia. The expression of transcripts encoding selected hypothalamic peptides associated with energy balance was attenuated in the *clock* mutant mice, suggesting that the circadian clock gene network plays an important role in mammalian energy balance [200]. Moreover, recent studies revealed that sleep loss in humans leads to metabolic disorders and an intriguing question would be the relation between a healthy biological clock and normal appetite and weight regulation [255]. More recent studies have shown that processes ranging from glucose transport to gluconeogenesis, lipolysis, adipogenesis, and mitochondrial oxidative phosphorylation are controlled through overlapping transcription networks that are tied to the clock and are thus time sensitive. Because disruption of tissue timing occurs when food intake, activity, and sleep are altered, understanding how these many tissue clocks are synchronized to tick at the same time each day, and determining how each tissue "senses time" set by these molecular clocks might open new insight into human disease, including diabetes and obesity [213]. Furthermore, a review of the anatomical evidence supports the proposal that an unbalanced autonomic nervous system output may lead to the simultaneous occurrence of diabetes type 2, dyslipidemia, hypertension, and visceral obesity [256]. It has been shown that the regulation of H_1 receptors is important for the control of energy metabolism, feeding rhythms, and obesity in rodents [207]. Therefore the hypothalamic H_1 receptor may be a novel therapeutic target for disrupting diurnal feeding rhythm and obesity.

Hepatic cholesterol synthesis also exhibits circadian rhythm [257, 258]. However, this rhythm varies according to individuals: there is a large variation in plasma mevalonate concentrations between subjects. Thus cholesterol synthesis is generally higher during the night than during daylight, and diurnal synthesis may represent up to 30–40% of daily cholesterol synthesis [259]. The metabolic flux may also influence the circadian rhythm. For instance, NADH/NAD$^+$ ratio has been suggested to regulate the CLK/CYC transcription factor [260]. Overall, ChrDDSs also offer the perspective of improved therapy for metabolic disorders such as obesity, diabetes, and hypercholesterolemia.

1.5.7 Biological Rhythms and Infectious Diseases

Biological rhythms have been reported for infectious diseases caused by viruses, bacteria, and parasites and even in the vectors of these diseases. The rhythm disturbances also characterize hematologic and immune related disease states, like, infection [261, 262]. For example, the aspects of chronobiology related to infectious diseases of the eye, particularly those that are caused by viral agents (e.g., herpes) were reviewed [263]. Another example of viral diseases with biological rhythm is acquired immune deficiency syndrome (AIDS) [264]. Since $CD4^+$ cells are known to exhibit diurnal variations and since it has been suggested that circulating virus concentrations also vary in a diurnal fashion, as well as nonperiodically, a mathematical model has been developed to provide the first demonstration of diurnal variations in AIDS patients [265]. These findings may also have implications for the future development of chrono-pharmaceutical systems against human immunodeficiency virus (HIV) [265].

Besides viral agents, circadian and other rhythms for parasites have been discussed by Hawkins [266]. In the case of malaria, the periodicity in the development of *Plasmodium* parasites in humans has been known for more than a century. This periodicity is a consequence of the synchronous matura-tion of the parasite during its intracellular development. The cyclic fever that characterizes malarial infections is the outward manifestation of parasite development [267]. For example, the duration of the schizogonic cycle of *P. v. vinckei* and *P. v. lentum*, two highly synchronous subspecies of *Plasmo-dium vinckei*, is 24 hours. With *P. v. lentum*, the timing of the schizogony and merozoites penetration into red blood cells depended on both the host's rhythm and the time of inoculation of frozen-thawed blood: schizogony occurred at 1800h if the inoculum was injected at 0600h or 1200h and at 0600h if injected at 1800h or 0001h [268]. Knowing that the merozoite is so far drug resistant, and that latent merozoites can maintain the infection for any length of time, it appears important to take into account these purely biological data, when studying the drug resistance of the human *P. falciparum* malaria to drugs such as chloroquine [269]. Drug administration during the medium size throphozoite (MT, most sensitive to chloroquine) stage phase-shifted the schizogonic cycle by 18 hours. Thus administration of two consecutive injections given 18 hours apart and timed to the overwhelming presence of the MT stage in the circulation gave the best therapeutic results [270]. Other parasites for a which a biological time series has been investigated and that are prevalent in some developing countries include *Trypanosoma brucei*, a central nervous system parasite [271], and *Giardia lamblia*, an intestinal parasite [272].

Moreover, biological rhythm has been observed in the mosquito vector of malaria (*Anopheles* (*An.*)). The peak indoor biting of *An. maculatus* occurred at 2130h while outdoor biting was higher after midnight. Outdoor biting of *An. barbirostris* and *An. sinensis* was observed throughout the night with several peaks after the second half of the night. Outdoor biting activities of *An. kochi* and *An. philippinensis* were primarily active after dusk and steadily declined after 2130h [273]. These observations with malaria vector suggest that under-standing the biological rhythm of the vector of major infectious diseases may lead to better and more effective prevention strategies. Overall, these observa-tions underscore the important concept of the kinetics of biomarkers that should also be elucidated for improved diagnosis and treatment in the context of chronotherapy [274]. Collectively, these findings suggest that biological rhythm should be taken into account early, not only in new drug research and development related to infectious diseases but also in their prevention strategies.

1.5.8 Biological Rhythms, Age, Race, Gender, and Socioeconomic Factors

The connection between gene and biological rhythms is now established. But the connection between these rhythms and age, race, gender, demographic, socioeconomic, and work factors may be important to the concept of effective and safe systems for chronotherapy and the prevention of diseases based on recent discussions on personalized medicine [275].

The concept of race-based therapeutics has been reported [276]. However, a recent discussion surrounded heart failure trials [277] and the morning/evening preference is largely independent of ethnicity, gender, and socioeconomic position, indicating that it is a stable characteristic that may be better explained by endogenous factors [278]. Moreover, a study compared the fibrinolytic variables between Caucasians (on a predominantly European diet) and Greenland Eskimos (on a traditional Inuit diet containing a substantial amount of fish and sea animals) and suggested that the circadian variation of fibrinolytic activators and inhibitors is a basic biologic phenomenon, which is not affected by life-style, dietary habits, or ethnic differences [279]. With respect to age, despite the limited number of experiments performed to date, it is already possible to state that a chronotherapeutic approach in pediatrics also provides better precision in pharmacologic study than the conventional approach not using time-related data [280]. For example, oral vitamin D [3] is usually administered to children with chronic renal failure in the morning. But it was reasonable to question if there was enough evidence that evening dosing is more beneficial with respect to suppression of parathyroid hormone and reduction of side effects such as hypercalcemia [281]. The treatment of intrinsic pediatric insomnia (a nonspecific impairing symptom) may additionally involve chronotherapy or medical management [282].

Age and gender impact the full repertoire of neurohormone systems, including most prominently the somatotropic, gonadotropic, and lactotropic axes. For example, the daily growth hormone production is approximately twofold higher in young women than men and varies by 20-fold by sexual developmental status and age [283]. It is also known that biological processes and functions in women are well organized in time and by the changes that occur with menarche, reproduction, and menopause. Therefore the therapeutic response and adverse effects of medications widely used by women can vary significantly with the time of treatment [284]. For example, the effect of selected cosmetic products in women has been shown to be time dependent. Namely, the evening application of Noctos (a generation of liposome made with nonionic lipid microspheres) was more efficient than the morning one and the magnitude of this beneficial effect was related both to age and to skin complexion [285]. Therefore to have more insights on this topic, future chronopharmaceutical system designs and trials may be more comprehensive and representative of women and men of different life stages, ethnicities, and likely times (morning vs. evening) of drug use.

1.5.9 Biological Rhythms and Pain

The chronobiology, chronopharmacology, and chronotherapeutics of pain have been extensively reviewed [286]. For example, there is a circadian rhythm in the plasma concentration of C-reactive protein [287] and interleukin-6 [288] in patients with rheumatoid arthritis. Increasingly, the arthritides have shown statistically quantifiable rhythmic parameters. Moreover, a number of drugs used to treat rheumatic diseases have varying therapeutic and toxic effects based on the timing of administration [289]. Patients with osteoarthritis tend to have less pain in the morning and more at night; while those with rheumatoid arthritis have pain that usually peaks in the morning and decreases throughout the day. Collectively, this knowledge also suggests that ChrDSSs and chronotherapy for all forms of arthritis using the appropriate drug should ensure that the highest blood levels of the drug coincide with peak pain.

1.5.10 Biological Rhythms and Surgery

The importance of biological rhythm and surgery may be viewed in terms of the psychosis, the efficacy of patient recovery, and the time of administration of the recommended drugs (e.g., immunosuppressive drugs). A significant correlation was observed between intensive care unit (ICU) psychosis and an irregular melatonin circadian rhythm. Supplementation with melatonin, or acceleration of melatonin secretion, may protect patients from development of ICU psychosis and may promote recovery to a normal mental state [290]. Preclinical study suggests that the degree of circadian alteration following surgery is positively related to the time required for recovery and reentrainment of rhythmicity [291]. Clinical study also indicated positive linear trends in activity and circadian activity periods related to better functioning and shorter length of stay [292]. There are variations in antithrombin activity in plasma after major surgery [293]. The correct use of immunosuppressive drugs has a considerable influence on the prognosis of patients with organ transplants. These observations were supported by the cyclosporine total body clearance and elimination half-lives in the morning, which were, on average, higher and shorter, respectively, than those in the evening. In addition, the disposition of tacrolimus was determined by the time of administration. The tacrolimus C_{max} and AUC after the morning dose were significantly higher than those after the evening dose. These results suggest that more careful consideration be given to the chronopharmacokinetics of tacrolimus and cyclosporine in order to obtain better results with fewer adverse effects [294]. Collectively, these findings also suggest that biological rhythms are important considerations for effective surgery and recovery from surgerical operations.

1.6 CLASSIFICATION OF CHRONOPHARMACEUTICAL SYSTEMS

From the abundance of research and published data, it is clear that chronopharmaceutical approaches to disease management have clinical advantages across all medical disciplines. Clearly, a pattern of real-time drug input at different release rates would be preferred to that of a constant rate. This drug delivery objective may be achieved by stimuli-sensitive and pulsatile drug delivery systems [11, 12, 295–302]. Based on their physicochemical properties, different classifications have been provided for such drug delivery systems. However, for practical reasons, it may be reasonable to classify ChrDDSs based on the main routes of drug administration (parenteral, oral, and transdermal).

1.6.1   Chronopharmaceutical Drug Delivery Systems for Parenteral Route

One of the earliest chronopharmaceutical delivery systems for parenteral administration was reported by Lynch et al. [303]. The system allowed the infusion of an aqueous solution of melatonin, mixed with a dye, or of an immiscible fluid lacking melatonin or dye to rats. They observed a 24-hour rhythm in melatonin urinary excretion which corresponded to the times of its infusion by the apparatus [303].

An excellent review of systems for triggered, pulsed, and programmed drug delivery is also available in the literature [295]. To our knowledge, infusion pumps on the market that have been referred to as chronomodulating for drug delivery application include the Melodie® [304], programmable Synchromed® [305], Panomat® V5 infusion [306], and Rhythmic® pumps. The portable pumps are usually characterized by a light weight (300–500 g) for easy portability and precision in drug delivery. For example, in the United States, the Synchromed® (Medtronic, USA) infusion system may be used for chronomodulated drug delivery [131, 307–311]. The Melodie® pump has been used successfully in cancer chemotherapy in different countries such as France [304], Germany [312, 313], Italy [314–319], Belgium [320], and Japan [321], indicating that the chronopharmaceutical systems for the parenteral route are important alternatives for effective and safe cancer therapy. However, chronomodulated infusion seemed to be more expensive, requiring dedicated electronic pumps and several disposable materials. In fact, further studies showed that the major material cost of chronochemotherapy devices was balanced by a better tolerability profile [318, 322].

The concept of chemical oscillators has also been explored in the search of chronopharmaceutical systems [323]. Based on the same principle, evidence was provided that low concentrations of acidic drugs can attenuate and ultimately quench chemical pH oscillators, by a simple buffering mechanism [324]. Moreover, taking advantage of a pH oscillator system whose periodicity is slower than that of previously considered oscillators, it was shown that multiple, periodic pulses of drug flux across a membrane could be achieved when the concentration of drug is sufficiently low [325]. A prototype gel oscillator that functions by dissipating the chemical energy of glucose by an enzyme-mediated reaction was also proposed [326]. The chemical oscillators as ChrDDSs are reviewed in greater detail in Chapter 4.

More recently, an alternative method to achieve pulsatile or chronopharmaceutical drug release involves using microfabrication technology [327]. For example, a hydrogel-based microfluidic control system may utilize a very small hydrogel based on phenylboronic acid to control the flow of an insulin solution in response to changes in glucose concentration [328, 329]. Further application of microfabrication technology such as the Microchips® technology is reviewed in greater detail in Chapter 9. The concept of a triggerable liposome [330] and a molecular machine for drug delivery [21, 198, 331] may be viewed as early attempts to design biological rhythm-guided nanomedicine for future chronotherapy.

1.6.2 Chronopharmaceutical Drug Delivery Systems for Oral Route

Ideal oral chronopharmaceutical drug delivery systems would allow agents that previously had to be administered two to four times daily to be administered once each day. However, their potential disadvantages (to be circumvented by ideal oral systems) include delayed attainment of pharmacodynamic effect, unpredictable or reduced bioavailability, enhanced first-pass hepatic metabolism (compared to the parenteral route), possibility of dose dumping in case of technological failure, sustained toxicity, dosing inflexibility, and increased cost (compared to conventional dosage forms). Their potential advantages include reduced dosing frequency, enhanced compliance and convenience, reduced toxicity, instantaneous drug level matching exact biological and physiological needs to treat the disease at each time point, drug effect matching body need to treat diseases, and decreased total required therapeutic or preventive dose. Currently, the key technologies in chronopharmaceutics for oral delivery include Diffucaps® (Chapter 5), Chronotopic™ technology (Chapter 6), Egalet® (Chapter 7), OROS® or Chronset™ (Chapter 8), the Contin™, Codas™, Ceform™, GeoClock™, and Port™ systems, Three Dimensional Printing™ (3DP), and the TIMERx™ technology. We have previously reviewed some of these technologies and their applications [12]. We now review their basic principles with appropriate references for readers who wish to learn more on each technology.

In the *Diffucaps*® technology [332] (for more details, see Chapter 5), a unit dosage form, such as a capsule for delivering drugs into the body in a circadian release fashion, is comprised of one or more populations of drug-containing particles (beads, pellets, granules, etc.). Each bead population exhibits a predesigned rapid or sustained release profile with or without a predetermined lag time of 3–5 hours. The active core of the dosage form may comprise an inert particle or an acidic or alkaline buffer crystal (e.g., cellulose ethers), which is coated with an API-containing film-forming formulation and preferably a water-soluble film-forming composition (e.g., hydroxypropylmethylcellulose, polyvinylpyrrolidone) to form a water-soluble/dispersible particle. The active core may be prepared by granulating and milling and/or by extrusion and spheronization of a polymer composition containing the API. Such a ChrDDS is designed to provide a plasma concentration–time profile, that varies according to physiological need during the day, that is, mimicking the circadian rhythm and severity/manifestation of a cardiovascular disease, predicted based on pharmacokinetic and pharmacodynamic considerations and in vitro/in vivo correlations.

The *Chronotopic*™ technology (for more details, see Chapter 6) is basically composed of a drug-containing core provided with an outer release-controlling coating. Both single and multiple-unit dosage forms, such as tablets and capsules or minitablets and pellets, have been employed as the inner drug formulation. Cores either meant for an immediate or a prolonged liberation of the active ingredient have been proposed. However, the main focus has so far been on the accomplishment of a rapid and transient delayed release, which is generally considered the most challenging and appealing pulsatile delivery mode. The outer barrier consists of swellable hydrophilic polymers of different viscosity grade, typically hydroxypropylmethylcellulose (HPMC), by exploiting a variety of methods. When exposed to aqueous fluids, these polymers undergo a glassy-rubbery transition. In the hydrated state, they are subject to permeability increase, dissolution, and/or mechanical erosion phenomena, which delay the delivery of drugs from the core. The system has been shown to provide the pursued pulsatile release behavior in vitro as well as in vivo, with programmable lag phases followed by drug release according to the core characteristics. In principle, it is possible to finely modulate the lag time by relying on different coating materials and coating thickness values. Moreover, depending on such variables, diverse mechanisms have been hypothesized and, in some instances, demonstrated to be involved in the control of release. When proper modifications have been introduced into the system design, the Chronotopic technology yields oral time-dependent colon delivery as well.

The *Egalet*® technology (for more details, see Chapter 7) offers a delayed-release form consisting of an impermeable shell with two lag plugs, enclosing a plug of active drug in the middle of the unit. After the inert plugs have eroded, the drug is released, thus a lag-time occurs. Time of release can then be modulated by the length and composition of the plugs. The shells are made of (slowly) biodegradable polymers (such as ethylcellulose) and include plasticizers (such as cetostearyl alcohol), while the matrix of the plugs is comprises a mixture of pharmaceutical excipients including polymers like polyethylene oxide (PEO).

Chronset^{TM} (for more details, see Chapter 8) is a proprietary OROS® delivery system that reproducibly delivers a bolus drug dose ($>80\%$ drug release within 15 minutes) in a time- or site-specific manner to the gastrointestinal tract (GIT). Using the Chronset technology, the drug formulation is completely protected from chemical and enzymatic degradation in the GIT before release, and the timing of release is unaffected by GIT contents. By specifically balancing the osmotic engine, the semipermeable membrane, and the other attributes of the system configuration, drug release onset times varying from 1 to 20 hours can be achieved. The design of Chronset, its operation mechanism, the control features, and in vivo performance in human volunteers are described.

The *Ceform*^{TM} technology [333] allows the production of uniformly sized and shaped microspheres of pharmaceutical compounds. This approach is based on "melt-spinning", which means subjecting solid feedstock (i.e., biodegradable polymer/bioactive agent combinations) to a combination of temperature, thermal gradients, mechanical forces, flow, and flow rates during processing. The microspheres obtained are almost perfectly spherical, having a diameter that is typically 150–180 μm, and allow for high drug content. The microspheres can be used in a wide variety of dosage forms, including tablets, capsules, suspensions, effervescent tablets, and sachets. The microspheres may be coated for controlled release with an enteric coating or may be combined into a fast/slow release combination.

In the *Codas*^{TM} (Chronotherapeutic Oral Drug Absorption System) technology [334], there is a multiparticle system designed for bedtime drug dosing, incorporating a 4–5-hour delay in drug delivery. This delay is introduced by the level of nonenteric release-controlling polymer applied to drug-loaded beads. The release-controlling polymer is a combination of water-soluble and water-insoluble polymers. As water from the gastrointestinal tract comes into contact with the polymer-coated beads, the water-soluble polymer slowly dissolves and the drug diffuses through the resulting pores in the coating. The water-insoluble polymer continues to act as a barrier, maintaining the controlled release of verapamil [335]. The rate of release is essentially independent of pH, posture, and food.

In the *Contin*^{TM} technology, molecular coordination complexes are formed between a cellulose polymer and a nonpolar solid aliphatic alcohol optionally substituted with an aliphatic group by solvating the polymer with a volatile polar solvent and reacting the solvated cellulose polymer directly with the aliphatic alcohol, preferably as a melt. This constitutes the complex having utility as a matrix in controlled release formulations since it has a uniform porosity (semi permeable matrixes) that may be varied [336].

The *GeoClock*^{TM} technology is based on the Geomatrix^{TM} technology. In the *Geomatrix technology,* a multi layer tablet design was initially proposed for constant drug release. It consists of a drug-free barrier layer on one or both bases of an active core (hydrophilic matrix). The partial coating modulates the core hydration process and reduces the surface area available for drug release. During dissolution, the swellable barrier swells and gels, but is not eroded, thus acting as a modulating membrane during the release process. The erodible barrier, instead, was progressively removed by the dissolution medium, exposing in time an increasing extent of the planar surface(s) of the core to interaction with the outer environment and to drug release [337]. Quite recently, this technology has been used to develop Lodotra^{TM}, a prednisone-containing chronopharmaceutical formulation for rheumatoid arthritis management.

With this new ChrDDS, the drug can be taken at bedtime, but the active substance only gets released in the early hours of the morning, the optimum time point to treat morning symptoms such as stiffness and pain due to the inhibition of inflammatory cytokines.

The *Port^{TM} (Programmable Oral Release Technologies)* [338] uses a uniquely coated, encapsulated system that can provide multiple programmed release of drug. The basic design of the Port technology tablet consists of a polymer core matrix coated with a semi permeable, rate-controlling polymer. Poorly soluble drugs can be coated with proprietary solubilization agents to ensure uniform controlled release from the dosage form. The basic design of the Port system of capsule consists of a hard gelatin capsule coated with a semi permeable, rate-controlling polymer. Inside the coated capsule is the osmotic energy source, which normally contains the therapeutic agent to be delivered. The capsule is sealed with a water-insoluble lipid separator plug. An immediate release dosage can be added above the plug to complete the dosing options.

Three Dimensional Printing™ (3DP) technology is used in the fabrication of complex oral dosage delivery pharmaceuticals based on solid free-form fabrication methods. It is possible to engineer devices with complicated internal geometries, varying densities, diffusivities, and chemicals [339]. Different types of complex oral drug delivery devices have been fabricated using the 3DP process: immediate–extended release tablets, pulse release, breakaway tablets, and dual pulsatory tablets. The enteric dual pulsatile tablets were constructed of one continuous enteric excipient phase into which diclofenac sodium was printed into two separated areas. These samples showed two pulses of release in vitro with a lag time between pulses of about 4 hours [340]. This technology is the basis of the TheriForm^{®} technology [341]. The latter is a microfabrication process that works in a manner very similar to an "inkjet" printer. It is a fully integrated computer-aided development and manufacturing process. Products may be designed on a computer screen as three-dimensional models before actual implementation of their preparation process.

The *TIMERx™* technology [342] is a very versatile hydrogel-based controlled release technology. The unique nature of TIMERx intermolecular physical chemistry was described in relation to the technology's potential to provide any one of a number of different release profiles, ranging from zero order to chronotherapeutic release. The authors claimed that the "molecular engine" replaces the need for complex processing or novel excipients and allows desired drug release profiles to be "factory set" following a simple formulation development process [343]. Basically, this technology [342] combines primarily xanthan and locust bean gums mixed with dextrose. The physical interaction between these components works to form a strong, binding gel in the presence of water. Drug release is controlled by the rate of water penetration from the gastrointestinal tract into the TIMERx™ gum matrix, which expands to form a gel and subsequently releases the active drug substance.

Other controlled release systems that may find future applications in chronotherapy include *e*rodible polymers in different forms [297], programmable pulsatile release capsule devices [297], guar gum-based matrix tablets [344], sigmoidal release systems [345, 346], and self exploding microparticles [347].

1.6.3 Chronopharmaceutical Drug Delivery Systems for Transdermal Route

The transdermal route is a potential alternative for drug administration for chronotherapy. For that goal, the technologies that have been or are being investigated include crystal reservoir, automated transdermal drug delivery (ChronoDose™ system), and other advanced transdermal drug delivery technologies.

Use of a crystal reservoir system was first reported by Kato et al. [348] as a transdermal system for chronotherapy that was expected to provide more effective and safe treatment of asthma and related diseases not only in adults but also in children. The superiority of the transdermal formulation of tulobuterol over the oral formulations was indicated by its excellent pharmacokinetic profile and was confirmed by the results of clinical trials [348]. A thermoresponsive membrane was also developed by entrapping a single or binary liquid crystal to achieve an on–off switching drug delivery for transdermal application via the externally repeated cycle of temperature change, which may simulate the dosing time of therapeutic needs for the human body [301]. Specifically in this case, a thermoresponsive membrane embedded with the binary mixture of 36% cholesteryl oleyl carbonate and 64% cholesteryl nonanoate was developed to achieve a rate-controlled and time-controlled drug release in response to the skin temperature of the human body [349].

The ChronoDose system is a revolutionary drug delivery device, worn like a wristwatch, which can be preprogrammed to administer drug doses into the body automatically, at different times of the day and with varying dose sizes. It automatically turns on and off to release drugs at preset times in preset amounts while the person is asleep or awake. The system is capable of precisely tailoring drug delivery where noninvasive, automated "time and dose precise" drug administration was previously impossible. This automated transdermal system is protected by a U.S. patent [350]. Basically, the system is a device for delivering a medicament, which has a membrane with at least one area permeable to the medicament and a reservoir space that contains a solvent and the medicament at least partially dissolved therein. An adjustable and/or deformable control element is disposed on the side of the membrane facing the reservoir space; access of the medicament from the reservoir space to at least one permeable area of the membrane can be changed. In addition an electronic device is provided whose control element can automatically be activated via a motor. The device permits the periodic alteration of the delivery rate of medicament, which is advantageous in many cases, including chronopharmaceutical applications.

In the future, advances in transdermal drug delivery systems [145, 351, 352] (e.g., iontophoresis, sonophoresis, electroporation, and microneedle) may be used either alone or in combination with nanoengineering tools in the search for novel ChrDDSs for this route.

1.6.4 Chronoprevention Systems of Diseases: Chronotheranostics

The term *theranostics* is a hybrid of the words therapeutics and diagnostics. It represents the integration of diagnostic and therapeutic products. It helps scientists develop better drugs, tailor the right therapy for individual patients, and make treatment more cost effective. Using theranostics, physicians are better able to select the right combination of drugs, in the right dose and at the right time. Instead of using standard dosing, doctors can personalize medicine, thereby greatly enhancing prospects for improving patients' lives. Drug companies and diagnostic test developers are increasingly teaming up to produce theranostics [353, 354]. Therefore chronotheranostics would be the integration of diagnostics in the design of ChrDDSs and chronotherapy. Understanding of the chronobiological basis of diseases suggests that the engineering of novel therapeutic systems not only for treating but also for real-time screening, diagnosis, monitoring, and/or prevention of diseases (for more details see chapter 11) would be advantageous and life saving. Therefore the bioengineering and health profession communities need to develop cost-effective, fully unobtrusive, truly ambulatory systems for the surveillance and treatment of key vital parameters such as blood pressure heart rate, blood glucose, and cholesterol. To illustrate this concept, we focus on the case of vaccines, cardiovascular diseases, diabetes, and hypercholesterolemia.

In the area of vaccination and immunotherapy, the various components of the immune system are characterized by a multifrequency time structure. The organization of the immune system along the yearly scale may influence the seasonal incidence of numerous infectious diseases and can affect the success/failure of immunotherapy [355].

In the cardiovascular aspect, advanced diagnostic technologies using ambulatory blood pressure monitoring (ABPM) and electrocardiogram have also allowed researchers to study the effects of varying the timing of administration or delivery of a concentration of a drug on endpoints, such as changes in blood pressure, heart rate, or intensity of angina [245]. The ABPM devices such as Spacelabs models have been shown to be accurate enough for routine clinical use in a variety of patients. Factors such as age, weight, gender, and severity of hypertension are statistically associated with greater device error but the differences are small enough to be unlikely to affect clinical practice [356]. The devices have to meet the Association for the Advancement of Medical Instrumentation's standards [357, 358]. It is even now possible to document the circadian hyperamplitude tension (CHAT) defined as a week-long overall increase in the circadian amplitude or otherwise-measured circadian variability of blood pressure above a mapped threshold [359]. Recently, it has been shown that chronobiology predicts actual and proxy outcomes when dipping fails [360].

For diabetes, using ABPM, it was reported that in persons with type 1 diabetes mellitus (DM1), an increase in systolic blood pressure during sleep precedes the development of microalbuminuria. In those whose blood pressure during sleep decreases normally, the progression from normal albumin excretion to microalbuminuria appears to be less likely [184]. It was also found that the accuracy and precision of the FreeStyle Navigator continuous glucose monitoring system (CGMS) in children with type 1 diabetes has the potential to be an important adjunct to treatment of youth with type 1 diabetes [361]. Moreover, a CGMS can detect postprandial hyperglycemia and unrecognized hypoglycemia in type 1 diabetes mellitus patients, and improve therapeutic management [362].

Nearly two-thirds of patients diagnosed with dyslipidemia and enrolled in a pharmacist-managed lipid clinic (LC) had low density lipoprotein cholesterol levels at or below the National Cholesterol Education Panel–Adult Treatment Panel III (NCEP ATP III) target goal compared with 16% of dyslipidemia patients who received usual care (UC) from their primary care provider. The pharmacist-managed LC patients were also twice as likely (83% vs. 41%) to have attained the total cholesterol target goal, but there was no difference between the two groups in the proportion of patients who attained either triglyceride or high density lipoprotein target goals [363]. Similar successful results from other pharmacist-managed LCs indicated that LCs can be developed and integrated into a primary care medical clinic. Pharmacists can effectively manage lipid-lowering therapy, helping to achieve LDL goals [364]. This successful human monitoring model in dyslipidemia suggested that a chronotheranostic approach in this case would also be beneficial.

Collectively, these studies suggest that the identification and real-time monitoring of rhythmic biomarkers may be useful in choosing the most appropriate time of day for administration of drugs and may increase their therapeutic effects and/or reduce their side effects [180, 365]. In the current era of genomics/proteomics, it has become clearer that most diseases are due to some form of chemical imbalance within the body. Traditional disease treatment has attempted to correct those chemical imbalances regardless of the physiological timing. With recent advances and knowledge in chronogenetics and epidemiology, we are beginning to understand that simple correction of the disease with a constant amount of chemical is not enough for optimal therapy. For optimum disease therapy, the time factor (kinetics) should be taken into account not only at the early stage of drug discovery and development but also during the use and delivery of the medication. Moreover, technologies that allow timely monitoring in an ambulatory setting and/or the prevention of disease such as diabetes, hypertension, and hypercholesterolemia will increase human lifespan in the future.

1.7 RESOURCES FOR CHRONOPHARMACEUTICAL DRUG DELIVERY RESEARCH

One of the bottlenecks to the advances in innovative sciences and technologies for chronotherapeutics application is the lack of information on current resources available to researchers in this emerging field. For didactic purposes, the relevant chronopharmaceutical resources may be divided among (1) formulation, (2) chronopharmacokinetics/chronopharmacodynamics, (3) chronogenetics/molecular biology resources, and (4) regulatory/ethical resources.

1.7.1 Chronopharmaceutical Drug Formulation Resources

The formulation of effective and safe chronopharmaceutical drug delivery systems may be based on emerging information from evidence-based medicine (EBM) and current advances in modeling delivery rhythmic processes. EBM stresses the examination of evidence from clinical research as an important basis for the practice of medicine. EBM is an approach that is intuitively reasonable and is increasingly taught in medical schools and incorporated into practice [366]. The use of EBM in the education of scientists and health care professionals involved in chronopharmaceutical drug development and delivery and prevention of diseases will be an important asset for effective formulation and drug delivery in the context of chronotherapy in the future. For example, a simple model for an autonomous pulsing drug delivery system was introduced by Li and Siegel [367]. Depending on system parameters and external driving substrate concentration, the qualitative dynamics of this model permit, two separate single steady state, double steady state, and permanently alternating (oscillatory) behaviors [367]. Other modeling and rationalization of biological rhythm data treatment have occurred at all levels: from the system engineering aspect (Siegel), to the molecular [368–372], cellular [373], and organismic levels [369, 372–375].

At the cellular level, for example, it was shown that a constant duration of the dosing interval yields higher survival rates in mice treated by cytarabine, as compared with random dosing intervals. Minimal myelotoxicity was exerted when the dosing interval was an exact multiple of the intermitotic time of bone marrow stem cells and erythroid progenitors (i.e., 7 h). Survival was significantly lower in mice treated every 8 h or its multiple, as compared with that of mice treated at a 7-h or 10-h dosing interval [376]. At the tissue level, the theoretical and experimental aspect of the resonance effect in self-renewing tissues was analyzed using a mathematical model to describe the kinetics of cell populations under periodic treatment by high doses of a phase-specific cytotoxic agent with blocking effect. That study provided excellent agreement between theoretical and experimental results and the estimations of cycle parameters of the drug; cryptogenic and transit cells of mice intestine epithelium were obtained [374].

The need for biologic models that account for the interaction of three or more periodic entities was indicated, documented and illustrated, with emphasis on the cephaloadrenal network of rodents [377]. Clearly, various mathematical models have been used to assess the suitability of periodic functions associated with biological rhythms. The most common approach is that of "cosinor rhythmometry," in which a linear least squares regression is used to fit a sinusoidal curve to time-series data [378–380]. Although these curve-fitting techniques can be helpful, they are not suitable for right-censored failure time data. To bridge the knowledge gap in this respect, a method to estimate the time to achieve minimum hazard along with its associated confidence interval has been presented [381]. The model was then used to predict the optimal day in the menstrual cycle for breast cancer surgery (i.e., day associated with the lowest recurrence rate) in premenopausal women. Perhaps this newer model will enhance the prediction power of chronotherapy and chronointerventions. Recently, the possibility to engineer rhythms has been demonstrated [6–8], suggesting future integration between engineering and biology (in the emerging concept of system biology) would perhaps provide additional foundation for chonopharmaceutics.

1.7.2 Chronopharmacokinetic and Chronopharmacodynamic Resources

Chronopharmacokinetics (discussed in detailed in Chapter 3) deals with the study of the temporal changes in absorption, distribution, metabolism, and elimination and thus takes into account the influence of time of administration on these different steps [140, 239, 382]. A mathematical model for area under the curve (AUC) determination was proposed by Hecquet [383], taking into account the circadian variation of cisplatin protein binding. The model can be applied to other drugs that are irreversibly bound to proteins or irreversibly bound to other plasma components if the binding rate depends on the time of day [384, 385]. Modelization also shows up the complex relationship between a temporally structured organism and an exogenous substance that has not been designed to be integrated into a set of biological rhythms [386].

Far more drugs are shown to display significant daily variations in their effects (chronopharmacodynamics [387]) even after chronic application or constant infusion [388]. Overall, there is clear evidence that the dose/concentration–response relationship of drugs can be significantly dependent on the time of day. Thus circadian time has to be taken into account as an important variable influencing a drug's pharmacokinetics and/or its effects or side effects [388].

A new approach for describing the input function in indirect response models with biorhythmic baselines of physiologic substances was recently introduced [389]. That approach used the baseline (placebo) response $R_b(t)$ to recover the equation for a periodic time-dependent production rate, $k_{in}(t)$. A computer program was developed to perform the square L2-norm approximation technique [389]. Theoretical equations and methods of data analysis were developed and simulations were also provided to demonstrate expected response behavior based on biexponential response dissipation. Such a model was subsequently applied for inhibition of circadian cortisol secretion by prednisolone [390]. Recently, the integrated models based on a two-harmonic function were able to capture the circadian expression patterns of plasma cortisol and glucocorticoid receptor and glutamine synthetase in normal rat skeletal muscle showing a dependence of tissue gene expression on plasma cortisol [391]. These data indicate that novel approaches in pharmacokinetics and pharmacodynamics are needed in the era of chrono-pharmaceutics to better capture the biological rhythm expression patterns.

1.7.3   Genetics and Molecular Biology Resources

The chronogenetic aspects as a solid foundation for chronopharmaceutics are discussed in detail in Chapter 2. Briefly, different genetic models have been used to elucidate the genetic basis of biological rhythms including zebrafish [392, 393], simple protozoans and unicellular algae (e.g., cyanobacterial strain [394–398]), *Drosophila* brain [183, 185], mammalian cells [190, 192, 393, 399], tissue-based circadian oscillators [195, 197, 400], and mouse [144, 159].

It is important to underscore that the convergence of data from microarray studies, quantitative trait locus analysis, and mutagenesis screens have demonstrated the pervasiveness of circadian regulation in biological systems [401]. The microarray studies [402–406] have been extensively used in chronogenetics research. Along with the improvement of the assay as a laboratory examination method, cDNA microarray would facilitate the integration of diagnosis and therapeutics, and the introduction of individual medicines [407]. The recent development in protein microarrays using reverse phase [209] has been referred to as one of the cornerstones in the future development of chronotheranostics [408]. The quantitative trait loci (QTLs) can be identified in several ways, but is there a definitive test of whether a candidate locus actually corresponds to a specific QTL [409]? A quantitative trait is one that has measurable phenotypic variation owing to genetic and/or environmental influences. Peleman et al. [410] presented an alternative method that significantly speeds up QTL fine mapping by using one segregating population [410]. A genetic screen (often shortened to screen) is a procedure or test to identify and select individuals who possess a phenotype of interest. Mutant alleles that are not tagged for rapid cloning are mapped and cloned by positional cloning [148]. Random mutagenesis screens for recessive phenotypes require three generations of breeding, using either a backcross or intercross strategy. Using a probabilistic approach, it was possible to contrast, for a range of experimental designs, the cost per mutation screened and to maximize the number of mutations that one can expect to screen in a given experiment [411].

1.7.4 Ethical and Regulatory Resources

The regulatory issue for modified drug delivery systems has been discussed extensively [412]. Nanomedicine is a science that uses nanotechnology to maintain and improve human health at the molecular scale. This emerging field has current and potential applications ranging from research involving diagnostic devices and drug delivery vehicles to enhanced gene therapy and tissue engineering procedures [413]. If a ChrDDS is a nanomedicine, it is important to underscore the regulatory challenges facing the FDA in regulating nanomedical products [414]. First, the FDA will have trouble fitting the products into the agency's classification scheme (nomenclature issue). Second, it will be difficult for the FDA to maintain adequate scientific expertise in the field. It is recommended that the FDA consider implementing several reforms now to ensure that it is adequately prepared to regulate nanomedicine including those related to chronotherapy. The value of quantitative thinking in drug development and regulatory review is increasingly being appreciated. Modeling and simulation of data pertaining to pharmacokinetics, pharmacodynamics, and disease progression is often referred to as pharmacometrics analysis [415]. There is a need for early interaction between the FDA and drug makers to plan development more efficiently by appreciating the regulatory expectations for drug products intended for chronotherapy and chronoprevention of diseases, due to the new nature of the field. It is also important to keep in mind that the draft guidance for industry related to extended-release solid oral dosage forms—the development, evaluation, and application of in vitro–in vivo correlations [416]—may be important resources in this respect. A biopharmaceutic drug classification scheme for correlating the invitro drug product dissolution and in vivo bioavailability for immediate release (IR) products has been proposed [417]. Further developments raised the issue of whether the biopharmaceutic classification has relevance to extended release (ER) products. In contrast to IR products, drugs selected for use in ER products should have good gastrointestinal permeability and an extended site of absorption. Of particular relevance to both permeability and solubility is the degree of ionization of the drug. Residence time at each site, pH changes, and the potential for drug degradation at different sites (the latter resulting in a restricted absorption window) will influence the time frame over which an in vitro and in vivo (IVIV) relationship is possible [418]. The practice of comparing rate of absorption from ER dosage forms using steady-state C_{max} is inappropriate due to lack of sensitivity [419]. Thus to develop and validate internally an IVIVC for a hydrophilic matrix extended release metoprolol tablet, the f_2 metric (similarity factor) was used to analyze the dissolution data, and the relatively low prediction errors for C_{max} and AUC observed strongly suggested that the metoprolol IVIVC models are valid [420]. Similar work and models remained to be demonstrated for ChrDDSs.

Demonstrating to regulatory agencies that a new drug product is safe, effective, and of acceptable quality (the first three hurdles) is no longer sufficient. The fourth hurdle is commonly described as what has to be done to gain market access and reimbursement for a pharmaceutical, medical technology, or biotech product. Drug product manufacturers must often now demonstrate both clinical effectiveness as well as costeffectiveness in order to assure success in the marketplace [421]. For example, patent and regulatory hurdles combined with low returns on investment have impacted the antibiotic R&D in the pharmaceutical industry [422]. These regulatory hurdles may be particularly important for ChrDDSs for which the benefits are not always obvious due to the long history of medical and pharmaceutical practice based on the obsolete notion of zero-order release. Despite notable steps in recent years to lower regulatory barriers and speed approvals, especially for products for life-threatening conditions, the FDA is under great pressure from Congress, industry, and patients to do more [423].

The basic expectations for the methods of human and animal biological rhythm research, both from the perspective of the fundamental criteria necessary for quality chronobiology investigation and from the perspective of humane and ethical research on human beings and animals, have been extensively reviewed [424]. All chronopharmaceutical and chronotherapy studies should conform to the respective policy and mandates of the Declaration of Helsinki and the Guide for the Care and Use of Laboratory Animals following the standards of good research practice. The foregoing information suggests that updated regulatory concern may be needed for chronopharmaceutical systems.

1.8 CONCLUSION AND FUTURE PERSPECTIVES

Applications of chronopharmaceutical drug products are now better understood for selected disease such as cancer and hypertension. But increasing resources will be required to achieve the chronopharmaceutical advantages of this emerging approach to disease therapy and prevention for other major human diseases. The ultimate outcomes would be a more effective and better quality medicine/pharmaceutical product or device for real-time and/or ambulatory disease monitoring systems. Although current technology is still in its infancy, it is speculated that the future integration of emerging technologies and engineering concepts with biology (e.g., system biology), and the ongoing education of health care providers (nurse, physician, and pharmacist) and patients on future developments in this field will play an important role in the achievement of these ideal disease prevention and treatment objectives. Efforts to expand the understanding and use of chronotherapy must include a basic research phase (to elucidate the temporal and molecular basis of diseases), a drug development phase (to increase product robustness, safety, efficacy, portability, flexibility, and artificial intelligence; to increase the number of active pharmaceutical ingredients; and to determine the diseases to be targeted by a given system), and an education phase (to increase the awareness for health care providers and patients).

REFERENCES

1. Smolensky MH, D'Alonzo GE. *Am J Med.* 1988; 85: 34.
2. Smolensky MH, Portaluppi F. *Am Heart J.* 1999; 137: S14.
3. Smolensky MH, Peppas NA. *Adv Drug Delivery Rev.* 2007; 59: 823.
4. Silver R, LeSauter J, Tresco PA, Lehman MN. *Nature.* 1996; 382: 810.
5. Bates DW, et al. *JAMA.* 1997; 277: 307.
6. Kiss IZ, Rusin CG, Kori H, Hudson JL. *Science.* 2007; 316: 1886.
7. Bongard J, Lipson H. *Proc Natl Acad Sci USA.* 2007; 104: 9943.
8. Kath WL, Ottino JM. *Science.* 2007; 316: 1857.
9. Moore-Ede M, Fuller C, Sulzman F. *The Clocks That Time Us.* Boston: Commonwealth Fund Publications, Havard University Press; 1982: 448.
10. Pittendrigh C, Aschoff J. In: Schmitt FO, Worden FG, eds. *Neurosciences Third Study Program.* Cambridge, MA: MIT Press; 1974: 437–458.
11. Bussemer T, Otto I, Bodmeier R. *Crit Rev Ther Drug Carrier Syst.* 2001; 18: 433.
12. Youan BB. *J Control Release.* 2004; 98: 337.
13. Reinberg AE, Lewy H, Smolensky M. *Chronobiol Int.* 2001; 18: 173.
14. Aschoff J. *Science.* 1965; 148: 1427.
15. Benzer S. *JAMA.* 1971; 218: 1015.
16. Wheeler DA, et al. *Science.* 1991; 251: 1082.
17. Young M, Ziman J. *Nature.* 1971; 229: 91.
18. Rosbash M, Takahashi JS. *Nature.* 2002; 420: 373.
19. Halberg F, et al. *J Circadian Rhythms.* 2003; 1: 2.
20. Langer R. *Acc Chem Res.* 2000; 33: 94.
21. Youan BB. *Nanomedicine.* 2008; 3: 401.
22. Chamberlain D. *Arethusa.* 1999; 32: 263.
23. Lassere F. *Les Belles Lettres.* Paris: Association Guillaume Bude; 1958 XXIV–XXVI.
24. Davenport G. *Carmina Archilochi: The Fragments of Archilochus.* Berkeley: University of California Press; 1964.
25. Bretzl H. *Botanische Forschungen des Alexanderzuges.* Leipzig: Teubner; 1903: 120–132.
26. de Mairan J. *Observation botanique.* Paris: Histoire de l'Académie Royale des Sciences; 1729: pp. 35–36.
27. de Mairan J. Traite physique et historique de l'Aurore Boréale. Par M. de Mairan. Suite des Mémoires de l'Académie Royale des Sciences, Année M. DCCXXXI (Physical and historical treatise of the Aurora Borealis. By M. De Mairan. Series of the Memoirs of the Royal Academy of Sciences, for the year 1731). Paris: Royal Printing Office; 1733: 570 pp. Second edition, 1754.

28. Hufeland CW. *Makrobiotik: The Art of Prolonging Life*. London: Bell; 1797 Second English translation, p 201.

29. Virey JJ. *Ephémérides de la vie humaine ou recherches sur la révolution journalière et la périodicité de ses phénomènes dans la santé et les maladies*. Paris: Thése Fac. Médecine; 1814.

30. AP de Candolle. *Physiologie végétale, ou, Exposition des forces et des fonctions vitales des végétaux pour servir de suite a l'organographie végétale, et d'introduction a la botanique géographique et agricole*. Paris: Bechet; 1832.

31. Vollot J, Sardou G, Faure M. De l'influence des taches solaires: sur les accidents aigus des maladies chroniques. *Gazette des Hôpitaux*. 1922: 904–905 (18 et 20 juillet).

32. Chizhevsky AL. In: Piéry M, ed. *Traité de Climatologie: Biologique et médicale*. Paris: Masson et Cie; 1934: 662–673.

33. Chizhevsky AL. Paper presented at the Verhandlungen, Zweiten Konferenz der Internationalen Gesellschaft für Biologische Rhythmusforschung, Utrecht, Holland, 1940.

34. Chizhevsky AL, Fedynsky VV, eds. *The Earth in the Universe*. (Translated from Russian and edited by IRST staff). NASA TT F-345. Jerusalem: Israel Program for Scientific Translations. (Available from US Department of Commerce, Clearinghouse for Federal Scientific and Technical Information, Springfield, Virginia, 1968, p. 280.

35. Sigel F. *Schuld ist die Sonne*. Frankfurt am Main: Harri Deutsch; 1979: 215.

36. T Düll, B Düll. *Virchows Arch*. 1934; 293: 272.

37. T Düll, B Düll. *Dtsch Med Wochenschr*. 1935; 61: 95.

38. Johnson MS. *J Exp Zool*. 1939; 82: 315.

39. Jores A. *Hippokrates (Stutt)*. 1939; 10: 1185.

40. Halberg F, Visscher MB. *Proc Soc Exp Biol*. 1950; 75: 846.

41. Halberg F, Visscher MB, Flink EB, Berge K, Bock F. *Lancet*. 1951; 71: 312.

42. Halberg F, Engel R, Halberg E, Gully RJ. *Fed Proc*. 1952; 11: 62.

43. Halberg F, Visscher MB. *Endocrinology*. 1952; 51: 329.

44. Halberg F. *J Pharmacol Exp Ther*. 1952; 106: 135.

45. Halberg F. *Lancet*. 1953; 73: 20.

46. Halberg F, Visscher MB, Bittner JJ. *Am J Physiol*. 1953; 174: 109.

47. Halberg F, Visscher MB, Bittner JJ. *Am J Physiol*. 1954; 179: 229.

48. Halberg F, Bittner JJ, Gully RJ, Albrecht PG, Brackney EL. *Proc Soc Exp Biol Med*. 1955; 88: 169.

49. Halberg F, Spink WW, Albrecht PG, Gully RJ. *J Clin Endocrinol*. 1955; 15: 887.

50. Menzel W. *Medizinische*. 1956; 1521.

51. Halberg F, Bittner JJ, Smith D. *Z Vitamin-, Hormon Fermentforsch*. 1957; 9: 69.

52. Halberg F, Jacobsen E, Wadsworth G, Bittner JJ. *Science*. 1958; 128: 657.

53. Halberg F, Barnum CP, Silber RH, Bittner JJ. *Proc Soc Exp Biol Med*. 1958; 97: 897.

54. Engel R, Halberg F, Dassanayake WL, J De Silva. *Nature*. 1958; 181: 1135.

55. Halberg F. *Int Z Vitaminforsch Beih*. 1959; 10: 225.

56. Halberg F, Haus E, Stephens A. *Fed Proc*. 1959; 18: 63.

57. Halberg F, Halberg E, Barnum CP, Bittner JJ. In: Withrow RB, ed. *Photoperiodism and Related Phenomena in Plants and Animals*, vol. 55. Washington DC: AAAS; 1959: 803–878.

58. Halberg F. *Cold Spring Harb Symp Quant Biol*. 1960; 25: 289.

59. Halberg F. *Am J Ment Defic*. 1960; 65: 156.

60. T Hellbrügge. *Cold Spring Harb Symp Quant Biol*. 1960; 25: 311.

61. Brown FAJ. *Cold Spring Harb Symp Quant Biol*. 1960; 25: 57.

62. Marte E, Halberg F. *Fed Proc*. 1961; 20: 305.

63. Halberg F, et al. *Experientia*. 1961; 17: 282.

64. Halberg F, Conner RL. *Proc Minn Acad Sci*. 1961; 29: 227.

65. Halberg F, Adkins G, Marte E, Jones F. *Fed Proc*. 1962; 21: 347.

66. Ungar F, Halberg F. *Science*. 1962; 137: 1058.

67. Ertel RJ, Ungar F, Halberg F. *Fed Proc*. 1963; 22: 211.

68. Ertel RJ, Halberg F, Ungar F. *J Pharmacol Exp Ther*. 1964; 146: 395.

69. Jones F, Haus E, Halberg F. *Proc Minn Acad Sci*. 1963; 31: 61.

70. Halberg F. *Monatskurse Aerztl Fortbild*. 1964; 14: 67.

71. Galicich JH, Halberg F, French LA. *Nature*. 1963; 197: 811.

72. Halberg F, Engeli M, Hamburger C, Hillman D. *Acta Endocrinol (Kbh)*. 1965; 50: 5.

73. Spoor RP, Jackson DB. *Science*. 1966; 154: 782.

74. Halberg F, Tong YL, Johnson EA. In: Mayersbach HV, ed. *The Cellular Aspects of Biorhythms, Symposium on Biorhythms*. New York: Springer-Verlag; 1967: 20–48.

75. Colin J, Houdas Y, Boutelier C, Timbal J, Siffre M. *J Physiol (Paris)*. 1967; 59: 380.

76. Krieger DT, Krieger HP. *Science*. 1967; 155: 1421.

77. Matthews JH, Marte E, Halberg F. In: Fink BR, ed. *Toxicity of Anesthetics*. Baltimore: Williams and Wilkins; 1968: 197–208.

78. Weimann BJ, Lohrmann R, Orgel LE, Schneider-Bernloehr H, Sulston JE. *Science*. 1968; 161: 387.

79. Scheving LE, Vedral DF, Pauly JE. *Nature*. 1968; 219: 621.

80. Passouant P, Halberg F, Genicot R, Popoviciu L, Baldy-Moulinier M. *Rev Neurol (Paris)*. 1969; 121: 155.

81. Halberg F. *Annu Rev Physiol*. 1969; 31: 675.

82. Cardoso SS, Scheving LE, Halberg F. *Pharmacologist*. 1970; 12: 302 (abstract) .

83. Haus E, et al. *Science*. 1972; 177: 80.

84. Halberg F, et al. *Experientia (Basel)*. 1973; 29: 909.

85. Scheving LE, Burns ER, Pauly JE, Halberg F, Haus E. *Cancer Res*. 1977; 37: 3648.

86. Halberg F, et al. *Cancer Treat Rep*. 1979; 63: 1428.

87. Halberg F. Paper presented at the Conference on Science and the International Man: The Computer, Chanea, Crete, June 1970.

88. Hastings JW. *N Engl J Med*. 1970; 282: 435.

89. Moore JG, Englert E Jr. *Nature*. 1970; 226: 1261.

90. Halberg F. In: *Encyclopædia of Occupational Health and Safety*, vol 1. Geneva: International Labour Office; 1971: 177–179.

91. Nelson W, Kupferberg H, Halberg F. *Toxicol Appl Pharmacol*. 1971; 18: 335.

92. Krieger DT. *Science*. 1972; 178: 1205.

93. Halberg F, Johnson EA, Nelson W, Runge W, Sothern R. *Physiol Tchr*. 1972; 1: 1.

94. Smolensky M, Halberg F, Sargent F. In: Itoh S, Ogata K, Yoshimura H, eds. *Advances in Climatic Physiology*. Tokyo: Igaku Shoin Ltd; 1972: 281–318.

95. Halberg F. In: Mills JN, ed. *Biological Aspects of Circadian Rhythms*. New York: Plenum Press; 1973: 1–26.

96. Simpson H, et al. Paper presented at the Workshop 2 on Chronobiology and Allergy, Tokyo, 1973.

97. Nelson W, Cadotte L, Halberg F. *Proc Soc Exp Biol (NY)*. 1973; 144: 766.

98. Sundararaj BI, Vasal S, Halberg F. *Int J Chronobiol*. 1973; 1: 362.

99. Rosene G, Lee J, Kühl JFW, Halberg F, Grage TB. *Int J Chronobiol*. 1973; 1: 354.

100. Pittendrigh CS, Daan S. *Science*. 1974; 186: 548.

101. Aschoff J. In: Aschoff J, Ceresa F, Halberg F, eds. *Chronobiological Aspects of Endocrinology*, vol. 1 (Suppl 1). Stuttgart: FK Schattauer Verlag; 1974: 483–495.

102. Ehret CF, Potter VR, Dobra KW. *Science*. 1975; 188: 1212.

103. Yates CA, Herbert J. *Nature*. 1976; 262: 219.

104. Turek FW, McMillan JP, Menaker M. *Science*. 1976; 194: 1441.

105. Langer R, Folkman J. *Nature*. 1976; 263: 797.

106. Halberg F. Biological as well as physical parameters relate to radiology. Guest Lecture, Paper presented at the 30th Annual Congress on Radiology, Post-Graduate Institute of Medical Education and Research, Chandigarh, India, January 1977: 8 pp.

107. Morin LP, Fitzgerald KM, Zucker I. *Science*. 1977; 196: 305.

108. Corrent G, McAdoo DJ, Eskin A. *Science*. 1978; 202: 977.

109. Handler AM, Konopka RJ. *Nature*. 1979; 279: 236.

110. Czeisler CA, Weitzman E, Moore-Ede MC, Zimmerman JC, Knauer RS. *Science*. 1980; 210: 1264.

111. Barnes P, FitzGerald G, Brown M, Dollery C. *N Engl J Med*. 1980; 303: 263.

112. Halberg F, Nelson WL, Haus E. In: Vernadakis A, Timiras PS, eds. *Hormones in Development and Aging*. New York: Spectrum Publications; 1981: 451–476.

113. Czeisler CA, Moore-Ede MC, Coleman RH. *Science*. 1982; 217: 460.

114. Takahashi JS, Zatz M. *Science*. 1982; 217: 1104.

115. Redman J, Armstrong S, Ng KT. *Science*. 1983; 219: 1089.

116. Eskin A, Takahashi JS. *Science*. 1983; 220: 82.

117. Zumoff B, et al. *N Engl J Med*. 1983; 309: 1206.

118. Earnest DJ, Turek FW. *Science*. 1983; 219: 77.

119. Garrick NA, Tamarkin L, Taylor PL, Markey SP, Murphy DL. *Science*. 1983; 221: 474.

120. Albers HE, Ferris CF, Leeman SE, Goldman BD. *Science*. 1984; 223: 833.

121. Takahashi JS, DeCoursey PJ, Bauman L, Menaker M. *Nature*. 1984; 308: 186.

122. Hrushesky WJ. *Science*. 1985; 228: 73.

123. Swann JM, Turek FW. *Science*. 1985; 228: 898.

124. Muller JE, et al. *N Engl J Med*. 1985; 313: 1315.

125. Turek FW, Losee-Olson S. *Nature*. 1986; 321: 167.

126. Czeisler CA, et al. *Science*. 1986; 233: 667.

127. Tofler GH, et al. *N Engl J Med*. 1987; 316: 1514.

128. Roenneberg T, Nakamura H, Hastings JW. *Nature*. 1988; 334: 432.

129. G Cornélissen, Halberg F. In: Goldson AL, ed. *Cancer Growth and Progression*. Dordrecht: Kluwer Academic Publisher; 1989: 103–133.

130. Turek FW, Losee-Olson S. *Endocrinology*. 1988; 122: 756.

131. Hrushesky WJ. *Prog Clin Biol Res*. 1990; 341A: 1.

132. Czeisler CA, et al. *N Engl J Med*. 1990; 322: 1253.

133. Levi F, Canon C, Dipalma M, Florentin I, Misset JL. *Ann N Y Acad Sci*. 1991; 618: 312.

134. Halberg F, G Cornélissen, Bingham C, Fujii S, Halberg E. *In vivo*. 1992; 6: 403.

135. Takahashi JS. *Science*. 1992; 258: 238.

136. Zaslavskaya RM. *Chronodiagnosis and Chronotherapy of Cardiovascular Diseases*, 2nd ed Translation into English from Russian Moscow: Medicina; 1993 397.

137. G Cornélissen, Halberg F. *Introduction to Chronobiology. Medtronic Chronobiology Seminar #7* 1994: p 52.

138. Takahashi JS, Pinto LH, Vitaterna MH. *Science*. 1994; 264: 1724.

139. Vitaterna MH, et al. *Science*. 1994; 264: 719.

140. Lemmer B. *Ciba Found Symp*. 1995; 183: 235.

141. Halberg F, G Cornélissen. *Fairy Tale or Reality? Medtronic Chronobiology Seminar #8*. Belgium: Brussels; 1995.

142. Myers MP, Wager-Smith K, Wesley CS, Young MW, Sehgal A. *Science*. 1995; 270: 805.

143. Sehgal A, et al. *Science*. 1995; 270: 808.

144. Gekakis N, et al. *Science*. 1995; 270: 811.

145. Mitragotri S, Blankschtein D, Langer R. *Science*. 1995; 269: 850.

146. Myers MP, Wager-Smith K, Rothenfluh-Hilfiker A, Young MW. *Science*. 1996; 271: 1736.

147. G Cornélissen, Halberg F, Hawkins D, Otsuka K, Henke W. *J Med Eng Technol*. 1997; 21: 111.

148. King DP, et al. *Cell*. 1997; 89: 641.

149. Antoch MP, et al. *Cell*. 1997; 89: 655.

150. Sun ZS, et al. *Cell*. 1997; 90: 1003.

151. Tei H, et al. *Nature*. 1997; 389: 512.

152. Shearman LP, Zylka MJ, Weaver DR, Kolakowski LF Jr, and Reppert SM. *Neuron*. 1997; 19: 1261.

153. Albrecht U, Sun ZS, Eichele G, Lee CC. *Cell*. 1997; 91: 1055.

154. Ikeda M, Nomura M. *Biochem Biophys Res Commun*. 1997; 233: 258.

155. Balsalobre A, Damiola F, Schibler U. *Cell*. 1998; 93: 929.

156. Schibler U. *Nature*. 1998; 393: 620.

157. Takumi T, et al. *Genes Cells*. 1998; 3: 167.

158. Takumi T, et al. *EMBO J*. 1998; 17: 4753.

159. Gekakis N, et al. *Science*. 1998; 280: 1564.

160. Zylka MJ, Shearman LP, Weaver DR, Reppert SM. *Neuron*. 1998; 20: 1103.

161. Zylka MJ, et al. *Neuron*. 1998; 21: 1115.

162. Koike N, et al. *FEBS Lett*. 1998; 441: 427.

163. Sangoram AM, et al. *Neuron*. 1998; 21: 1101.

164. Jones CR, et al. *Nat Med*. 1999; 5: 1062.

165. Tischkau SA, et al. *J Neurosci*. 1999; 19: RC15.

166. Takahashi JS. *Science*. 1999; 285: 2076.

167. Takumi T, et al. *Genes Cells*. 1999; 4: 67.

168. Griffin EA Jr., Staknis D, Weitz CJ. *Science*. 1999; 286: 768.

169. van der Horst GT, et al. *Nature*. 1999; 398: 627.

170. Okamura H, et al. *Science*. 1999; 286: 2531.

171. Santini JT Jr, Cima MJ, Langer R. *Nature*. 1999; 397: 335.

172. Yamazaki S, et al. *Science*. 2000; 288: 682.

173. Levi F. *Novartis Found Symp*. 2000; 227: 119.

174. Lowrey PL, et al. *Science*. 2000; 288: 483.

175. Bunger MK, et al. *Cell*. 2000; 103: 1009.

176. Balsalobre A, et al. *Science*. 2000; 289: 2344.

177. Krishnan B, et al. *Nature*. 2001; 411: 313.

178. Davis S, Mirick DK, Stevens RG. *J Natl Cancer Inst*. 2001; 93: 1557.

179. Toh KL, et al. *Science*. 2001; 291: 1040.

180. Ohdo S, Koyanagi S, Suyama H, Higuchi S, Aramaki H. *Nat Med*. 2001; 7: 356.

181. Yagita K, Tamanini F, van Der Horst GT, Okamura H. *Science*. 2001; 292: 278.

182. Schibler U, Ripperger JA, Brown SA. *Science*. 2001; 293: 437.

183. Panda S, et al. *Cell*. 2002; 109: 307.

184. Lurbe E, et al. *N Engl J Med*. 2002; 347: 797.

185. Panda S, Hogenesch JB, Kay SA. *Nature*. 2002; 417: 329.

186. Storch KF, et al. *Nature*. 2002; 417: 78.

187. Ueda HR, et al. *Nature*. 2002; 418: 534.

188. Fu L, Pelicano H, Liu J, Huang P, Lee C. *Cell*. 2002; 111: 41.

189. Schibler U, Sassone-Corsi P. *Cell*. 2002; 111: 919.

190. Schibler U. *Science*. 2003; 302: 234.

191. Yamaguchi S, et al. *Science*. 2003; 302: 1408.

192. Matsuo T, et al. *Science*. 2003; 302: 255.

193. Etchegaray JP, Lee C, Wade PA, Reppert SM. *Nature*. 2003; 421: 177.

194. Preitner N, et al. *Cell*. 2002; 110: 251.

195. Fu L, Lee CC. *Nat Rev Cancer*. 2003; 3: 350.

196. Zaslavskaya RM, et al. *Neuroendocrinol Lett*. 2003; 24: 238.

197. Hastings MH, Reddy AB, Maywood ES. *Nat Rev Neurosci.* 2003; 4: 649.

198. Benenson Y, Gil B, Ben-Dor U, Adar R, Shapiro E. *Nature.* 2004; 429: 423.

199. Kaasik K, Lee CC. *Nature.* 2004; 430: 467.

200. Turek FW, et al. *Science.* 2005; 308(5724): 1043–1045.

201. Gorbacheva VY, et al. *Proc Natl Acad Sci USA.* 2005; 102: 3407.

202. Xu Y, et al. *Nature.* 2005; 434: 640.

203. Koh K, Zheng X, Sehgal A. *Science.* 2006; 312: 1809.

204. Schwartzkopff O, et al. Paper presented at the International Conference on the Frontiers of Biomedical Science: Chronobiology, Chengdu, China, September 24–26, 2006.

205. Maywood ES, O'Neill J, Wong GK, Reddy AB, Hastings MH. *Prog Brain Res.* 2006; 153: 253.

206. van Mark A, Spallek M, Kessel R, Brinkmann E. *J Occup Med Toxicol.* 2006; 1: 25.

207. Masaki T, Yoshimatsu H. *Trends Pharmacol Sci.* 2006; 27: 279.

208. Manev H, Uz T. *Trends Pharmacol Sci.* 2006; 27: 186.

209. Eisenstein M. *Nature.* 2006; 444: 959.

210. Bhattacharjee Y. *Science.* 2007; 317: 1488.

211. Xu Y, et al. *Cell.* 2007; 128: 59.

212. Bentivoglio M, Kristensson K. *Trends Neurosci.* 2007; 30: 645.

213. Kohsaka A, Bass J. *Trends Endocrinol Metab.* 2007; 18: 4.

214. Mignot E, Takahashi JS. *Cell.* 2007; 128: 22.

215. Gooneratne NS. *Clin Geriatr Med.* 2008; 24: 121.

216. Misra S, Malow BA. *Clin Geriatr Med.* 2008; 24: 15.

217. Green CB, Takahashi JS, Bass J. *Cell.* 2008; 134: 728.

218. Belden WJ, Dunlap JC. *Cell.* 2008; 134: 212.

219. Asher G, et al. *Cell.* 2008; 134: 317.

220. Fuller PM, Lu J, Saper CB. *Science.* 2008; 320: 1074.

221. O'Neill JS, Maywood ES, Chesham JE, Takahashi JS, Hastings MH. *Science.* 2008; 320: 949.

222. Harrisingh MC, Nitabach MN. *Science.* 2008; 320: 879.

223. Mendez-Ferrer S, Lucas D, Battista M, Frenette PS. *Nature.* 2008; 452: 442.

224. Rajaratnam SM, Arendt J. *Lancet.* 2001; 358: 999.

225. Wagner DR. *Neurol Clin.* 1996; 14: 651.

226. Mignot E, Taheri S, Nishino S. *Nat Neurosci.* 2002; 5(Suppl), 1071.

227. Taheri S, Mignot E. *Lancet Neurol.* 2002; 1: 242.

228. Ziegler MC, Lake CR, Wood JH, Ebert MH. *Nature.* 1976; 264: 656.

229. Arendt J, Skene DJ, Middleton B, Lockley SW, Deacon S. *J Biol Rhythms.* 1997; 12: 604.

230. Skene DJ, Lockley SW, Arendt J. *Biol Signals Recept.* 1999; 8: 90.

231. Lockley SW, Brainard GC, Czeisler CA. *J Clin Endocrinol Metab.* 2003; 88: 4502.

232. Hattar S, Liao HW, Takao M, Berson DM, Yau KW. *Science.* 2002; 295: 1065.

233. Berson DM, Dunn FA, Takao M. *Science*. 2002; 295: 1070.

234. Cermakian N, et al. *Curr Biol*. 2002; 12: 844.

235. Martin RJ, Banks-Schlegel S. *Am J Respir Crit Care Med*. 1998; 158: 1002.

236. Smolensky MH, Reinberg A, Queng JT. *Ann Allergy*. 1981; 47: 234.

237. Reinberg A, et al. *Presse Med*. 1986; 15: 581.

238. Reinberg A, et al. *J Allergy Clin Immunol*. 1988; 81: 51.

239. Lemmer B. *Semin Perinatol*. 2000; 24: 280.

240. Smolensky MH, Reinberg A, Labrecque G. *J Allergy Clin Immunol*. 1995; 95: 1084.

241. Haus E. *Pathol Biol (Paris)*. 1996; 44: 618.

242. Green CB. *Proc Natl Acad Sci USA*. 2005; 102: 3529.

243. Muller JE, Tofler GH, Willich SN, Stone PH. *J Cardiovasc Pharmacol*. 1987; 10: S104.

244. Lobenberg R, Kim JS, Amidon GL. *Eur J Pharm Biopharm*. 2005; 60: 17.

245. Anwar YA, White WB. *Drugs*. 1998; 55: 631.

246. Carter BL. *Am J Health Syst Pharm*. 1998; 55(suppl 3), S17.

247. Casetta I, Granieri E, Portaluppi F, Manfredini R. *JAMA*. 2002; 287: 1266.

248. Poirel C, Ennaji M. *Psychol Rep*. 1991; 68: 783.

249. Poirel C, Ennaji M. *Encephale*. 2000; 26: 57.

250. G van Luijtelaar, et al. *Epilepsy Res*. 2001; 46: 225.

251. Harper DG, et al. *Arch Gen Psychiatry*. 2001; 58: 353.

252. Volicer L, Harper DG, Manning BC, Goldstein R, Satlin A. *Am J Psychiatry*. 2001; 158: 704.

253. Priori A, et al. *Exp Neurol*. 2004; 189: 369.

254. Thaut MH, Kenyon GP, Schauer ML, McIntosh GC. *IEEE Eng Med Biol Mag*. 1999; 18: 101.

255. Block G. *Sci Aging Knowledge Environ*. 2005; 13.

256. Buijs RM, Kreier F. *J Neuroendocrinol*. 2006; 18: 715.

257. Hulcher FH, Reynolds J, Rose JC. *Biochem Int*. 1985; 10: 177.

258. Mayer D. *Arch Toxicol*. 1976; 36: 267.

259. Pappu AS, Illingworth DR. *Atherosclerosis*. 2002; 165: 137.

260. Rutter J, Reick M, Wu LC, McKnight SL. *Science*. 2001; 293: 510.

261. Sothern RB, et al. *Prog Clin Biol Res*. 1990; 341A: 67.

262. Swoyer J, et al. *Prog Clin Biol Res*. 1990; 341A: 437.

263. Romano A, Ashkenazi IE. *Metab Pediatr Syst Ophthalmol*. 1987; 10: 68.

264. Paglieroni TG, Holland PV. *Transfusion*. 1994; 34: 512.

265. Zeichner SL, Mueller BU, Pizzo PA, Dimitrov DS. *Pathobiology*. 1996; 64: 289.

266. Hawkins F. *Adv Parasitol*. 1975; 13: 123.

267. Garcia CR, Markus RP, Madeira L. *J Biol Rhythms*. 2001; 16: 436.

268. Gautret P, Deharo E, Chabaud AG, Ginsburg H, Landau I. *Parasite*. 1994; 1: 235.

269. Landau I, Chabaud AG. *Parasite*. 1994; 1: 105.

270. Cambie G, et al. *Ann Parasitol Hum Comp*. 1991; 66: 14.

271. Schultzberg M, Ambatsis M, Samuelsson EB, Kristensson K, N van Meirvenne. *J Neurosci Res*. 1988; 21: 56.

272. Hermida RC, Ayala DE, Arroyave RJ. *Chronobiol Int*. 1990; 7: 329.

273. Hassan AA, Rahman WA, Rashid MZ, Shahrem MR, Adanan CR. *J Vector Ecol*. 2001; 26: 70.

274. Verhagen H, et al. *Mutat Res*. 2004; 551: 65.

275. Ginsburg GS, Konstance RP, Allsbrook JS, Schulman KA. *Arch Intern Med*. 2005; 165: 2331.

276. Bloche MG. *N Engl J Med*. 2004; 351: 2035.

277. Schmitz N. *Jaapa*. 2007; 20: 24.

278. Paine SJ, Gander PH, Travier N. *J Biol Rhythms*. 2006; 21: 68.

279. Johansen LG, Gram J, Kluft C, Jespersen J. *Chronobiol Int*. 1991; 8: 352.

280. Reinberg A, Hallek M, Levi F, Touitou Y, Smolensky M. *Prog Clin Biol Res*. 1987; 227B: 249.

281. Sanchez CP. *Pediatr Nephrol*. 2004; 19: 722.

282. Younus M, Labellarte MJ. *Paediatr Drugs*. 2002; 4: 391.

283. Veldhuis JD, Bowers CY. *J Endocrinol Invest*. 2003; 26: 799.

284. Smolensky MH, Hermida RC, Haus E, Portaluppi F, Reinberg A. *J Womens Health (Larchmt)*. 2005; 14: 38.

285. Reinberg A, et al. *Chronobiol Int*. 1990; 7: 69.

286. Auvil-Novak SE. *Annu Rev Nurs Res*. 1999; 17: 133.

287. Herold M, Gunther R. *Prog Clin Biol Res*. 1987; 271.

288. Arvidson NG, et al. *Ann Rheum Dis*. 1994; 53: 521.

289. Vener KJ, Reddy A. *Semin Arthritis Rheum*. 1992; 22: 83.

290. Miyazaki T, et al. *Surgery*. 2003; 133: 662.

291. Farr LA, Campbell-Grossman C, Mack JM. *Nurs Res*. 1988; 37: 170.

292. Redeker NS, Mason DJ, Wykpisz E, Glica B, Miner C. *Nurs Res*. 1994; 43: 168.

293. Olsson P. *Acta Chir Scand*. 1963; 126: 24.

294. Baraldo M, Furlanut M. *Clin Pharmacokinet*. 2006; 45: 775.

295. Theeuwes F, Yum SI, Haak R, Wong P. *Ann N Y Acad Sci*. 1991; 618: 428.

296. Maroni A, Zema L, Cerea M, Sangalli ME. *Expert Opin Drug Deliv*. 2005; 2: 855.

297. Ross AC, MacRae RJ, Walther M, Stevens HN. *J Pharm Pharmacol*. 2000; 52: 903.

298. Sershen S, West J. *Adv Drug Deliv Rev*. 2002; 54: 1225.

299. Stubbe BG, De Smedt SC, Demeester J. *Pharm Res*. 2004; 21: 1732.

300. Peppas NA, Leobandung W. *J Biomater Sci Polym Ed*. 2004; 15: 125.

301. Lin SY. *Curr Drug Deliv*. 2004; 1: 249.

302. Kost J, Langer R. *Adv Drug Deliv Rev*. 2001; 46: 125.

303. Lynch HJ, Rivest RW, Wurtman RJ. *Neuroendocrinology*. 1980; 31: 106.

304. Levi F, Zidani R, Misset JL. *Lancet*. 1997; 350: 681.

305. von Roemeling R, Hrushesky WJ. *J Clin Oncol*. 1989; 7: 1710.

306. Tzannis ST, Hrushesky WJ, Wood PA, Przybycien TM. *Proc Natl Acad Sci USA.* 1996; 93: 5460.

307. Delhaas EM, Verhagen J. *Paraplegia.* 1992; 30: 527.

308. Vaidyanathan S, et al. *BMC Urol.* 2003; 3: 3.

309. Keene KS, et al. *Int J Radiat Oncol Biol Phys.* 2005; 62: 97.

310. Roemeling RV, Hrushesky WJ. *Prog Clin Biol Res.* 1987; 227B: 357.

311. Vogelzang NJ, Ruane M, DeMeester TR. *J Clin Oncol.* 1985; 3: 407.

312. Adler S, et al. *Cancer.* 1994; 73: 2905.

313. Merkel U, Wedding U, Roskos M, Hoffken K, Hoffmann A. *Exp Toxicol Pathol.* 2003; 54: 475.

314. Giacchetti S. *Chronobiol Int.* 2002; 19: 207.

315. Giacchetti S, et al. *J Clin Oncol.* 2006; 24: 3562.

316. Falcone A, et al. *Oncology.* 1999; 57: 195.

317. Garufi C, et al. *J Infus Chemother.* 1995; 5: 134.

318. Tampellini M, et al. *Tumori.* 2004; 90: 44.

319. Terzoli E, et al. *J Cancer Res Clin Oncol.* 2004; 130: 445.

320. Focan C, et al. *Anticancer Drugs.* 1999; 10: 385.

321. Sagawa T, et al. *Gan To Kagaku Ryoho.* 2003; 30: 537.

322. Focan C. *Chronobiol Int.* 2002; 19: 289.

323. Giannos SA, Dinh SM, Berner B. *J Pharm Sci.* 1995; 84: 539.

324. Misra GP, Siegel RA. *J Pharm Sci.* 2002; 91: 2003.

325. Misra GP, Siegel RA. *J Control Release.* 2002; 79: 293.

326. Leroux JC, Siegel RA. *Chaos.* 1999; 9: 267.

327. Staples M, Daniel K, Cima MJ, Langer R. *Pharm Res.* 2006; 23: 847.

328. Ziaie B, Baldi A, Lei M, Gu Y, Siegel RA. *Adv Drug Deliv Rev.* 2004; 56: 145.

329. Siegel RA, Ziaie B. *Adv Drug Deliv Rev.* 2004; 56: 121.

330. Thompson DH, Gerasimov OV, Wheeler JJ, Rui Y, Anderson VC. *Biochim Biophys Acta.* 1996; 1279: 25.

331. Benenson Y, et al. *Nature.* 2001; 414: 430.

332. Percel P, Vishnupad K, Venkatesh G. Eurand Pharmaceuticals Ltd, United States, 2002; p 13.

333. Fuisz, R. Fusz Technologies Ltd, United States, 1996; p 34.

334. Panoz D, Geoghegan E. Elan Corporation, United States, 1989; p 49.

335. Prisant LM, Devane JG, Butler J. *Am J Ther.* 2000; 7: 345.

336. Leslie S. Euroceltique SA, United States, 1982; p 20.

337. Conte U, Maggi L. *Biomaterials.* 1996; 17: 889.

338. Crison JR, Vieira ML, Amidon GL. In: Rathbone MJ, Hadgraft J, Roberts MS, eds. *Modified-Release Drug Delivery Technology*, vol. 126. New York: Marcel Dekker; 2003: 249–256.

339. Katstra WE, et al. *J Control Release.* 2000; 66: 1.

340. Rowe CW, et al. *J Control Release.* 2000; 66: 11.

341. Monkhouse D, Yoo J, Sherwood J, Cima M, Bornancini E. Therics, Inc, United States, 2003; p 19.

342. Baichwal A, Staniforth J. Penwest Pharmaceuticals Co., United States, 2002; p 19.

343. Staniforth JN, Baichwal AR. *Expert Opin Drug Deliv*. 2005; 2: 587.

344. Altaf SA, Yu K, Parasrampuria J, Friend DR. *Pharm Res*. 1998; 15: 1196.

345. Narisawa S, et al. *Pharm Res*. 1994; 11: 111.

346. Narisawa S, Nagata M, Hirakawa Y, Kobayashi M, Yoshino H. *J Pharm Sci*. 1996; 85: 184.

347. BG De Geest, et al. *Biomacromolecules*. 2006; 7: 373.

348. Kato H, Nagata O, Yamazaki M, Suzuki T, Nakano Y. *Yakugaku Zasshi*. 2002; 122: 57.

349. Lin SY, Ho CJ, Li MJ. *J Control Release*. 2001; 73: 293.

350. Strausak S, Leuenberger H. Inventors; Asulab, SA, USA, assignee. U.S. Patent, 5,370,635, 1994.

351. Mitragotri S. *Adv Drug Deliv Rev*. 2004; 56: 555.

352. Mitragotri S. *Nat Rev Drug Discov*. 2005; 4: 255.

353. Picard FJ, Bergeron MG. *Drug Discov Today*. 2002; 7: 1092.

354. Hooper JW. *MLO Med Lab Obs*. 2006; 38: 22.

355. Pati AK, et al. *Cell Immunol*. 1987; 108: 227.

356. Pang TC, Brown MA. *Am J Hypertens*. 2006; 19: 801.

357. Baumgart P, Kamp J. *Blood Press Monit*. 1998; 3: 303.

358. Belsha CW, Wells TG, H Bowe Rice, Neaville WA, Berry PL. *Blood Press Monit*. 1996; 1: 127.

359. Halberg F, et al. *Biomed Instrum Technol*. 2002; 36: 89.

360. Cornelissen G, Halberg F, Otsuka K, Singh RB, Chen CH. *Hypertension*. 2007; 49: 237.

361. Wilson DM, et al. *Diabetes Care*. 2007; 30: 59.

362. Maia FF, Araujo LR. *Diabetes Res Clin Pract*. 2007; 75: 30.

363. Mazzolini TA, Irons BK, Schell EC, Seifert CF. *J Manag Care Pharm*. 2005; 11: 763.

364. Cording MA, Engelbrecht-Zadvorny EB, Pettit BJ, Eastham JH, Sandoval R. *Ann Pharmacother*. 2002; 36: 892.

365. Ohdo S. *Yakugaku Zasshi*. 2002; 122: 1059.

366. Laupacis A. *Can J Clin Pharmacol*. 2001; 8(suppl A), 6A.

367. Li B, Siegel RA. *Chaos*. 2000; 10: 682.

368. Dibrov BF, Zhabotinsky AM, Kholodenko BN. *J Math Biol*. 1982; 15: 51.

369. Agur Z, Abiri D, Van der Ploeg LH . *Proc Natl Acad Sci USA*. 1989; 86: 9626.

370. Locke JC, Millar AJ, Turner MS. *J Theor Biol*. 2005; 234: 383.

371. Xie Z, Kulasiri D. *J Theor Biol*. 2007; 245: 290.

372. Tsumoto K, Yoshinaga T, Iida H, Kawakami H, Aihara K. *J Theor Biol*. 2006; 239: 101.

373. Kurosawa G, Goldbeter A. *J Theor Biol*. 2006; 242: 478.

374. Dibrov BF. *J Theor Biol.* 1998; 192: 15.

375. Refinetti R. *J Theor Biol.* 2004; 227: 571.

376. Agur Z, Arnon R, Schechter B. *Eur J Cancer.* 1992; 28A: 1085.

377. Halberg F, Guillaume F, S Sanchez de la Pena, Cavallini M, Cornelissen G. *Chronobiologia.* 1986; 13: 137.

378. Nelson W, Tong YL, Lee JK, Halberg F. *Chronobiologia.* 1979; 6: 305.

379. Bingham C, Arbogast B, Guillaume GC, Lee JK, Halberg F. *Chronobiologia.* 1982; 9: 397.

380. Ayala DE, Hermida RC. *Prog Clin Biol Res.* 1990; 341B: 209.

381. Elkum NB, Myles JD. *J Circadian Rhythms.* 2006; 4: 14.

382. Bruguerolle B, Lemmer B. *Life Sci.* 1993; 52: 1809.

383. Hecquet B. *Chronobiol Int.* 1986; 3: 149.

384. Hecquet B, Sucche M. *J Pharmacokinet Biopharm.* 1986; 14: 79.

385. Hecquet B. *C R Acad Sci III.* 1986; 302: 293.

386. Hecquet B. *Pathol Biol (Paris).* 1987; 35: 937.

387. Reinberg AE. *Annu Rev Pharmacol Toxicol.* 1992; 32: 51.

388. Lemmer B. *Acta Physiol Pharmacol Bulg.* 1999; 24: 71.

389. Krzyzanski W, Chakraborty A, Jusko WJ. *Chronobiol Int.* 2000; 17: 77.

390. Krzyzanski W, Jusko WJ. *J Pharmacokinet Pharmacodyn.* 2001; 28: 57.

391. Yao Z, DuBois DC, Almon RR, Jusko WJ. *Pharm Res.* 2006; 23: 670.

392. Delaunay F, Thisse C, Marchand O, Laudet V, Thisse B. *Science.* 2000; 289: 297.

393. Delaunay F, Laudet V. *Trends Genet.* 2002; 18: 595.

394. Earnest DJ, Liang FQ, Ratcliff M, Cassone VM. *Science.* 1999; 283: 693.

395. Iwasaki H, et al. *Cell.* 2000; 101: 223.

396. Kondo T, et al. *Science.* 1994; 266: 1233.

397. Kondo T, et al. *Science.* 1997; 275: 224.

398. Schmitz O, Katayama M, Williams SB, Kondo T, Golden SS. *Science.* 2000; 289: 765.

399. Brown SA, et al. *Science.* 2005; 308: 693.

400. Hastings MH, et al. *Novartis Found Symp.* 2003; 253: 203.

401. Lowrey PL, Takahashi JS. *Annu Rev Genomics Hum Genet.* 2004; 5: 407.

402. Ziauddin J, Sabatini DM. *Nature.* 2001; 411: 107.

403. Zhu H, et al. *Science.* 2001; 293: 2101.

404. Perou CM, et al. *Nature.* 2000; 406: 747.

405. Outinen PA, et al. *Biochem J.* 1998; 332(Pt 1), 213.

406. Kadota K, et al. *Physiol Genomics.* 2001; 4: 183.

407. Miyachi H, et al. *Rinsho Byori.* 2002; 50: 161.

408. Marshall E. *Science.* 2003; 302: 588.

409. Abiola O, et al. *Nat Rev Genet.* 2003; 4: 911.

410. Peleman JD, et al. *Genetics.* 2005; 171: 1341.

411. Silver JD, Hilton DJ, Bahlo M, Kile BT. *Mamm Genome.* 2007; 18: 5.

412. Marroum PJ. In: Rathbone MJ, Hadgraft J, Roberts MS, eds. *Modified-Release Drug Delivery Technology*. New York: Marcel Dekker; 2003: 943–974.

413. Wagner V, Dullaart A, Bock AK, Zweck A. *Nat Biotechnol*. 2006; 24: 1211.

414. Miller J. *Columbia Sci Technol Law Rev*. 2003; 4: E5.

415. Bhattaram VA, et al. *AAPS J*. 2005; 7: E503.

416. Malinowski H, et al. *Adv Exp Med Biol*. 1997; 423: 269.

417. Amidon GL, Lennernas H, Shah VP, Crison JR. *Pharm Res*. 1995; 12: 413.

418. Corrigan OI. *Adv Exp Med Biol*. 1997; 423: 111.

419. Reppas C, Lacey LF, Keene ON, Macheras P, Bye A. *Pharm Res*. 1995; 12: 103.

420. Eddington ND, Marroum P, Uppoor R, Hussain A, Augsburger L. *Pharm Res*. 1998; 15: 466.

421. Paul JE, Trueman P. *Pharmacoepidemiol Drug Safety*. 2001; 10: 429.

422. Katz ML, Mueller LV, Polyakov M, Weinstock SF. *Nat Biotechnol*. 2006; 24: 1529.

423. Goodman CS, Gelijns AC. *Baxter Health Policy Rev*. 1996; 2: 267.

424. Touitou Y, Portaluppi F, Smolensky MH, Rensing L. *Chronobiol Int*. 2004; 21: 161.

CHAPTER 2

CHRONOGENETICS

FRANCK DELAUNAY

"We spend our lives on the run: we get up by the clock, eat and sleep by the clock, get up again, go to work—and then we retire. And what do they give us? A body clock."

— David Allen (1945–)

CONTENTS

Chronopharmaceutics: Science and Technology for Biological Rhythm-Guided Therapy and Prevention of Diseases, edited by Bi-Botti C. Youan
Copyright © 2009 John Wiley & Sons, Inc.

2.1   INTRODUCTION

Internal circadian clocks synchronize the physiology and behavior of most living organisms to the external light–dark cycle. The core element of these clocks located both in the suprachiasmatic nuclei of the hypothalamus and in peripheral organs is a cell-autonomous molecular oscillator. Molecular genetics and biochemical approaches have identified a group of clock genes as the essential components of circadian oscillators in all model systems from cyanobacteria to mammals. Clock genes define positive and negative elements that interact together to form interlocked transcriptional–translational auto-regulatory feedback loops that ultimately generate robust 24-hour gene expression rhythms. Synchronization to the environment involves the light regulation of specific clock genes in the hypothalamus. Clock genes in turn, rhythmically regulate, a variety of clock-controlled genes and thus associated biological processes through direct and indirect output pathways.

2.2   OVERVIEW

Since the beginning of life on Earth, most organisms have been exposed to the light–dark cycle. Consequently, endogenous time-keeping systems oscillating with a ~ 24-h (circadian) periodicity have evolved to provide adaptive mechanisms able to temporally coordinate and synchronize biological processes to the daily changes in the external environment. These internal circadian clocks are indeed found from cyanobacteria, fungi, and higher plants, to metazoans. Remarkably, although major phylogenetic differences exist in terms of complexity and molecular components, the same basic principles have been found to govern all known circadian clocks [1]. The core of any circadian clock is an assembly of positive and negative elements that form at least one feedback loop generating circadian oscillations. This molecular oscillator is synchronized to the environment through input pathways and regulates in turn rhythmic biological processes through output pathways. In complex organisms such as higher vertebrates, the circadian regulation of physiology and behavior is orchestrated by a plethora of oscillators present in virtually all cells and interacting to form an integrated circadian system. In mammals including humans, central to this system are the suprachiasmatic nuclei (SCN) of the hypothalamus, which contain neurons able to express in a cell-autonomous manner self-sustained circadian rhythms in electrical firing, cytosolic Ca^{2+}

concentration, and gene expression. The network formed by these unique neurons constitutes a central pacemaker that is reset by light through the retinohypothalamic tract and which, in turn, entrains and coordinates through ill-defined internal cues local oscillators present in most peripheral tissues [2]. These peripheral oscillators can also be reset by hormonal and metabolic time cues independently of the SCN [3, 4]. How mammalian central and peripheral oscillators work at the cellular and molecular level has been the focus of a tremendous research effort during the last 10 years. Collectively, these genetic and biochemical studies have identified clock genes as essential components and provided a comprehensive molecular framework for the mammalian circadian clock despite unraveling increasingly complex regulatory mechanisms as the list of clock genes extends. This is the focus of this chapter with emphasis on clock genes.

Following the initial evidence for a genetic control of circadian clocks, a major step toward the identification of clock molecular components was the demonstration almost 35 years ago that chemically induced mutations could affect circadian rhythms in *Drosophila*, *Neurospora*, and *Clamydomonas* [5–7]. Two of these studies paved the way for the discovery of the first clock genes, *Period* (*Per*) in *Drosophila* and *Frequency* in *Neurospora*. Subsequent analyses of the *Drosophila Per* mRNA and protein temporal expression profiles suggested a negative autoregulatory mechanism of the *Per* gene expression that could form the basis for a molecular circadian oscillator. The identification and analysis of *Timeless* (*Tim*), a second *Drosophila* clock gene, further supported this hypothesis [8]. Forward genetics then identified additional *Drosophila* clock genes whose products displayed biochemical properties compatible with the predicted transcriptional–translational feedback loop model. This principle has now been shown to be conserved in all organisms in which circadian clocks have been studied, most probably as a result of convergent evolution. While clock mechanisms seem to have appeared independently during evolution in bacteria, fungi, plants, and animals, circadian rhythms in *Drosophila* and vertebrates are generated by homologous clock genes, suggesting that all metazoans share a common ancestral circadian clock mechanism. Because the *Drosophila* model has been instrumental in establishing important concepts that are valid in the context of mammalian circadian clocks, a brief outline of the fruitflys clock mechanism is therefore presented first. This is followed by a more detailed description of the current molecular and genetic bases of mammalian circadian clocks.

2.3   THE *DROSOPHILA* CIRCADIAN CLOCK

The fruitfly *Drosophila melanogaster* shows prominent circadian rhythms of adult emergence (eclosion) and locomotor activity, two easily tractable phenotypes that have been extremely useful for the establishment of the genetic basis of circadian regulation in this organism and the subsequent identification of the molecular components of circadian clocks. An important step has been the isolation by Kanopka and Benzer [5] of the first three period mutants exhibiting either long (Per^L), short (Per^S), or arrythmic (Per^0) phenotypes in eclosion circadian rhythms. These three mutations were mapped to a single locus in the X chromosome and were shown 10 years latter to encode the first known clock gene, *Period* [9, 10]. Rhythmic expression of *Per* was then demonstrated at both the mRNA and protein levels and further expression studies revealed a group of approximately 30 lateral neurons in the fly's brain as the anatomic structure responsible for the generation of behavioral circadian rhythms [11]. The power of *Drosophila* genetics combined to biochemical approaches has since then progressively led to a comprehensive and relatively simple model as compared to the increasingly complex mechanism underlying the mammalian clock.

The current model for the *Drosophila* clock mechanisms is based on two interlocked feedback loops, each involving both positive and negative components [12]. The first described loop is composed of four core clock genes, two of which are positive elements while the two others act as negative regulators. The two positive elements encode the transcriptional regulators CLOCK (CLK) and CYCLE (CYC), which form a heterodimeric complex that recognizes specific DNA response elements termed E-boxes present in the promoter region of the two other clock genes, *Period* and *Timeless* [13–15]. This results in the activation of *Per* and *Tim* transcription and as PER and TIM proteins accumulate in the cytoplasmic compartment, they associate and translocate to the nucleus where they inhibit CLK:CYC-dependent transcriptional activity. This main feedback loop was found to be the subject of posttranslational regulation at several levels. The constitutively expressed protein kinase *CKIε* encoded by the gene *Doubletime* associates rhythmically with, and phosphorylates, PER [16–18]. Hyperphosphorylated PER is recruited by the E3 ligase SLIMB and targeted for degradation through the ubiquitin–proteasome pathway, thus delaying the nuclear entry of the PER:TIM complex [19, 20]. *Shaggy*, a gene previously known to be critical in the Wnt developmental signaling pathway and encoding the glycogen synthase protein kinase 3 (GSK-3), was recently found to promote TIM phosphorylation and translocation of the PER:TIM complex to the nucleus [21]. Recently, the casein kinase 2 (CK2), a well-known multifunctional kinase, was also shown to stimulate PER:TIM nuclear translocation possibly by acting as a priming kinase prior to DBT or GSK-3 action [22]. Finally, dephosphorylation and stabilization of PER by the heteromeric protein phosphatase PP2A is an additional posttranslational regulatory mechanism involved in the rhythmic expression and nuclear accumulation of PER [23]. The light entrainment of this core oscillator is conferred by the product of the *Cryptochrome* (*Cry*) gene, which is considered as a circadian photoreceptor and whose function is to promote the light-dependent proteasomal degradation of TIM [24, 25]. The CLK:CYC heterodimer also activates the transcription of the *Vrille* (*Vri*) and *PAR domain protein 1 ε* (*Pdp1ε*) genes, which encode two transcription factors binding to the same response elements within the *Clk* promoter but with antagonistic transcriptional activities and differential kinetics of accumulation [26–28]. This results in a second feedback loop required for the rhythmic transcription of *Clk* and normal circadian locomotor activity.

In summary, extensive forward genetics and additional molecular approaches have now identified a set of 10 clock genes essential to form a light entrainable circadian molecular oscillator in *Drosophila*. Interestingly, this mechanism is operative not only in the lateral neurons of the fly's brain that control rhythmic behavior but also in most peripheral organs where it may control specific physiological processes such as olfaction [29, 30]. More detailed description of the *Drosophila* circadian clock systems can be obtained in recent reviews [31–33].

2.4 MAMMALIAN CLOCK GENES

Circadian locomotor activity can be precisely, automatically, longitudinally, and easily monitored in mammals using wheel running, infrared beams, or telemetric devices. Thus, as for *Drosophila*, the prominent criteria for defining a clock gene in mammals remains the impairment of the circadian rhythm of locomotor activity in individuals carrying a mutation of that gene. The complexity of the mammalian genome with the presence of multiple functionally paralogous genes as well as the physiological diversity of the tissues containing a circadian clock mechanism is challenging this definition, influenced by the primacy of the SCN. Consequently, the current knowledge of the mammalian circadian system involving both systemic and more specific clock gene products suggests that a clock gene may now be defined as a gene that is directly involved in the clockwork mechanism of central and/or circadian oscillators rather than a gene specifically required for normal circadian behavior. Characteristics of mammalian clock genes and the phenotypic consequences of their mutation are summarized in Tables 2.1 and 2.2, respectively.

2.4.1 *Clock* and NPAS2

The search for mammalian clock genes was the subject of intense efforts during the late 1990s, resulting in the isolation and characterization of more than half of the presently known mammalian clock genes in less than 2 years. The most spectacular work was probably the cloning in 1997 of the mouse *Clock* gene using a forward genetics strategy by J. Takahashi and colleagues. This laboratory had previously identified during the course of a *N*-ethyl-*N*-nitrosourea mutagenesis in the mouse the *clock* mutation causing a range of circadian behavior aberrations from period lengthening to complete arrythmicity [34]. By combining a positional cloning and a transgenic rescue approach, it was subsequently established that the *Clock* gene encodes a transcription factor from the basic helix–loop–helix (bHLH)/PAS (PER-ARNT-SIM) family

Table 2.1. Mammalian Circadian Clock Genes

Family	Gene	Tissue Distribution	Amplitude of Cyclic Expression	Molecular Function
bHLH-PAS	*Clock*	SCN, periphery	Low	BMAL1 and BMAL2 partner, activation of *Per* genes, Rev-erbα and RORα
	NPAS2	Forebrain, periphery	Low	*Clock* paralog
	Bmal1	SCN, periphery	High	CLOCK and NPAS2 partner, activation of *Per* genes, Rev-erbα and RORα
	Bmal2	Periphery	Low	*Bmal1* paralog
PER-PAS	*Per1, Per2, Per3*	SCN, periphery	High	CRY partner, repression of CLOCK:BMAL1 activity
Flavoproteins	*Cry1, Cry2*	SCN, periphery	High (*Cry1*)	PER partner, repression of CLOCK:BMAL1 activity
Casein kinases	*CKIε, CKIδ*	SCN, periphery	No	Phosphorylation and nuclear translocation of PER proteins
Nuclear receptors	Rev-erbα, Rev-erbβ	SCN, periphery	High	Repression of *Bmal1*
	RORα	SCN, periphery	Low	Activation of *Bmal1*
	RORβ	SCN, pineal gland, retina	High	Activation of *Bmal1*
	RORγ	Muscle, thymus	High	Activation of *Bmal1*

[35, 36]. Important structural determinants in the CLOCK protein include an amino-terminal bHLH DNA binding domain, two PAS protein–protein interaction domains, and a glutamine-rich carboxy-terminal domain known to be important for transcriptional activation in other transcription factors. Accordingly, the *Clock* mutation was found to cause a 51 amino acid deletion in the glutamine-rich carboxy-terminal domain, resulting in a transcriptonally inactive protein. Consistent with a role in the mammalian circadian clock mechanism, *Clock* expression was observed in the SCN and the retina but also

Table 2.2. Effects of Clock Gene Mutations in Mammals

Family	Gene	Species	Mutation	Circadian Behavior Phenotype	Other Phenotypes	References
bHLH-PAS	*Clock*	Mouse	ENU induced	2 to 5 h longer free-running period, arrhythmic after 14 days in DD	Metabolic syndrome, reduced fertility	[35, 169, 170]
		Human	Polymorphism 3111C	Delayed morningness/eveningness preference		[38]
	NPAS2	Mouse	Targeted	Normal	Impaired cued and contextual memory	[40, 171]
	Bmal1	Mouse	Targeted	Immediately arrhythmic in DD	Impaired glucose homeostasis Arthropathy, increased sensitivity to cyclophosphamide	[55, 172–174]
PER-PAS	*Per1*	Mouse	Targeted	0.6–1 h shorter free-running period, arrhythmic after 10–14 days in DD (background)		[50, 51, 127]
	Per2	Mouse	Targeted	1.6 h shorter free-running period, arrhythmic after 2–18 days in DD	Cancer prone, abnormal bone function increased alcohol intake	[47, 50, 51, 175, 176]
		Human	Missense S662G	Familial Advanced Sleep Phase Syndrome		[49]

(Continued)

57

Table 2.2. Continued

Family	Gene	Species	Mutation	Circadian Behavior Phenotype	Other Phenotypes	References
	Per3	Mouse	Targeted	0.5 h shorter free-running period		[48]
Flavoproteins	*Cry1*	Mouse	Targeted	0.8–1.3 h shorter free-running period		[64, 65]
	Cry2	Mouse	Targeted	0.6–0.9 h longer free-running period		[61, 64, 65]
Casein kinases	*CKIε*	Hamster	*Tau*	4 h shorter free-running period		[76]
	CKIδ	Human	Missense T44A	Familial advanced sleep phase syndrome		[77]
Nuclear receptors	Rev-erbα	Mouse	Targeted	0.5 h shorter free-running period, increased response to light-induced phase shift	Cerebellum defects, dyslipidemia	[81, 83, 177]
	RORα	Mouse	*staggerer*, targeted	0.35 h shorter free-running period	Ataxia, artherosclerosis, apoalphalipoproteinemia	[84, 178, 179]
	RORβ	Mouse	Targeted	0.4 h longer free-running period	*Vacillans* phenotype, blind	[87]

DD: dark dark cycle (e.g., constant darkness).

in a number of peripheral tissues, yet at relatively constant levels in contrast to the oscillating *Drosophila Clock*. A highly conserved human ortholog of the mouse *Clock* gene was also identified and a polymorphism in the 3' flanking region of the gene was found to be associated with circadian related phenotypes or diseases [37–39]. Neuronal PAS domain protein 2 (NPAS2), a paralogous gene of *Clock* mainly expressed in the mammalian forebrain but not in the SCN, has also been identified in the mouse and proposed to be a functional equivalent of *Clock* in the frontal cortex, a region of the brain that is important for sensory processing and memory acquisition [40].

2.4.2 *Period* Genes

Simultaneously to the discovery of the mouse clock, the first mammalian ortholog of the *Drosophila Period* gene was isolated independently by two laboratories using different strategies [41, 42]. Both groups identified the *Per1* gene (previously named *Rigui* and *Per*) in mouse and human, and comparison of the deduced amino acid sequences with the *Drosophila* PER led Tei et al. [42] to the definition of five conserved regions including two PAS domains, an amino-terminal domain, a region immediately downstream of the *Drosophila Per^s* mutation, and a carboxy-terminal domain homologous to the threonine–glycine repeat containing region of the *Drosophila* PER. Expression of *Per1* was found to oscillate in the SCN and the retina, yet with phase differences between the two structures. Two paralogs of *Per1* have subsequently been identified by several laboratories using homology cloning approaches [43–46]. Both PER2 and PER3 proteins contain the domains that were initially found to be conserved in the *Drosophila* PER and mammalian PER1 and their mRNA are also expressed rhythmically in the SCN, in the retina, and in the periphery. While genetic studies have clearly established the essential role of *Per1* and *Per2* as core clock components, such a role for *Per3* could not be demonstrated as the null mutation of *Per3* only causes a very limited circadian phenotype, even in the context of *Per1* or *Per2* mutation mutant mice [47–51]. Unexpectedly, circadian patterns of *Per1*, *Per2,* and *Per3* gene expression were also observed in peripheral tissues such as the liver and muscle, suggesting that the clock function of these genes may not be restricted to the SCN.

2.4.3 *Bmal1* and *Bmal2*

Because heterodimerization between members of the bHLH/PAS family of proteins through their PAS domain is often observed, the finding that CLOCK was a novel bHLH/PAS factor immediately suggested that it may also heterodimerize with another bHLH/PAS factor. Using a two-hybrid strategy, the screening of a hamster hypothalamus cDNA library with CLOCK as a bait led to the identification of an interacting protein related to the aryl hydrocarbon receptor nuclear translocator (ARNT) protein and previously reported to be abundant in brain and muscle. This CLOCK partner, whose function was previously unknown, was termed brain and muscle ARNT like 1 (*Bmal1*) [52–54]. Rhythmic expression at the mRNA and protein levels of *Bmal1* as well as coexpression together with *Clock* and *Per1* in the SCN strongly suggested a role as a clock gene. Accordingly, disruption of the *Bmal1* gene in the mouse resulted in immediately and completely arrhythmic animals upon release in constant darkness [55]. As for *Clock*, a paralog of *Bmal1* named *Bmal2* was identified latter in mammals, yet this gene showed a more restricted expression pattern as compared to *Bmal1* [56].

2.4.4 *Cryptochrome* Genes

The mammalian clock genes *Cryptochrome 1* (*Cry1*) and *Cryptochrome 2* (*Cry2*) encode proteins that belong to the family of blue-light photoreceptors collectively termed cryptochromes and that despite a homology to photolyases display no DNA repair activity [58, 75]. Their prominent and oscillating expression pattern in the SCN and the retina first suggested that CRY1 and CRY2 could be the circadian photoreceptors involved in the light responsiveness of the mammalian clock in analogy to what is observed in the *Drosophila* clock system [59, 60]. However, conflicting data have been reported regarding the photoreceptive role of CRY1 and CRY2 [61–63]. Unexpectedly, loss of function experiments have in contrast provided compelling evidence that mammalian CRY1 and CRY2 are key molecular components of core circadian oscillators. Indeed, mice homozygous for null mutation of both *Cry1* and *Cry2* genes become immediately and completely arrhythmic when released in constant darkness and display an abnormal circadian expression pattern of *Per1* in light–dark cycle and *Per2* in constant darkness [64, 65]. Experiments reported by Kume et al. [66] indicated that a major role of CRY1 and CRY2 is to associate with PER proteins and repress CLOCK:BMAL1 transcriptional activity. These two genes have also been shown to be rhythmically expressed in numerous peripheral tissues.

2.4.5 *Timeless*

Genetic and biochemical studies have established a critical role for *Timeless* in the *Drosophila* clock mechanism, and the conservation of other clock components between *Drosophila* and mammals suggested that a mammalian homolog of the *Drosophila Tim* may exist. A mammalian timeless was indeed isolated in 1998 by several laboratories [67, 68]. Although this gene encodes a protein that interacts with PER1 and CRY proteins and inhibits CLOCK:BMAL1-dependent transcriptional activity, conflicting results regarding its circadian expression in the SCN, responsiveness to light, or role in the cellular localization of PER proteins have been reported and questioned the role of the mammalian *Tim* as a clock gene [66–71]. This gene may actually be the ortholog of a recently identified *Drosophila* gene of unknown function termed *Timeout or Timeless2* and which has a better sequence similarity to the mammalian *Tim* than the *Drosophila Tim* [72, 73]. To further complicate the situation, deletion of the mammalian *Tim* gene resulted in embryonic lethality, revealing an unanticipated role for this gene during development [72]. To circumvent this problem, Barnes et al. [74] have performed in vitro knockdown experiments using rat SCN explants cultured in the presence of *Tim* antisense oligonucleo-tides and showed that *Tim* was required for normal neuronal activity [74]. Interestingly, they also showed that the *Tim* gene encodes long and short isoforms but that only the long one is oscillating, which may explain some of the previously reported conflicting data. A conditional knockout approach should definitively test the hypothesis of a circadian role of the mammalian *Tim* in vivo.

2.4.6 Casein Kinases Iε and δ

The serine/theonine casein kinase encoded by the *Drosophila* gene *doubletime* has two paralogs in mammals, casein kinase Iε (*CKIε*) and casein kinase Iδ (*CKIδ*). Exceptionally, a critical role for these two enzymes in the mammalian clock mechanism has been demonstrated by the genetic analysis of naturally occurring mutations. The first one to be identified almost 20 years ago by Ralph and Menaker [75] is the *tau* mutation in the Syrian hamster, which results in a 4-h shortened free-running period. A comparative genomics approach led to the discovery that this phenotype was caused by a point mutation in the *CKIε* gene [76]. Independently and consistently, a human genetic analysis identified a form of familial advance sleep phase syndrome (FAPS) caused by a mutation of the conserved CKI phosphorylation site within the PER2 protein [49]. Another form of FAPS was recently shown to be the result of a mutation in the *CKIδ* gene [77]. The *CKIε* and *CKIδ* genes, which are ubiquitously and constitutively expressed, appear thus to encode key posttranslational regulators of the mammalian clock.

2.4.7 Rev-erbα and RORα Nuclear Receptors

Rev-erbα and RORα are orphan members of a superfamilly of nuclear hormone receptors [78, 79]. While Rev-erbα is considered a true orphan receptor, recent evidence indicates that cholesterol and cholesterol metabolites may be physiological ligands of RORα [80]. These two receptors, identified more than 10 years ago, were shown to be involved in multiple physiological processes such as differentiation, apoptosis, inflammation, and metabolism but have only very recently been recognized as components of the core clock mechanism [81, 82]. They act as antagonistic transcriptional regulators that bind in a mutually exclusive manner to specific DNA response elements termed RORE present in the promoter regions of their target genes including the clock genes *Clock*, *Bmal1*, and *Cry1* [83–85]. Consistent with their role in the clock mechanism, both genes are expressed in the SCN and peripheral organs. While the repressor Rev-erbα displays a robust and high amplitude oscillation of its expression, expression of the positive regulator RORα exhibits a more complex pattern with tissue-specific isoforms and oscillation patterns. Importantly, like many other nuclear receptors, Rev-erbα and RORα have paralogous genes, namely, Rev-erbβ, RORβ, and RORγ, which are all rhythmically expressed in the SCN and/or peripheral organs and which, given their biochemical characteristics, may also play a role in the circadian clock mechanism. Consistently in vitro and in vivo data indicate that these genes are additional candidates for the regulation of the molecular clock [86, 87].

2.5 BASIC PRINCIPLES OF THE MAMMALIAN CORE CIRCADIAN CLOCK MECHANISM

Elucidating how mammalian clock genes work together to generate robust and entrainable 24 h period oscillations has been a central issue of modern chronobiology. As in all other model systems studied so far, the current concept for the mammalian clock mechanisms is based on interlocked transcriptional–translational feedback loops [1, 31, 88, 89]. The key positive components are the CLOCK and BMAL1 transcription factors that heterodimerize through their PAS protein–protein interaction domains and transactivate the *Per1, Per2, Cry1,* and *Cry2* clock genes. The specific DNA response element recognized by the CLOCK:BMAL1 heterodimer is a hexanucleotide CACGTG termed E-box and found in the *Per1, Cry1,* and *Cry2* promoters [54]. The core E-box sequence is a widespread binding site in the genome that can respond to multiple signaling pathways, and experimental evidence suggests that flanking sequences may be critical to drive rhythmic transcription [53, 90]. CLOCK:BMAL1-dependent transactivation of the *Per2* gene occurs through a noncanonical E-box element [91]. Accordingly, expression of *Per1, Per2, Cry1,* and *Cry2* is severely impaired in *Clock* and *Bmal1* mutant mice [55, 92]. Furthermore, the phase relationship between the profiles of the PER1, PER2, CRY1, and CRY2 proteins and those of CLOCK and BMAL1 is consistent with a mechanism involving the coordinated transcriptional regulation of the *Per* and *Cry* genes by the CLOCK:BMAL1 heterodimer [93]. At low expression level, PER proteins are phosphorylated by the casein kinase Iε and then degraded through the proteasome pathway. Once the cytoplasmic concentration of PER proteins has reached a threshold level, phosphorylated PER proteins associate with CRY proteins to form a multimeric complex that translocates to the nucleus and suppresses the expression of their own genes by inhibiting CLOCK:BMAL1-dependent transcriptional activity [66, 94]. Thus the *Per* and *Cry* genes encode the negative components of the feedback loop. Importantly, there is genetic evidence showing that the repressive activity of the different PER/CRY complexes is dependent on their composition in PER and CRY proteins with PER1/CRY1 and PER2/CRY2 complexes having a significantly higher repressive potential than PER1/CRY2 and PER2/CRY1 complexes [95, 96]. Unexpectedly, *Per2* knockout mice displayed reduced *Bmal1* gene expression and the CLOCK:BMAL1 heterodimer represses the *Bmal1* promoter, suggesting a negative autoregulatory mechanism for *Bmal1* gene expression and the existence of additional components in the clockwork mechanism [97, 98]. Examination of the *Bmal1* proximal promoter revealed the presence of specific response elements for Rev-erbα, an orphan member of the nuclear receptor superfamily expressed with a robust circadian rhythm in liver [99, 100]. This expression pattern was also observed in the SCN, and mice with a disruption of the Rev-erbα gene exhibited elevated levels of *Bmal1*, establishing Rev-erbα as a critical negative regulator of *Bmal1* expression [83]. These observations led Preitner et al. [83] to propose Rev-erbα as a molecular link between the positive and negative limbs of mammalian circadian oscillators. Consistently, expression of Rev-erbα was found to be positively regulated by the CLOCK:BMAL1 heterodimer [83, 101]. A functional genomics approach subsequently identified RORα, another nuclear orphan receptor sharing the same response element as Rev-erbα, as a positive regulator of *Bmal1* in the SCN [84].

Although the above described transcriptonal–translational based mechanism can provide a comprehensive framework for mammalian circadian oscillators that relies on a limited number of clock genes and regulatory loops as shown in Figure 2.1, additional components, mechanisms, and interactions are likely to be required for the generation and maintenance of robust circadian rhythms. This issue has been addressed by Ueda et al. [102] using a system biology approach. By integrating expression, promoter analysis, and phase relationship data obtained for 16 clock and clock controlled genes, they could indeed propose implemented mechanistic rules that underlie the complexity of mammalian circadian clocks at the transcriptional level.

2.6 IMPORTANCE OF POSTTRANSLATIONAL REGULATION

The alternating rhythmic transcriptional activation and inhibition of specific clock genes, resulting in oscillating expression at the mRNA and protein levels, constitutes a basic mechanisms underlying the generation of circadian rhythm at the molecular level. To generate sustained 24-h oscillations, it is critical that products of the clock components involved in these transcriptional–translational feedback loops are not only regulated at the expression level but also undergo a fine-tuned posttranslational control. A well-established example of the importance of such regulation is that of casein kinases Iε and Iδ, which phosphorylate PER proteins and thereby control their degradation. Once a protein has been translated, there are in fact multiple pathways that may regulate its abundance and/or activity. This includes subcellular localization,

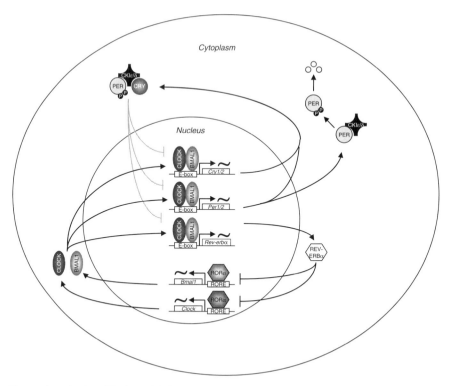

Figure 2.1. A simplified model for mammalian circadian oscillators. Shown are clock genes operative in the SCN. Peripheral oscillators may use the same or alternative paralog genes. This model is based on two interlocked transcriptional–translational autoregulatory loops that involved both activators and repressors, some of which undergo an important post translational control (see text for details).

modifications such as phosphorylation, ubiquination, and SUMOylation, as well as interactions with other proteins.

2.6.1 Subcellular Localization

Following their synthesis in the cytoplasm, PER and CRY proteins translocate to the nucleus, where they inhibit the CLOCK:BMAL1 transcriptional activity. In addition to the rhythmic expression of the mRNA and protein products of the *Per* and *Cry* genes, initial immunohistochemical studies have reported oscillating nuclear abundance of the PER1, PER2, CRY1, and CRY2 proteins [93]. This suggested that the dynamics of subcellular localization of clock proteins may play an important role in the clock mechanism in particular for maintaining the clock phase. Because all known mammalian clock proteins are larger than 50 kDa, their nuclear translocation is an active mechanism that requires the presence of one or several nuclear localization signals (NLSs) or alternatively their association with a partner containing a NLSs. Typical nuclear import sequences contain basic amino acids organized as monopartite (PKKKRKV) or bipartite (KRPX$_N$KKKK) NLSs. These sequences are recognized by the importin α and β that mediate the subsequent import through the nuclear pore in the presence of the small GTPase Ran [103]. Functional studies based on the use of deletion mutant proteins, chimeric proteins with a green fluorescent protein (GFP), or β-galactosidase moieties and point mutation mutant proteins in transfected cells have led to the identification of NLS motifs in a number of clock proteins including BMAL1, PER1, PER2, PER3, CRY1, CRY2, and REV-ERBα [104–107]. Similar to nuclear entry, nuclear export is mediated by specific motifs termed nuclear export sequence (NES) that trigger the active translocation from the nucleus to the cytoplasm. The consensus NES sequence is a Lx$_{(1-3)}$Lx$_{(2-4)}$LxL(V/I/M) motif that is recognized by the CRM1/exportin1 protein [108]. Three such NES motifs have been mapped in the PER1 and PER2 proteins [109, 110]. These NES motifs were shown to be required for the cytoplasmic localization of PER2 as the mutation of all of them or the treatment of the cells with leptomycin, a nuclear export inhibitor targeting CRM1/exportin1, resulted in an exclusively nuclear PER2. [110]. Importantly, heterokaryon nucleocytoplasmic shuttling assays, in which two cells are fused and thus have a common cytoplasm but two different nuclei, have demonstrated that PER2 is continuously shuttling between the cytoplasmic and nuclear compartments [110].

2.6.2 Phosphorylation and Ubiquitination

Phosphorylation is probably the most widespread posttranslational regulatory mechanism and it is estimated to impinge on up to one-third of all intracellular proteins [111]. Accordingly, many clock proteins have been shown to be phosphorylated by various kinases. Phosphorylation can affect subcellular localization, protein–protein interactions, protein stability, and activity. *CKIε* was the first kinase shown to play a critical role in the circadian clock mechanism. The *CKIε* proteins (DBT in *Drosophila*) are functionally equivalent as they both phosphorylate and destabilize PER proteins. In mammals, PER proteins are also substrates for *CKIδ*, a second kinase related to *CKIε* [70, 93, 112]. As a result of *CKIε*- and *CKIδ*-dependent phosphorylation, mammalian PER proteins are ubiquinated and targeted to the proteasome pathway for degradation. Consistently, proteasomal inhibition increases PER1 and PER2 abundance while overexpressing *CKIε* or *CKIδ* decreases their stability. BMAL1 and CRY proteins have also been shown to be substrates for *CKIε* [113]. Several core clock proteins including BMAL1, CRY1, and CRY2 have also been identified as targets of the mitogen activated protein (MAP) kinase pathway, which plays a role in the resetting of mammalian clocks [114–116]. Control of the clock phase also involves phosphorylation by mammalian ortholog of the *Drosophila* glycogen synthase kinase 3 β (GSK3β) [117–119].

2.6.3 SUMOylation

The covalent and reversible linking of small ubiquitin-related modifier protein (SUMO) to lysine residues is a reversible posttranslational modification termed SUMOylation that is similar to that operating through the ubiquitin pathway [120]. Transcriptional regulation has been shown to involve SUMOylation through numerous mechanisms. Highly conserved SUMOylation consensus motifs ΨKxE/D (Ψ is a hydrophobic residue and x any amino acid) are present in the BMAL1 protein, and lysine 259 of the mouse protein was recently shown to be a major SUMOylation site in vivo [121]. It was further shown that BMAL1 SUMOylation follows a circadian pattern that parallels transcriptional activity and requires the presence of the heterodimerization partner CLOCK. Importantly, rescue experiments using BMAL1 deficient mouse embryonic fibroblasts showed that wild-type BMAL1 could restore a normal pattern of circadian gene expression while a protein in which lysine 259 was changed to an arginine generated a shorter period as a result of defective SUMOylation and thus more stable BMAL1 protein. These recent data provide a novel regulatory mechanism for the control of circadian molecular clocks and may well apply to other core clock proteins.

2.6.4 Protein–Protein Interactions

Dimerization is a common theme in the mechanism of action of many transcription factors that function as homo- or heterodimers. A critical transcription activating complex in the mammalian clock is formed by the CLOCK:BMAL1 complex. CLOCK:BMAL1 heterodimerization induces, on the one hand, BMAL1 phosphorylation and, on the other hand, CLOCK nuclear accumulation and degradation through proteasome- dependent and -independent pathways [122]. The relevance of these dimerization-dependent posttranslational events to the clock mechanism was demonstrated by the absence of nuclear accumulation of CLOCK in serum shocked embryonic fibroblasts or in the liver of *Bmal1* deficient mice [122]. The activity of PER1, a protein of the negative limb of the clock, was also recently shown to be regulated by two associated proteins termed NONO and WDR5 [123]. NONO was previously characterized as a RNA- and DNA-binding protein, while WDR5 is a member of a histone methyltransferase complex. While NONO acts antagonistically to PER1, WDR5 promotes PER1 mediated repression. These antagonistic activities are thought to contribute to the robustness of the clock.

2.7 RESPONSE OF CLOCK GENES TO LIGHT

Light is a major and universal resetting signal of the circadian system (or zeitgeber) in all species. In mammals, the photic information is conveyed to the

SCN via the retino hypothalamic tract and is able to reset the internal clock only when light is normally not expected, that is, during the night. This occurs independently of the visual reception pathway, as mice or humans devoid of light perception still respond to light synchronization [31]. At the level of the retina, an important role in light-dependent entrainment of the circadian clock is played by a group of photoreceptive retinal ganglion cells that contain a recently discovered nonvisual pigment termed melanopsin [124]. How the SCN perceive the light information at the molecular level has been the subject of intense research and important clues have been obtained from studies investigating the response of clock genes to light pulses and the light resetting phenotype of clock mutant mice. Several of these studies have collectively led to the concept that *Per1* plays a critical role in the light responsiveness and entrainment of the SCN clock [43, 89, 125]. However, the involvement of *Per1* in the control of either phase advance or delay has not been fully clarified, as contradictory results have been reported by several laboratories possibly related to differences in loss of function approaches, modified alleles, light pulse duration, or genetic background [126–128]. Conversely, the role of *Per2* in light resetting seems to be clearly confined to the control of phase delay [128]. Consistently, patients who carry a mutation of the *CKIε* phosphorylation site in PER2 develop FASPS [49]. Mechanistically, photic induction of *Per1* and *Per2* seems to be associated with the dynamic remodeling of chromatin and mediated by cyclic AMP responsive element-binding protein (CREB) that binds to a cAMP responsive element located in the promoters of these two genes [129–132]. Importantly, to exert its action, CREB has to be phosphorylated at Ser142 in response to light [133]. Furthermore, CRE and E-box mediated regulation of *Per1* and *Per2* genes has been shown to be independent [134]. The BMAL1 protein has also been reported to be degraded in response to light in the rat SCN, yet this observation could not be extended to the mouse SCN, suggesting that a species-specific mechanism may be involved [135, 136]. Light regulation of the clock gene is not restricted to the SCN, as photic induction of *Per1* and *Per2* gene expression was recently demonstrated to occur in the adrenal glands via the SCN–sympathetic nervous system [137].

2.8   OUTPUTS OF CENTRAL AND PERIPHERAL CIRCADIAN OSCILLATORS

The mechanisms responsible for the generation and maintenance of circadian rhythms at the molecular level are becoming relatively well established in a number of model systems including mammals. Conversely, the pathways through which core circadian oscillations result in rhythmic behavior and physiology remain poorly understood. Because a continuously increasing number of physiological processes are being found to be under circadian control in mammals while a circadian component is recognized for major pathologies such as metabolic and cardiovascular diseases, sleep disorders, and cancer [138], the analysis of clock output pathways has become a central issue for chronobiology.

2.8.1   Functional Diversity, Tissue Specificity, and Coordination of Clock-Controlled Genes

Many clock genes encode transcriptional regulators including CLOCK, BMAL1, RORα, and REV-ERBα that function as DNA binding proteins. Clock proteins are thus expected to control rhythmically physiological processes through the direct or indirect transcriptional regulation of clock-controlled genes (CCGs) involved in these processes. Identifying CCGs is therefore an important step toward the understanding of output pathways of the mammalian clock. Until the year 2000, a handful of such CCGs were characterized, including the pineal aryl-alkyl-amino transferase and the liver P450 cytochrome 7 alpha-hydroxylase, two rate-limiting enzymes in the melatonin and cholesterol biosynthetic pathways, respectively [139, 140]. Importantly, questions related to the number of CCGs, their functions, and the tissue distribution of their circadian expression pattern were unanswered. At that time researchers started to use DNA microarrays to identify cycling transcripts in various model systems. With this technology, the expression level of thousands of genes can be analyzed simultaneously, thus providing a global approach to assess the extent and the function of CCGs on a genomic scale. In mammals, several groups have performed circadian expression screens in the SCN and peripheral organs as well as in synchronized cultured cells [84, 141–149]. In general, microarray experiments aiming at identifying cycling transcripts are performed with animals kept under free-running conditions or with serum shocked fibroblasts, and mRNA expression data sets are processed with a dedicated algorithm that detects circadian expression profiles. All these studies have demonstrated that circadian gene expression is extensive in all organs with several hundreds of genes being under circadian control, and a survey of all available data sets indicates that approximately 5–10% of the transcriptome in a given tissue is under circadian regulation [150]. Functional categorization of cycling transcripts has revealed that the circadian clock regulates a very wide variety of biological processes, including metabolism, transcription, translation, protein turnover, immune response, cell death, vesicle trafficking, ion transport, and signaling. Comparison of circadian gene expression in the SCN and the liver has been performed by two groups, and both showed that a maximum of 10% of the CCGs were oscillating in both tissues [143, 145]. Comparing the liver CCG data set with either the heart or aorta data sets showed that peripheral organs also share a minority of their rhythmic transcriptome [144, 149]. Altogether, these comparative analyses led to the conclusion that while clock genes are expressed and generate molecular rhythms in almost every tissue, they regulate downstream targets in a highly tissue-specific manner. Interestingly, this tissue specificity seems to operate at the level of the circadian regulation rather than the level of gene expression, since up to 50% of cycling transcripts in one tissue are expressed constitutively in another tissue. A well-documented analysis of the liver and SCN rhythmic transcriptomes performed by Panda et al. [143] has also revealed that key metabolic pathways such as cholesterol and glucose metabolism are under circadian control through the rhythmic transcription of multiple genes including those encoding rate-limiting step enzymes, suggesting a coordinated regulation.

2.8.2 Direct Regulation of Clock Outputs

Determining how clock proteins rhythmically regulate CCGs is crucial to understanding the temporal organization of mammalian physiology. The CLOCK:BMAL1 heterodimer is a key activating complex in the clockwork mechanism that recognized E-box sequences present in the promoter regions of other clock genes (*Per1*, *Per2*, Rev-erbα) but also in those from some CCGs, suggesting that these CCGs are potentially directly regulated by the CLOCK: BMAL1 activating complex. This has recently been shown to be the case for two physiological outputs from the SCN. The first example is the arginine vasopressin (AVP) gene that encodes a neuropeptide which is well known for its role in the control of the water and salt balance in the periphery. This function is performed by AVP originating from the paraventricular and supraoptic nuclei of the hypothalamus. SCN also produce and release AVP, but in contrast to other hypothalamic nuclei, this occurs with a circadian pattern. The SCN peptide acts locally by modulating the SCN neuronal activity as well as at a distance by conveying circadian information to other hypothalamic nuclei or extrahypothalamic sites. The circadian expression of AVP is totally abolished in the SCN but is not affected in other hypothalamic vasopressinergic nuclei of clock mutant mice, indicating that this gene is a target [92]. Analysis of the proximal promoter of the AVP gene revealed the presence of an E-box sequence that is conserved in the human, mouse, rat, and bovine genes. This response element was further shown to be activated by the CLOCK:BMAL1 heterodimer and repressed by the PER and TIM proteins, thus arguing for a direct mechanism regulating AVP circadian expression within the SCN.

Another example was provided by a recently identified cysteine-rich secreted protein termed prokineticin 2 (PK2) that was first shown to be a potent stimulator of the contraction of gastrointestinal smooth muscle. PK2 was identified as a SCN output molecule binding to G-protein-coupled receptor located in major target nuclei of the SCN efferent pathways and involved in the control of behavioral circadian rhythms [151]. Correspondingly, expression of PK2 was found to display a very robust oscillation in the SCN of normal mice, while circadian clock mutants exhibited virtually no expression. A molecular analysis of the 5′ flanking of the *PK2* gene showed that the four E-box elements present in the 3 kb upstream of the putative transcription start site were able to confer responsiveness to the CLOCK:BMAL1 heterodimer, indicating that PK2 is a direct target gene of clock transcription factors.

Consistently, CLOCK:BMAL1-dependent activation of the PK2 promoter is inhibited by PER and CRY proteins. One example of a direct clock output identified in the periphery is that of the plasminogen activator inhibitor-1 (PAI-1), whose activity follows a circadian rhythm with a peak in the morning, a feature that may account for the early morning prevalence of myocardial infarction as a result of reduced fibrinolysis activity [138]. The *PAI-1* gene was shown to be directly regulated by a heterodimer composed of BMAL2 (termed also CLIF or MOP9), a paralog of BMAL1 expressed in endothelial cells and neurons, and CLOCK through two E-box response elements located in the proximal promoter [56].

Additional direct clock targets in the SCN and in peripheral organs are likely to be discovered in the near future and this will undoubtedly be accelerated by the development of new functional genomic strategies such as the combination of chromatin immunoprecipitation to genome wide tiling microarrays technology that allow the unbiased identification of first-order targets on a genomic scale. However, as detailed later, evidence strongly indicates that direct regulation of clock outputs may not be the most prevalent mechanism in the circadian system.

2.8.3 Indirect Regulation of Clock Outputs

Accumulating evidence suggests that clock genes may regulate a large proportion of the rhythmic transcriptome through indirect mechanisms. Using a conditional expression system in *Drosophila* Schneider cells, it was first shown by McDonald and Rosbash [152] that as few as 7 out of 134 genes were directly regulated by CLOCK in the fly. Furthermore, the analysis of the promoter region of CCGs expressed in the mouse liver or the SCN revealed that very few contained the canonical E-box response element recognized by the CLOCK:BMAL1 heterodimer [143]. Finally, an increasing number of transcriptional regulators under circadian control and not primarily involved in the core circadian clock mechanism are being identified in the SCN and in peripheral tissues. Altogether, these observations argue for the existence of multiple and indirect pathways through which the clock controls physiological outputs.

A very well documented example is that of the three members of the PAR bZip (proline and acidic amino acid-rich basic leucine zipper) family of transcription factors, DBP (albumin D-element binding protein), HLF (hepatocyte leukemia factor), and TEF (thyrotroph embryonic factor) [153]. Following their isolation, these three genes were shown to display a robust circadian expression pattern at the mRNA and protein levels in the liver and other peripheral organs as well as in the SCN, while other brain regions show very low amplitude oscillations [154, 155]. DBP, the founding member of the PAR bZIP family, has been the most investigated and this has now provided a comprehensive mechanism explaining how clock genes can indirectly regulate specific outputs. The complete loss of DBP rhythmic expression in *clock* mutant mice together with the identification of several functional E-box response elements located in the first and second introns of the gene established DBP as a direct target of the circadian pacemaker [156, 157]. DBP regulates, in turn, the circadian expression of several genes involved in liver metabolism. These notably include the steroid 15α-hydroxylase (*Cyp2a4*), an enzyme involved in the catabolism of sex steroid, coumarin 7-hydroxylase (*Cyp2a5*) that encodes a detoxification enzyme [158], cholesterol 7α hydroxylase (*Cyp7a1*), another P450 enzyme catalyzing a rate-limiting step in the catabolism of cholesterol to bile acids [140], and pyridoxal kinase (*Pdxk*), an enzyme implicated in the metabolism of vitamin B_6. All these enzymes display a circadian rhythm at gene expression and activity levels that is altered in mice deficient for one or several of the three circadian PAR bZip factors. Because DBP, HLF, and TEF are partially redundant, the most dramatic circadian phenotypes are only observed in compound mutant mice, as exemplified by the complete loss of circadian expression of *Pdxk* in $Dbp^{-/-}Hlf^{-/-}Tef^{-/-}$ triple knockout mice, while more subtle change such as phase shift may be observed in single mutant animals, as in the case of the *Cyp7a1* expression in $Dbp^{-/-}$ mice. Interestingly, Gachon et al. [153] have demonstrated that, in contrast to the liver, low oscillations of PAR bZip factors in the brain may be a mechanism to protect the brain from pyridoxal deficiency induced epilepsies.

Another recently identified indirect mechanism for the regulation of clock outputs involves the two transcriptional repressors *Dec1* and *Dec2*, which are members of the bHLH-PAS family. *Dec1* was previously identified as a cell growth inhibitor required for normal immune function [159, 160], while the role of *Dec2* has not yet been clearly demonstrated; however, the expression of both genes is regulated by multiple signaling pathways including the circadian clock [161]. *Dec1* and *Dec2* circadian expression was demonstrated in the SCN and various peripheral tissues, and the promoter regions of both genes were shown to be regulated by the core clock transcriptional regulators through E-box elements [162–164]. The circadian expression pattern of *Dec1* and *Dec2* in the SCN, their biochemical characteristics, and the light responsiveness of *Dec1* in this key structure led to the hypothesis that *Dec1* and *Dec2* may encode additional components of the core clock mechanism [162]. Accordingly, in vitro biochemical experiments indicated that both proteins can suppress CLOCK:-BMAL1-mediated transcription by directly binding to E-box elements through their bHLH DNA binding domain and that DEC1 can also repress this activity through protein–protein interaction with BMAL1 [165, 166]. However, no circadian phenotype of the locomotor activity rhythm could be observed in mice carrying a null mutation for *Dec1*, while clock gene expression was found indistinguishable from controls in $Dec1^{-/-}$ mice [163]. Although *Dec2* may compensate for the absence of $Dec1^{-/-}$, this result strongly argues for a role as molecular link between clock genes and physiological output. This hypothesis was confirmed by the identification of 20 CCGs among 42 *Dec1* target genes in the mouse liver, indicating that a principal function of *Dec1* is to regulate circadian clock outputs [163]. Interestingly, the identification of several targets shared by other circadian transcriptional regulators such as DBP, yet acting antagonistically to DEC1, suggests circadian oscillators use complementary and alternating indirect pathways to finely tune the oscillation of physiological outputs [167, 168].

2.9 CONCLUSION

A considerable amount of information has been accumulated in recent years regarding the genetics and the molecular mechanisms underlying mammalian circadian clocks. This has now provided a comprehensive framework able to explain how the core molecular oscillator of central and peripheral clocks functions. Important challenges for the near future will be to decipher the upstream and downstream regulatory networks that interact with this timing mechanism at the cellular and the organism levels and the functional consequences of sequence variations in human clock genes.

ACKNOWLEDGMENT

Work in the author's laboratory is supported by Université de Nice, CNRS, ARC and the European Commission, LSHM-CT 2005-01865, and LSHG-CT 2006-037543.

REFERENCES

1. Dunlap JC. *Cell*. 1999; 96: 271–290.
2. Yoo S-H, et al. *Proc Nat Acad Sci USA*. 2004; 101: 5339–5346.
3. Damiola F, et al. *Genes Dev*. 2000; 14: 2950–2961.
4. McNamara P, et al. *Cell*. 2001; 105: 877–889.
5. Kanopka RJ and Benzer S. *Proc Nat Acad Sci USA*. 1971; 68: 2112–2116.
6. Bruce VG. *Genetics*. 1972; 70: 537–548.
7. Feldman JF, and Hoyle MN. *Genetics*. 1973; 75: 605–613.
8. Seghal A, Price JL, Man B, and Young MW. *Science*. 1994; 263: 1603–1606.
9. Bargiello TA, Jackson FR, and Young MW. *Nature*. 1984; 312: 752–754.
10. Reddy P. *Cell*. 1984; 38: 701–710.
11. Ewer J, Fridch B, Hamblen-Coyle MJ, Rosbash M, and Hall JC. *J Neurosc*. 1992; 12: 3321–3349.
12. Glossop NRJ, Lyons LC, and Hardin PE. *Science*. 1999; 286: 766–768.
13. Allada R, White NE, So WV, Hall JC, and Rosbash M. *Cell*. 1998; 93: 791–804.

14. Rutila JE, et al. *Cell*. 1998; 93: 805–814.

15. Darlington TK, et al. *Science*. 1998; 280: 1599–1603.

16. Kloss B, et al. *Cell*. 1998; 94: 97–107.

17. Price JL, et al. *Cell*. 1998; 94: 83–95.

18. Kloss B, Rothenfluh A, Young MW, and Saez L. *Neuron*. 2001; 30: 699–706.

19. Grima B, et al. *Nature*. 2002; 420: 178–182.

20. Ko HW, Jiang J, and Edery I. *Nature*. 2002; 420: 673–678.

21. Martinek S, Inonog S, Manoukian AS, and Young MW. *Cell*. 2001; 105: 769–779.

22. Akten B, et al. *Nat Neurosci*. 2003; 6: 251–257.

23. Sathyanarayanan S, Zheng X, Xiao R, and Seghal A. *Cell*. 2004; 116: 603–615.

24. Stanewsky R, et al. *Cell*. 1998; 95: 681–692.

25. Emery P, So WV, Kaneko M, Hall JC, and Rosbash M. *Cell*. 1998; 95: 669–679.

26. Blau J, and Young MW. *Cell*. 1999; 99: 661–671.

27. Cyran SA, et al. *Cell*. 2003; 112: 329–341.

28. Glossop NR, et al. *Neuron*. 2003; 37: 249–261.

29. Plautz JD, Kaneko M, Hall JC, and Kay SA. *Science*. 1997; 278: 1632–1635.

30. Krishnan B, Dryer SE, and Hardin PE. *Nature*. 1999; 400: 375–378.

31. Panda S, Hogenesh JB, and Kay SA. *Nature*. 2002; 417: 330–335.

32. Stanewsky R. *J Neurobiol*. 2003; 54: 111–147.

33. Hardin PE. *Cur Biol*. 2005; 15: R714–R722.

34. Vitaterna MH, et al. *Science*. 1994; 264: 719–725.

35. King DP, et al. *Cell*. 1997; 89: 641–653.

36. Antoch MP, et al. *Cell*. 1997; 89: 655–667.

37. Steeves TDL, King DP, Zhao Y, Sangoram AM, and Du F. *Genomics*. 1999; 57: 189–200.

38. Katzenberg D, et al. *Sleep*. 1998; 21: 569–576.

39. Benedetti F, et al. *Am J Med Genetics*. 2003; 123: 23–26.

40. Reik M, Garcia JA, Dudley C, and McKnight SL. *Science*. 2001; 293: 506–509.

41. Sun ZS, et al. *Cell*. 1997; 90: 1003–1011.

42. Tei H, Okamura H, Shigeyoshi Y, Fukuhara C, and Osawa R. *Nature*. 1997; 389: 512–516.

43. Albrecht U, Sun H, Eichele G, and Lee CC. *Cell*. 1997; 91: 1055–1064.

44. Shearman LP, Zylka MJ, Weaver DR, Kolakowski LF, and Reppert SM. *Neuron*. 1997; 19: 1261–1269.

45. Zylka MJ, Shearman LP, Weaver DR, and Reppert SM. *Neuron*. 1998; 20: 1103–1110.

46. Takumi T, et al. *EMBO J*. 1998; 17: 4753–4759.

47. Zheng B, et al. *Nature*. 1999; 400: 169–173.

48. Shearman LP, Jin X, Lee C, Reppert SM, and Weaver DR. *Mol Cell Biol*. 2000; 20: 6269–6275.

49. Toh KL, et al. *Science*. 2001; 291: 1040–1043.

50. Zheng B, et al. *Cell*. 2001; 105: 683–694.

51. Bae K, et al. *Neuron*. 2001; 30: 525–536.

52. Ikeda M, and Nomura M. *Biochem Biophys Res Com*. 1997; 233: 258–264.

53. Hogenesch JB, Gu YZ, Jain S, and Bradfield CA. *Proc Nat Acad Sci USA*. 1998; 95: 5474–5479.

54. Gekakis N, et al. *Science*. 1998; 280: 1564–1569.

55. Bunger MK, et al. *Cell*. 2000; 103: 1009–1017.

56. Maemura K, et al. *J Biol Chem*. 2000; 275: 36847–36851.

57. Cashmore AR. *Cell*. 2003; 114: 537–543.

58. Sancar A. *J Biol Chem*. 2004; 279: 34079–34082.

59. Miyamoto K, and Sancar A. *Proc Nat Acad Sci USA*. 1998; 95: 6097–6102.

60. Miyamoto K, and Sancar A. *Brain Res Mol Brain Res*. 1999; 71: 238–243.

61. Threshner RJ, et al. *Science*. 1998; 282: 1490–1494.

62. Okamura H, et al. *Science*. 1999; 286: 2531–2534.

63. Selby CP, Thompson C, Therese SM, VanGelder RN, and Sancar A. *Proc Nat Acad Sci USA*. 2000; 97: 14697–14702.

64. van derHorst GTJ, et al. *Nature*. 1999; 398: 627–630.

65. Vitaterna MH, et al. *Proc Nat Acad Sci USA*. 1999; 96: 12114–12119.

66. Kume K, et al. *Cell*. 1999; 98: 193–205.

67. Zylka MJ, et al. *Neuron*. 1998; 21: 1115–1122.

68. Sangoram AM, et al. *Neuron*. 1998; 21: 1101–1113.

69. Hastings MH, Field MD, Maywood ES, Weaver DR, and Reppert SM. *J Neurosci*. 1999; 19(RC11): 1–7.

70. Vielhaber EL, Eide EJ, Rivers A, Gao ZH, and Virshup DM. *Mol Cell Biol*. 2000; 20: 4888–4899.

71. Field MD, et al. *Neuron*. 2000; 25: 437–447.

72. Gotter AL, Manganaro T, Weaver DR, Kolakowski LF, and Possidente B. *Nat Neurosci*. 2000; 3: 755–756.

73. Benna C, et al. *Cur Biol*. 2000; 10: R512–R513.

74. Barnes JW, et al. *Science*. 2003; 302: 439–442.

75. Ralph MR, and Menaker M. *Science*. 1988; 293: 1225–1227.

76. Lowrey PL, et al. *Science*. 2000; 288: 483–492.

77. Xu Y, et al. *Nature*. 2005; 434: 640–644.

78. Giguère V. *Endocr Rev*. 1999; 20: 689–725.

79. Gronemeyer H, Gustafsson J-A , and Laudet V. *Nat Rev Drug Discov*. 2004; 3: 950–964.

80. Kallen JA, et al. *Structure*. 2002; 10: 1697–1707.

81. Chomez P, et al. *Development*. 2000; 127: 1489–1498.

82. Boukhtouche F, Mariani J, and Tedgui A. *Arterioscl Thromb Vasc Biol*. 2004; 24: 637–643.

83. Preitner N, et al. *Cell*. 2002; 110: 251–260.

84. Sato TK, et al. *Neuron*. 2004; 43: 527–537.

85. Akashi M , and Takagi Y. *Nature Strucutral Biology*. 2005; 12: 441–448.

86. Guillaumond F, Dardente H, Giguere V, and Cermakian N. *J Biol Rhythms*. 2005; 20: 391–403.

87. André E, et al. *EMBO J*. 1998; 17: 3867–3877.

88. Young MW, and Kay SA. *Nat Rev Genetics*. 2001; 2: 702–715.

89. Reppert SM , and Weaver DR. *Nature*. 2002; 418: 935–941.

90. Munoz E, Brewer M, and Baler R. *J Biol Chem*. 2002; 277: 36009–36017.

91. Yoo S-H, et al. *Proc Nat Acad Sci USA*. 2005; 102: 2608–2613.

92. Jin X, et al. *Cell*. 1999; 96: 57–68.

93. Lee C, Etchegaray J-P, Cagampang FRA, Loudon ASI, and Reppert SM. *Cell*. 2001; 107: 855–867.

94. Sato, TK, et al. *Nat Genetics*. (2006); 38: 312–319.

95. Oster H, Yasui A, Gijsbertus TJ, van derHorst GTJ, and Albrecht U. *Genes Dev*. 2002; 16: 2633–2638.

96. Oster H, Baeriswyl S, Van DerHorst GT, and Albrecht U. *Genes Dev*. 2003; 17: 1366–1379.

97. Shearman LP, et al. *Science*. 2000; 288: 1013–1019.

98. Yu W, Nomura M, and Ikeda M. *Biochem Biophys Res Com*. 2002; 290: 933–941.

99. Balsalobre A, Damiola F, and Schibler U. *Cell*. 1998; 93: 929–937.

100. Pineda Torra I, et al. *Endocrinology*. 2000; 141: 3799–3806.

101. Triqueneaux G, et al. *J Mol Endocrinol*. 2004; 33: 585–608.

102. Ueda HR, et al. *Nat Genetics*. 2005; 37: 187–192.

103. Moroianu J. *J Cell Biochem*. 1999; (Suppl 32–33): 76–83.

104. Yagita K, et al. *Genes Dev*. 2000; 14: 1353–1563.

105. Miyazaki K, Mezaki M, and Ishida N. *Mol Cell Biol*. 2001; 21: 6651–6659.

106. Hirayama J, Nakamura H, Ishikawa T, Kobayashi Y, and Todo T. *J Biol Chem*. 2003; 278: 35620–35628.

107. Chopin-Delannoy S, et al. *J Mol Endocrinol*. 2003; 30: 197–211.

108. Stade K, Ford CS, Guthrie C, and Weis K. *Cell*. 1997; 90: 1041–1050.

109. Vielhaber EL, Duricka D, Ullman KS, and Virshup DM. *J Biol Chem*. 2001; 276: 45921–45927.

110. Yagita K, et al. *EMBO J*. 2002; 21: 1301–1314.

111. Johnson SA , and Hunter T. *Nat Methods*. 2005; 1: 17–25.

112. Akashi M, Tsuchiya Y, Yoshino T, and Nishida E. *Mol Cell Biol*. 2002; 22: 1693–1703.

113. Eide EJ, Vielhaber EL, Hinz WA, and Virshup DM. *J Biol Chem*. 2002; 277: 17248–17254.

114. Sanada K, Okano T, and Fukada Y. *J Biol Chem*. 2002; 277: 267–271.

115. Sanada K, Harada Y, Sakai M, Todo T, and Fukada Y. *Genes Cells*. 2004; 9: 697–708.

116. Akashi M, and Nishida E. *Genes Dev*. 2000; 14: 645–649.

117. Iitaka C, Miyazaki K, Akaike T, and Ishida N. *J Biol Chem*. 2005; 280: 29397–29402.

118. Harada Y, Sakai M, Kurabayashi N, Hirota T, and Fukada Y. *J Biol Chem*. 2005; 280: 31714–31721.

119. Yin L, Wang J, Klein PS, and Lazar MA. *Science*. 2006; 311: 1002–1005.

120. Gill G. *Cur Opin Gen Dev*. 2005; 15: 536–541.

121. Cardone L, et al. *Science*. 2005; 309: 1390–1394.

122. Kondratov RV, et al. *Genes Dev*. 2003; 17: 1921–1932.

123. Brown SA, et al. *Science*. 2005; 308: 693–696.

124. Panda S, et al. *Science*. 2002; 298: 2213–2216.

125. Shigeyoshi Y, et al. *Cell*. 1997; 91: 1043–1053.

126. Akiyama M, et al. *J Neurosci*. 1999; 19: 1115–1121.

127. Cermakian N, Monaco L, Pando MP, Dierich A, and Sassone-Corsi P. *EMBO J*. 2001; 20: 3967–3974.

128. Albrecht U, Zheng B, Larkin D, Sun ZS , and Lee CC. *J Biol Rhythms*. 2001; 16: 100–104.

129. Crosio C, Cermakian N, Allis CD, and Sassone-Corsi P. *Nat Neurosci*. 2000; 3: 1241–1247.

130. Travnickova-Bendova Z, Cermakian N, Reppert SM, and Sassone-Corsi P. *Proc Nat Acad Sci USA*. 2002; 99: 7728–7733.

131. Tischkau SA, Mitchell JW, Tyan SH, Buchanan GF, and Gillette MU. *J Biol Chem*. 2003; 278: 718–723.

132. Naruse Y, et al. *Mol Cell Biol*. 2004; 24: 6278–6287.

133. Gau D, et al. *Neuron*. 2002; 34: 245–253.

134. Shearman LP, and Weaver DR. *Neuroreport*. 1999; 10: 613–618.

135. Tamaru T, et al. *J Neurosci*. 2000; 20: 7525–7530.

136. vonGall C, Noton E, Lee C, and Weaver DR. *Eur J Neurosci*. 2003; 18: 125–133.

137. Ishida A, et al. *Metabolism Cell*. 2005; 2: 297–307.

138. Hastings MH, Reddy AB, and Maywood ES. *Nat Rev Neurosci*. 2003; 4: 649–661.

139. Foulkes NS, Borjigin J, Snyder SH, and Sassone-Corsi P. *Proc Nat Acad Sci USA*. 1996; 93: 14140–14145.

140. Lavery DL, and Schibler U. *Genes. Dev*. 1993; 10: 1871–1884.

141. Grundschober C, et al. *J Biol Chem*. 2001; 276: 46751–46758.

142. Duffield GE, et al. *Cur Biol*. 2002; 12: 551–557.

143. Panda S, et al. *Cell*. 2002; 109: 307–320.

144. Storch K-F, et al. *Nature*. 2002; 417: 78–83.

145. Ueda HR, et al. *Nature*. 2002; 418: 534–539.

146. Akhtar RA, et al. *Cur Biol*. 2002; 12: 540–550.

147. Kita Y, et al. *Pharamacogenetics*. 2002; 12: 55–65.

148. Martino T, et al. *J Mol Med*. 2004; 82: 256–264.

149. Rudic RD, et al. *Circulation*. 2005; 112: 2716–2724.

150. Delaunay F, and Laudet V. *Trends in Genetics*. 2002; 18: 595–597.

151. Cheng MY, et al. *Nature*. 2002; 417: 405–410.

152. McDonald MJ, and Rosbash M. *Cell*. 2001; 107: 567–578.

153. Gachon F, et al. *Genes Dev*. 2004; 18: .

154. Falvey E, Fleury-Olela F, and Schibler U. *EMBO J*. 1995; 14: 4307–4317.

155. Fonjallaz P, Ossipow V, Wanner G, and Schibler U. *EMBO J*. 1996; 15: 351–362.

156. Ripperger JA, Shearman LP, Reppert SM, and Schibler U. *Genes Dev*. 2000; 14: 679–689.

157. Ripperger J, and Schibler U. *Nat Genetics*. 2006; 38: 369–374.

158. Lavery DL, et al. *Mol Cell Biol*. 1999; 19: 6488–6499.

159. Sun H, and Taneja R. *Proc Nat Acad Sci USA*. 2000; 97: 4058–4063.

160. Sun H, Lu B, Li R-Q, Flawell RA, and Taneja R. *Nat Immunol*. 2001; 2: 1040–1047.

161. Yamada K, and Myamoto K. *Front Biosci*. 2005; 10: 3151–3171.

162. Honma S, et al. *Nature*. 2002; 419: 841–844.

163. Grechez-Cassiau A, et al. *J Biol Chem*. 2004; 279: 1141–1150.

164. Hamaguchi H, et al. *Biochem J*. 2004; 382: 43–50.

165. Li Y, et al. *Biochem J*. 2004; 382: 895–904.

166. Sato F, et al. *Eur J Biochem*. 2004; 271: 4409–4419.

167. Fraser DJ, Zumsteg A, and Meyer UA. *J Biol Chem*. 2003; 278: 39392–39401.

168. Noshiro M, et al. *Genes to Cells*. 2004; 9: 317–329.

169. Miller BH, et al. *Cur Biol*. 2004; 14: 1367–1373.

170. Turek FW, et al. *Science*. 2005; 308: 1043–1045.

171. Garcia JA, et al. *Science*. 2000; 288: 2226–2230.

172. Rudic RD, et al. *PLOS Biol*. 2004; 2: 1893–1899.

173. Bunger MK, et al. *Genesis*. 2005; 41: 122–132.

174. Gorbacheva VY, et al. *Proc Nat Acad Sci USA*. 2005; 102: 3407–3412.

175. Fu L, Pelicano H, Liu J, Huang P, and Lee CC. *Cell*. 2002; 111: 41–50.

176. Spanagel R, et al. *Nat Med*. 2005; 11: 35–42.

177. Raspe E, et al. *J Lipid Res*. 2002; 43: 2172–2179.

178. Steinmayr M, et al. *Proc Nat Acad Sci USA*. 1998; 95: 3960–3965.

179. Mamontova A, et al. *Circulation*. 1998; 98: 2738–2743.

CHAPTER 3

CHRONOPHARMACOKINETICS

BERNARD BRUGUEROLLE

"An inch of time is an inch of gold. But an inch of gold can't buy an inch of time.... With time and patience the mulberry leaf becomes a silk gown."

— *Chinese Proverb*

CONTENTS

3.1   INTRODUCTION

Novel drug delivery systems have recently been developed in order to better deliver drugs. These procedures involve and depend on pharmacokinetics principles. Compared to "classical" drug delivery, they allow one to "delay" the moment of administration of the drug. According to the existence of biological rhythms and data from chronopharmacology, it is of particular importance to take into account the hour of administration [1–3]. This naturally leads to chronopharmacokinetics or chronokinetics, which studies

Chronopharmaceutics: Science and Technology for Biological Rhythm-Guided Therapy and Prevention of Diseases, edited by Bi-Botti C. Youan
Copyright © 2009 John Wiley & Sons, Inc.

the influence of the time of administration of a drug on its pharmacokinetics (e.g., absorption, distribution, metabolism, and elimination) [4–11].
Thus knowledge of chronobiology may be used in order to optimize efficacy
and safety of novel drug delivery systems, which constitutes chronopharmaceutics [12].

For several years, chronokinetic studies have been reported for many drugs
both to partly explain chronopharmacodynamic phenomena and to demonstrate that the time of administration of a drug is a possible factor of variation
of its kinetics. Many chronokinetic studies have been reviewed elsewhere [1–11],
describing kinetic changes according to several periodicities, for example, time
of day (circadian) as well as day of the month (infradian, menstrual): the
present chapter only focuses on circadian time-dependent changes in kinetics.

More than simply describing chronokinetics, the aim of this chapter is to
define and present principles, methods, and applications of chronopharmacokinetics in order to better understand the influence of biological rhythms on
drug delivery systems and to evaluate how chronopharmacokinetics knowledge
can contribute to the rational design and evaluation of chronopharmaceutical
drug delivery systems [12].

3.2 PRINCIPLES OF CHRONOPHARMACOKINETICS

"To produce its characteristic effects, a drug must be present in appropriate
concentration at its sites of action" [13]. Thus after introduction into the
organism, a drug is absorbed, distributed (most frequently by protein binding)
in order to diffuse into tissues and act on specific receptors to produce its
pharmacological effects, and then is metabolized and eliminated. This "classical" scheme may be modified according to the existence of biological rhythms:
it is now well established that the fate of the drug in the organism depends on
its moment of administration: this constitutes chronopharmacokinetics (or
chronokinetics), which postulates that the different steps in pharmacokinetics
(e.g., absorption, distribution, metabolism, and elimination) are influenced by
different physiological functions of the body which may vary with time of day
(Figure 3.1). Thus pharmacokinetic parameters characterizing bioavailability,
distribution, and elimination, which are conventionally considered to be
constant in time, are circadian time dependent [10]. Chronokinetic studies
have been reported for many drugs in order to partly explain chronopharmacodynamic phenomena and to demonstrate that the time of administration of a
drug is a possible factor of variation of its kinetics. Many chronokinetic studies
have been reviewed elsewhere [1–8].

As an illustrative example, chronopharmacokinetics of local anesthetics
have been reported [14–18]: the different studies have shown that local
anesthetic agents, such as lidocaine and bupivacaine, showed a two times
higher peak drug concentration (C_{max}) and shorter time to peak concentration
(T_{max}) after dosing at 2200h in rodents (middle of the active period) compared

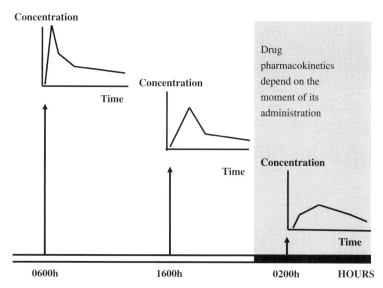

Figure 3.1. Chronopharmacokinetics: different kinetic patterns of drug plasma concentrations according to time of administration.

to 0400 h [15–17]. Figure 3.2 illustrates the chronopharmacokinetics of bupivacaine in mice according to the hour of administration (1000, 1600, 2200 or 0400h). In humans chronokinetic differences were also demonstrated, with higher plasma levels documented after dosing in the afternoon (middle of the active period), which agree well with the opposite synchronization between humans and rodents [18].

Table 3.1 represents a list of drugs that show chronokinetic changes. As representative examples of chronokinetic studies, Table 3.2 summarizes the main chronokinetic changes of nonsteroidal anti-inflammatory drugs in humans [19–33].

From these studies it appears that, in humans, (1) bioavailability of many drugs taken orally is higher when the drug is taken in the morning (e.g., theophylline, salicylates, benzodiazepines, digoxin, nonsteroidal anti-inflamatory drugs); (2) temporal variations are more often observed and marked for liposoluble compounds; (3) sustained released forms decrease chronokinetics; and (4) the route of administration may be involved in a chronokinetic change.

3.2.1 Biological Rhythms Involvement in Kinetics of Drugs

Many biological factors are involved in drug kinetics: for example, gastric emptying, gastric pH, gastrointestinal motility, cutaneous permeability, posture, blood flow, tissue perfusion, plasma protein binding, metabolizing enzyme

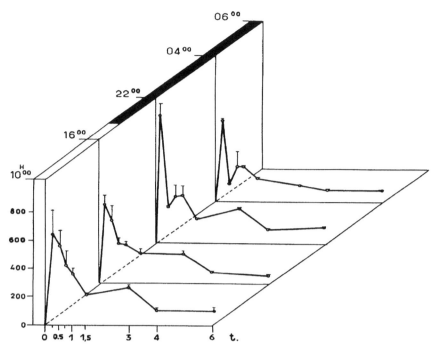

Figure 3.2. Bupivacaine chronokinetics in mice (20 mg/kg/IP): plasma levels according to time when the drug is injected at four different clock hours, that is, 1000h, 1600h, 2200h, and 0400h.

activity, renal perfusion, glomerular filtration, and urinary pH (Figure 3.3). As previously mentioned, many of these factors may be circadian time dependent (as well as ultradian or infradian) and thus may be involved in the different steps of the fate of the drug in the organism, leading to chrono-pharmacokinetics.

3.2.2 Mechanisms Involved in Chronokinetics

Possible mechanisms involved in such chronopharmacokinetic variations may be illustrated at different steps, that is, resorption, distribution, metabolism, and elimination of the drug.

Temporal Variations in Drug Absorption The oral route is the most often used route of drug administration. Among the different mechanisms by which a drug may be absorbed (e.g., passive or facilitated diffusion, active transport), passive diffusion is the most important process. Many factors may have pronounced effects on drug absorption and the variability of absorption processes: the physicochemical properties of the drug (lipophilicity

Table 3.1. Some of the Drugs that Show Chronokinetics in Humans

Analgesic and Anti-inflammatory	Antibiotic and Antiinfectious	Anticancer	Cardiovascular	Nervous System	Miscellaneous
Acetaminophen	Amikacin	Busulfan	Atenolol	Amitriptyline	Bezafibrate
Acetylsalicylic acid	Cefodizime	Carboplatin	Digoxin	Carbamazepine	Cyclosporine
Antipyrine	Ciprofloxacin	Cisplatin	Diltiazem	Diazepam	Ferrous sulfate
Cortisol	Gentamycin	Doxorubicin	Enalapril	Lithium	Mequitazine
Dexamethasone	Isepamicin	5-Fluorouracil	Isosorbide dinitrate	Lorazepam	5-Methoxypsoralen
Diclofenac	Nelfinavir	Folinic acid	Dipyridamole	Midazolam	Nicotine
Dipyridamole	Netilmycin	Irinotecan	Methyldigoxin	Nortryptiline	Nizatidine
Ibuprofen	Rifampicin	Methotrexate	Nifedipine	Oxcarbazepine	Phenylpropanolamine
Indomethacin	Sulfamethoxazole	Oxaliplatin	Nitrindipine	Sertraline	Pravastatin
Ketoprofen	Sulfanilamide	Vindesine	Pentoxifylline	Sumatriptan	Terbutaline
Ketorolac	Sulfasymazine		Propanolol	Trazodone	Theophylline
Lignocaine	Vancomycin		Verapamil	Triazolam	
Morphine				Valproic acid	
Methamphetamine					
Pranoprofen					
Prednisolone					
Sodium salicylate					

83

Table 3.2. Chronopharmacokinetic Changes of Nonsteroidal Anti-inflammatory Drugs in Humans

Drug	Number and Types of Subjects	Administration/Dosing/Hours	Major Significant Findings ($p < 0.05$)	References
5-Aminosalicylic acid	$n = 12$, young healthy males	$1.5\,g \times 3$ PO every 7 hours Enteric-coated tablets Immediately after meal or 1 h after meal	Diurnal effect: rise of 5-ASA concentrations in early morning	[19]
Diclofenac	$n = 10$, healthy	Single oral dose 50 mg at 0700, 1900h	Highest peak at 0700h (32% change); highest AUC (23% change); no significant difference in T_{max} and $T_{1/2}$	[20]
Ibuprofen	$n = 5$, healthy	Morning versus evening Single oral 300-mg dose Immediate or sustained released forms, food influence	No significant difference for immediate release form; longest T_{max} (50%change) and lower bioavailability after morning intake; major influence of food	[21]
Indomethacin	$n = 9$, healthy	Single oral dose 100 mg at 0700, 1100, 1500, 1900, 2300h	Highest peak at 0700h and 1100h (52%change); $T_{1/2\beta}$ highest at 1900h	[22]
Indomethacin slow release	$n = 16$, Patients (osteoarthritis)	Single oral dose 75 mg at 0800, 1200, 2000h	Highest C_{max} at 1200h (25% change); highest AUC and highest $T_{1/2}$ at 2000h (10% change)	[23, 24]

(Continued)

Drug	n	Protocol	Result	Ref.
Indomethacin slow release	$n = 10$, elderly volunteers	Single oral dose 75 mg at 0900, 1200, 2100h	T_{max} highest at 2100h (38% change)	[25]
Ketoprofen	$n = 8$, healthy	Single oral dose 100 mg at 0700, 1300, 1900, 0100h	Highest C_{max} (50% change) and AUC at 0700h (58% change); highest $T_{1/2 \, \beta}$ at 01.00 (60% change)	[26]
Ketoprofen slow release	$n = 10$, healthy	Single oral dose 200 mg at 0700, 1900h	Shortest T_{max} at 0700h (24% change)	[27]
Ketoprofen constant infusion	$n = 8$, patients (sciatica)	Constant IV infusion 5 mg/kg/day during 24 hours, sampling every 2 hours	Circadian variations of plasma levels with a peak at 2100h (48% change)	[28]
Ketorolac	$n = 12$, healthy	Single oral dose 30 mg at 0700, 1300, 1900, 0100h	AUC higher and Cl lower at 1900 and 0100h, respectively (10% change)	[29]
Pranoprofen	$n = 7$, healthy	Single oral dose 75 mg at 1000, 2200h	T_{max} shorter at 1000h; no significant difference of AUC, $T_{1/2 \, \beta}$, Cl.	[30]
Salicylic acid	$n = 6$, healthy	Single oral dose 1 g, at 0600, 1000, 1800, 2200h	Highest C_{max} (20% change), AUC (17% change), and $T_{1/2 \, \beta}$ (20% change) at 0600h	[31]
Salicylic acid	$n = 6$, healthy	Single oral dose 1 g at 0700, 1100, 1500, 1900, 2300h	Urinary elimination longest at 0700h (22% change)	[32]
Sulindac	$n = 10$, healthy	400 mg/ 8 days at 0800, 2000h	After morning dosing, highest 24-h urinary amount (76% change)	[33]

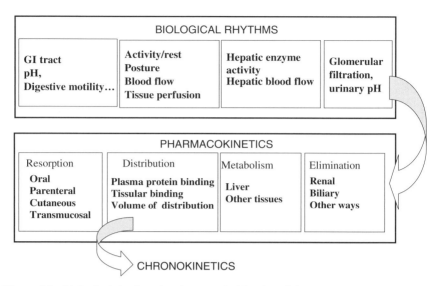

Figure 3.3. Biological rhythms involvement in kinetics of drugs: different physiological factors, varying according to time, possibly involved in the different steps of drug pharmacokinetics.

or hydrophilicity), the structure of the biomembrane, gastric emptying time, pH, motility, gastrointestinal blood flow [8], the drug formulation, and the posture and feeding conditions (e.g., possible influence of food). Most of these factors, such as gastric acid secretion and pH, motility, gastric emptying time and gastrointestinal blood flow, vary along the 24-hour scale, and it is not surprising that many studies have reported temporal variations of drug absorption [1–8]. Such variations may be predicted by physicochemical properties of a drug since most of the lipophilic drugs seem to be absorbed faster when the drug is taken in the morning as compared to evening dosing. At the opposite end, the absorption processes of highly water-soluble drugs were not demonstrated to change according to time of day. The underlying mechanisms of the chronokinetic pattern of lipophilic drugs involve a faster gastric emptying time and a higher gastrointestinal perfusion in the morning [34]. Shiga et al. [35] documented differences of chronopharmacokinetic profiles between propranolol, a lipophylic beta-blocker and atenolol, a hydrophylic beta-blocker, in patients with hypertension, showing that propranolol, but not atenolol, is absorbed more rapidly after morning administration compared to evening administration.

Elsewhere, physiological factors such as posture may play a role in temporal variations in drug absorption by influencing, for instance, gastric emptying time. Variations of posture related to usual life conditions may partly explain why gastric emptying time of solids is faster in the morning than during the evening in humans.

The qualitative and quantitative influence of food must not be neglected in chronokinetics studies involving ingestion by the oral route. We reported several years ago on circadian variations in carbamazepine kinetics when the drug was given orally to rats [36]. A circadian time-dependent variation in drug absorption, as estimated by the C_{max}/T_{max} ratio, was demonstrated in non-fasting animals. Under fasting conditions, the same experiment confirmed and amplified this variation, demonstrating that food influence is not the only factor involved in the circadian change in drug absorption (Figure 3.4). Ohdo et al. [37] reported for valproic acid that meal composition may influence circadian variations: significant differences in the kinetics of valproate were demonstrated, depending on morning or evening dosing under usual life conditions (light meal as breakfast and heavy meal as dinner). When the same conditions (e.g. same size and content of breakfast and dinner) were applied, no significant circadian changes were detected between morning and evening. This points out the necessity to control and take into account in chronokinetic studies the feeding habits of the patients enrolled in the trials. As an illustrative example, the influence of food and time of administration were documented for sertraline, a serotonin reuptake inhibitor [38]: the kinetics of sertraline were not influenced by the time of administration with or without food. This does not eliminate, obviously, a chronokinetic influence but means that under fasting or nonfasting conditions, kinetics of sertraline are similar after morning and evening dosing. This point will be further underlined as far as methodological aspects of a chronokinetic study are concerned. The above

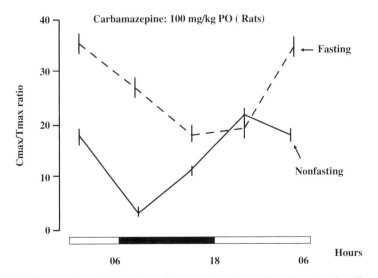

Figure 3.4. Temporal variations in carbamazepine absorption in rats: circadian time-dependent changes in C_{max}/T_{max} ratio in rats receiving carbamazepine orally according to fasting conditions.

chronopharmacological reported data involving the oral route of drug administration must be kept in mind when novel drug delivery devices are to be used.

Drug formulation is also an important factor that may introduce a supplementary variability in drug absorption. As far as chronokinetics are concerned, it is of particular interest to control the drug galenic presentation since it may determine whether or not chronokinetics are present.

Drug resorption by other routes of administration may also be influenced by biological rhythms [39]. For instance, skin penetration of a eutectic mixture of lidocaine and prilocaine was reported to depend on the time of administration: lidocaine plasma levels were higher after evening application as compared to morning in children, while the opposite was demonstrated in rats [40]. Circadian dosing time dependency in the skin penetration of hydrophylic methylnicotinate and lipophylic hexylnicotinate was also demonstrated [41]. Elsewhere, circadian variations were demonstrated in the ocular absorption of topically applied timolol [42].

Thus to conclude whether or not chronokinetics of a drug are present can only be documented when all factors, including route of administration, feeding conditions, posture, and galenic formulation, are controlled and taken into account.

Temporal Variations in Drug Distribution   Drug distribution changes may be implicated in kinetic variability. Daily variations for drug protein binding have been reported both in animals and in humans [43, 44]. As reviewed elsewhere [7, 8], the free plasma levels of many drugs were documented for drugs such as bupivacaine [17], carbamazepine [47], cisplatin [48], diazepam [49, 50], etidocaine [17], mepivacaine [17], phenytoin [51], and valproic acid [52, 53] (Table 3.3).

Drug protein binding may depend on the amount of plasma proteins, which are known to be circadian time dependent [43–46], more than on the temporal changes in the affinity of the proteins. As an illustrative example, a chronokinetic study in rats has documented circadian time-dependent kinetics of carbamazepine, an antiepileptic drug [36]. Among the possible mechanisms involved, plasma protein binding was demonstrated, with higher values occurring in the middle of the dark active phase compared to the lowest values occurring at the beginning of the light resting period. A parallel variation of albumin, the main plasma protein involved in carbamazepine binding, was also observed, with highest values observed at the same hour.

These changes may also depend on many factors, such as temperature, pH, and physicochemical properties of the particular drug, which may possibly be subject to temporal variations.

More recently, Ando et al. [54] reported on the diurnal variations of P-glycoprotein (Pgp), a multidrug transporter that contributes to renal, biliary, and intestinal elimination of drugs: these authors have documented daily variations of Pgp expression levels.

Table 3.3. Temporal Variations in Drug Distribution (Protein Binding)

Drug	Species	Main Results	Reference
Bupivacaine	Mouse	Maximum protein binding at 1600 h	[17]
Carbamazepine	Rat	Minimum free fraction at 0400 h when albumin is highest	[36]
Carbamazepine	Human	Higher free fraction at 1700h	[47]
Cisplatin	Human	Maximum protein binding at 1600h	[48]
Diazepam	Human	Higher bound fraction at 0900h	[49]
Diazepam	Human	Higher bound fraction at 0930h	[50]
Etidocaine	Mouse	Maximum protein binding at 1000h and 2200h	[17]
Lidocaine	Rat	Maximum free fraction at 1600h	[15]
Mepivacaine	Mouse	Maximum protein binding at 0400h	[17]
Phenytoin	Human (epileptics)	Maximum free fraction during daytime when VPA associated	[51]
Valproïc acid	Human	Maximum free fraction between 0200h and 0800h	[52]
Valproïc acid	Human	Free fraction clearance higher in the morning	[53]

It is well established that clinically significant consequences of temporal changes in drug binding are relevant only for drugs that are highly bound (more than 80%). Thus temporal variations in plasma drug binding may have clinical implications only for drugs characterized by a high protein binding and a small volume of distribution. Nevertheless, to our knowledge, clinical consequences due to circadian variations in plasma proteins have not yet been demonstrated.

Some drugs may also bind to red blood cells. We have reported circadian time-dependent changes in the passage of drugs such as local anesthetics (lidocaine, bupivacaine, etidocaine, and mepivacaine), indomethacin, and theophylline into red blood cells [6–8].

Finally, temporal variations in drug distribution may also proceed from circadian time-dependent changes in blood flow and in tissue blood flow as documented in animals as well as in humans [56].

Temporal Variations in Drug Metabolism   Drug metabolism is generally assumed to depend on enzyme activity and/or blood flow, which were both shown to be circadian time dependent as far as the liver is concerned. Circadian variations in enzyme activity also documented in many other animal tissues, such as liver, kidney, and brain [57–59] can explain some time-dependent changes in the kinetics of drugs [59, 60]. The hepatic metabolism of hexobarbital as well as the hypnotic effect has been shown to be circadian time dependent depending on the circadian rhythm of hexobarbital oxydase in rats. This study was the first work documenting a temporal correlation between the metabolism and the effect of a drug. Temporal variations have been detected in various oxidative reactions catalyzed by the microsomal monooxygenase systems for compounds such as aniline, benzphetamine, and benzo[*a*]pyrène in rodents. Time-dependent changes in nonoxidative pathways of drug metabolism (reduction, hydrolysis, and conjugation) were also documented in animals.

In humans, indirect evidence of circadian changes in enzymatic activity was documented. Several clinical chronopharmacological studies have indirectly investigated temporal variations in hepatic drug metabolism capacity by demonstrating chronokinetics of drugs and their metabolites. Thus conjugation, hydrolysis, and oxidation were shown to be circadian time dependent [2–8]. More recently, circadian variations in cytochrome P450 3A activity, mainly involved in drug metabolism, were assessed by establishing daily variations of the urinary 6β-hydrocortisol to cortisol ratio, a noninvasive index of human CYP3A activity, in humans [61].

Concerning metabolic phenotype determination, Shaw et al. [62] have shown the effect of diurnal variation on debrisoquine metabolic phenotyping, with the slowest metabolism during daytime.

In recent years, research on the molecular mechanisms of circadian oscillation and rhythmic transcription of clock output regulators such as an enzyme of the cytochrome P450 superfamily in liver has progressed. Recently, Tada et al. [63] reported in renal transplant patients that, despite a lack of statistical difference in pharmacokinetics of tacrolimus between 0900h and 2100h, lower nighttime AUC corresponded to the occurrence of clinical acute rejection of transplants.

The hepatic blood flow is of particular importance for drugs with a high hepatic extraction ratio ($E > 0.7$). Temporal variations in the clearance of these drugs are explained by changes in liver perfusion, dependent on circadian variations in hepatic blood flow. A circadian rhythm in hepatic blood flow estimated by indocyanine green clearance was reported in healthy subjects with higher values at 0800h [56]: this provides strong arguments for circadian time-dependent metabolism of drugs with a high hepatic extraction ratio.

Temporal Variations in Drug Elimination Most drugs (particularly hydrophilic ones) are eliminated by the kidneys. As illustrated in Figure 3.1, many physiological factors involved in renal elimination of drugs (e.g., glomerular filtration, renal blood flow, urinary pH, tubular resorption) have been shown to be circadian time dependent, with higher values during daytime in humans [64]. Thus the urinary excretion of many drugs depends on these rhythmic variations [8]. The physicochemical properties of the drug are of particular importance in this field; renal elimination of hydrophilic drugs (mainly excreted unchanged by the kidneys) has been shown to be circadian time dependent (related to the above mentioned circadian rhythms in renal functions). Elsewhere, the ionization of drugs is of particular importance in the renal elimination of drugs: thus temporal changes in urinary pH may modify ionization and explain why acidic drugs are excreted faster after an evening than a morning administration, as described for sodium salicylate [32] and sulfasymazine [65], for instance. As an illustrative example, time-dependent variations in the duration of excretion of sodium salicylate in healthy subjects were documented [32], salicylate excretion being quicker when urine pH was more alkaline and vice versa. More recently, the influence of food on chronokinetics of antibiotics was documented, showing that feeding restriction may modify the chronokinetic pattern of antimicrobial agents [66].

Recently, the chronokinetics of norfloxacin [67] and ceftriaxone [68], two antimicrobial agents, were documented in rats showing a higher elimination during the activity period (e.g., during the nighttime). As far as ciprofloxacin is concerned, these results are in good agreement with data obtained in humans. These results are of particular importance for determination of the in vivo efficacy: daily variations in kinetics may account for impairment in the chemotherapeutic effects as demonstrated for ciprofloxacin [69].

3.3 METHODOLOGICAL ASPECTS OF A CHRONOKINETIC STUDY

3.3.1 When and Why a Chronokinetic Study May Be Indicated?

As previously mentioned, the aim of such a study may be realized (1) for a theoretical aspect in order to document possible chronokinetic changes, (2) for a registration study of a new drug, or (3) simply as a complementary study seeking to identify the possible involvement of time of administration in the observed variability.

As mentioned previously, the moment of administration of a drug is one possible factor inducing chronokinetic changes, but many other factors may interfere with the kinetics of a drug and thus must be controlled and /or taken into account before starting a chronokinetic study. These factors depend on drug and patient characteristics.

3.3.2 Drug Delivery Conditions

As previously mentioned, different formulation procedures developed elsewhere in this book make it possible to deliver the drug at a definite time, which is the goal of chronotherapy, in order to ameliorate the efficacy and tolerance of the treatment. Thus novel drug delivery systems provide very useful tools for chronotherapy, allowing doctors to choose the best time of administration according to chronopharmacological findings. This point will be developed further, but we want to emphasize here the importance of considering the drug formulation procedure: as previously noticed, chronokinetic differences demonstrated for a standard form may not be observed for the same drug when presented as a sustained released form. This was demonstrated for isosorbide-5-mononitrate [70] and nifedipine [34].

Chronotherapy may involve asymmetric delivery of drugs on the 24-hour scale: as mentioned in other chapters, external or surgically implantable pumps allow delivery of drugs according to programmable rates [71], taking into account possible chronokinetic characteristics of the drugs.

3.3.3 Sampling Conditions

A chronokinetic study may be realized according to different goals, inducing differences in the protocol. Such a study may be done under daily practice conditions if the drug must be administrated two times daily: the aim of this chronokinetic study may be to search for a possible kinetic difference between morning or evening intake. On the other hand, in order to conduct a real chronokinetic study (i.e., the search for a circadian time-dependent change), several time points (dosing times) are needed [7]. For ethical (number of samples), financial, galenic (once-a-day formulation), or practical reasons (daily life conditions), many chronokinetic clinical studies are often done by determining only two time points. This must also be interpreted, since the timing of drug administration with respect to meals is a usual fact in drug prescription, while not scientifically justified. Such a protocol may miss a circadian variation while in fact it exists but would detect the variation if two more time points are included in the study. A preliminary experiment is necessary, if only two time points are possible, in order to justify and choose these points according to the peak or trough time of a biological marker, for instance.

New specific sampling methods have been developed recently. Among them, microdialysis is a bioanalytical sampling technique allowing continuous monitoring of chemical events that are occurring at the tissue level [72]. This procedure allows one to monitor endogenous or exogenous compounds (e.g., drugs, neurotransmitters, amino acids) in several tissues, including blood, of the same animal and thus are of particular interest in pharmacological and pharmacokinetics studies. However, surprisingly, very few chronobiological studies were conducted using this technique [73, 74] until now. This technique is also available for clinical use and would be of great interest as a "continuous sampling" tool in chronokinetic studies.

3.3.4 Characteristics of the Patients

Chronokinetics may vary according to many physiopathological factors, such as fasting or feeding habits, posture, gender, pathology, mode of synchronization, type of meal, meal timing, working habits, sleeping times, or age. As previously mentioned [7] these factors of variability must be strictly controlled in setting up a study design. Since they all participate to the intrasubject variability, it is of particular importance to control and standardize them in a chronokinetic study. Most of these factors are often not taken into account in inclusion/noninclusion criteria of clinical studies, which may introduce a bias or at least an increased variability.

3.3.5 Specific Data Analysis in Chronokinetics

The description of the fate of a drug in the organism and its characterization proceed from either noncompartmental analysis or compartmental analysis. Noncompartmental pharmacokinetics involves physiological models with usually determined kinetic parameters summarizing bioavailability (e.g., C_{max}, T_{max}, AUC, MRT), distribution (e.g., volume of distribution), drug protein binding characteristics, and elimination (e.g., clearance and elimination half-life). Compartmental analysis implies the use of models with compartments that model the fate of the drug in the organism. The influence of time of administration of a drug on its kinetics may be assumed as a covariable among other factors of variability, which is rarely done [75]. In other words, for a given drug and a given subject, the influence of the time of administration may imply a different kinetic pattern, leading to a different kinetic model related to time of administration [76]. Specific methods may be used for modeling of the chronopharmacokinetic pattern: this has been attempted by Hecquet [76] and Gries et al. [77]. As an illustrative example, Aranson et al. [78] developed a chronokinetic model involving cosine wave time-variant parameters [78] in order to reanalyse some previously reported chronokinetic studies related to nonsteroidal anti-inflammatory drugs.

In order to simulate the drug concentration at its site of action and thus to better characterize its concentration–effects relationships, there is a growing interest in specific analysis methods allowing pharmacokinetic/pharmacodynamic (PK/PD) modeling [75]. As far as chronokinetics are concerned, very few chronopharmacological studies have been conducted using such models [79–81]. However, use of PK/PD modeling in chronokinetic studies may not be useful when chronokinetic changes are not the main mechanism responsible for the chronopharmacological changes observed. For example, the chronokinetics of cardiovascular drugs, while significantly detected, do not represent the main mechanism implicated in their circadian time-dependent effects [82], as demonstrated, for instance, with propranolol [34].

Another analytic approach for characterizing changes in drug clearance throughout the day was proposed by Gries et al. [77] for nicotine. For studying the possible influence of meals and circadian rhythms on nicotine clearance, they described a modeling technique by use of nonparametric incorporation of discrete events; the use of a spline function seems to represent a more realistic model than the parametric one. Once again, this study illustrates the intricate implications of food and circadian variations in kinetics.

Finally, methods used for population pharmacokinetics may be applied to chronokinetic studies in order to reduce the number of samples in a defined subject. Chronokinetic changes may be analyzed with such methods by considering time of administration as a covariable component of the intrasubject variability.

3.4 APPLICATIONS: CHRONOPHARMACOKINETICS, A BASIS FOR CHRONOPHARMACEUTICS

We mentioned in introduction that "to produce its characteristic effects, a drug must be present in appropriate concentration at its sites of action." We may now add to this assertion that this must be done also "at the right moment" related to chronopharmacological effects. Thus chronopharmacology and chronokinetics may be considered as a basis for chronotherapy by justifying the choice of the best moment of administration of the drug. Obviously, choosing the moment of administration of a drug sometimes may seem to be incompatible with usual daily habits and usual drug formulation: for instance, taking a pill in the middle of the night when the patient is sleeping may be problematic! Thus specific tools designed for a timed and delayed delivery are necessary.

Most of the different available novel devices releasing the drug at the chosen site at the chosen time are detailed in this book. We only underline the interest in some of them in relation to chronokinetics findings.

The main novel delivery systems involved are:

- Electronically controlled systems permitting a chronomodulated delivery pattern (i.e., the delivery of a precise dose of drug at precise time—pulse or sinusoidal delivery)
- Diffusion-controlled systems where the controlled diffusion and the lag time are governed mainly by the rate of water penetration into the system
- Chemically activated systems based on changes in the property of the matrix
- Compartmental systems allowing drug release at a predetermined time from different compartments

All of these novel drug delivery systems allow a timed administration: they permit delivery at a fixed, determined clock hour according to a time-dependent delivery. Thus chronopharmaceutics allows using intelligently novel drug delivery systems.

Nevertheless, most of the systems using the oral route introduce an additional chronobiological factor. The system itself may depend on chronobiological factors: the delivery lag time may change according to pathological and physicochemical rhythmic changes. For instance, as far as diffusion-controlled systems are concerned, the time-dependent delivery may vary according to the hour of application: related to circadian variations of gastric pH, gastrointestinal tract mobility, and other possible factors (e.g., osmotic process may not be similar according to time of application). Thus drug release (lag time and duration) from timed delivery systems must take into account the hour of administration along the 24-hour scale. Specific studies are needed to better characterize chronobiological release from drug delivery systems.

Nevertheless, chronopharmaceutics provide useful and powerful tools for chronopharmacology and thus chronotherapy. The sinusoidal delivery pattern of anticancer drugs has optimized their efficacy and safety in cancer patients: this is achieved by internal or external programmable infusion pumps that deliver the drug intravenously or subcutaneously. To our knowledge, new delivery drug devices do not permit such delivery patterns for the oral route: this is needed for future chronotherapeutic studies. Data from chronokinetics contribute to a better understanding of the fate of a drug in an organism according to biological rhythms and thus provide a basis for chronopharmaceutics.

Future experimental and clinical studies will take advantage of the convergence of pharmaceutics and chronobiology, permitting an optimization of medical practices.

REFERENCES

1. Reinberg A. *Ann Rev Pharmacol Toxicol.* 1992; 32: 51.
2. Bruguerolle B. In: Touitou Y, Haus E, eds. *Biological Rhythms in Clinical and Laboratory Medicine.* Paris: Springer-Verlag; 1992: 114–137.
3. Bruguerolle B. In: Touitou Y, ed. *Biological Clocks: Mechanisms and Applications.* Paris: Elsevier Pergamon North Holland; 1998: 437–443.
4. Reinberg A, Smolensky M. *Clin Pharmacokinet.* 1982; 7: 401.
5. Bruguerolle B. *Pathol Biol.* 1987; 35: 925.
6. Lemmer B. *J Pharm Pharmacol.* 1999; 51: 887.
7. Bruguerolle B, Lemmer B. *Life Sci.* 1993; 2: 1809.
8. Lemmer B, Bruguerolle B. *Clin Pharmacokinet.* 1994; 26: 419.
9. Labrecque G, Belanger P. *Pharmacol Ther.* 1991; 52: 95.
10. Belanger P, Bruguerolle B, Labrecque G. In: Redfern PH, Lemmer B, eds. *Physiology and Pharmacology of Biological Rhythms.* Heidelberg: Springer-Verlag; 1997: 177–204.
11. Bruguerolle B. *Clin Pharmacokinet.* 1998; 35: 83.
12. Youan B. *J Control Release.* 2004; 98: 337.
13. Hardman JG, Limbird LE, Gilman AG, eds. *Goodman and Gilman's. The Pharmacological Basis of Therapeutics,* 10th edition New York: McGraw-Hill; 2001.
14. Bruguerolle B. In: Lemmer B, ed. *Chronopharmacology, Cellular and Biochemical Interactions.* New York: Marcel Dekker; 1989: 581–596.
15. Bruguerolle B, Valli M, Bouyard L, Jadot G, Bouyard P. *Eur J Drug Metab Pharmacokinet.* 1983; 8: 233.
16. Bruguerolle B, Prat M. *Annu Rev Chronopharmacol.* 1988; 5: 227.

17. Bruguerolle B, Prat M. *Chronobiol Int.* 1992; 9: 448.

18. Bruguerolle B, Isnardon R. *Ther Drug Monit.* 1985; 7: 369.

19. Demey C, Meineke I. *Br J Clin Pharmacol.* 1992; 33: 17.

20. Mustofa M, Suryawati S, Dwiprahasto I, Santoso B. *Br J Clin Pharmacol.* 1991; 32: 246.

21. Halsas M, Hietala J, Veski P, Jurjenson H, Marvola M. *Int J Pharm.* 1999; 189: 179.

22. Clench J, Reinberg A, Dziewanowska Z, Ghata J, Smolensky M. *Eur J Clin Pharmacol.* 1981; 20: 359.

23. Guissou P, Cuisinaud G, Llorca G, Lejeune E, Sassard J. *Eur J Clin Pharmacol.* 1983; 24: 667.

24. Bruguerolle B, Desnuelle C, Jadot G, Valli M, Acquaviva PC. *Rev Int Rhum.* 1983; 13: 263.

25. Bruguerolle B, Barbeau G, Belanger P, Labrecque G. *Annu Rev Chronopharmacol.* 1986; 3: 425.

26. Ollagnier M, et al. *Clin Pharmacokinet.* 1987; 12: 367.

27. Reinberg A, et al. *Annu Rev Chronopharmacol.* 1986; 3: 317.

28. Decousus H, Ollagnier M, Cherrah Y, Queneau P. *Annu Rev Chronopharmacol.* 1986; 3: 321.

29. Srinivasu P, Rambhau D, Rao R. *Clin Drug Invest.* 1995; 10: 110.

30. Fujimura A, et al. *J Clin Pharmacol.* 1989; 29: 786.

31. Markiewicz A, Semenowicz K. *Int J Clin Pharmacol Biopharm.* 1979; 17: 409.

32. Reinberg A, et al. *C R Acad Sci.* 1975; 280: 1697.

33. Couet W, et al. *Semin Hop Paris.* 1986; 62: 2677.

34. Lemmer B, Scheidel B, Behne S. *Ann NY Acad Sci.* 1991; 618: 166.

35. Shiga T, Fujimura A, Tateishi T, Ohashi K, Ebihara A. *J Clin Pharmacol.* 1993; 33: 756.

36. Bruguerolle B, Valli M, Bouyard L, Jadot G, Bouyard P. *Eur J Drug Metab Pharmacokinet.* 1981; 6: 189.

37. Ohdo S, Nakano S, Ogawa N. *J Clin Pharmacol.* 1992; 32: 822.

38. Ronfeld RA, Wilner KD, Baris BA. *Clin Pharmacokinet.* 1997; 32: 50.

39. Gries JM, Benowitz N, Verotta D. *J Pharmacol Exp Ther.* 1998; 285: 457.

40. Bruguerolle B, Giaufre E, Prat M. *Chronobiol Int.* 1991; 8: 277.

41. Reinberg A, et al. *Life Sci.* 1995; 57: 1507.

42. Ohdo S, Grass GM, Lee VH. *Invest Ophthalmol Vis Sci.* 1991; 32: 2790.

43. Reinberg A, Schuller E, Deslanerie N, Clench J, Helary M. *Nouv Presse Med.* 1977; 6: 3819.

44. Valli M, Jadot G, Bruguerolle B, Bussiere H, Bouyard P. *J Physiol (Paris).* 1979; 75: 811.

45. Bruguerolle B. In: Vandendriessche T, ed. *Membranes and Circadian Rhythms.* Heidelberg: Springer-Verlag; 1996: 159–167.

46. Bruguerolle B. In: Redfern PH, Lemmer B, eds. *Physiology and Pharmacology of Biological Rhythms.* Heidelberg: Springer-Verlag; 1997: 607–618.

47. Riva R, et al. *Epilepsia.* 1984; 25: 476.

48. Hecquet B, Sucche M. *J Pharmacokinet Biopharm*. 1986; 14: 79.

49. Naranjo CA, Sellers EM, Giles HG, Abel. JG. *Br J Clin Pharmacol*. 1980; 9: 265.

50. Nakano S, Watanabe H, Nagai K, Ogawa N. *Clin Pharmacol Ther*. 1984; 36: 271.

51. Riva R, et al. *Neurology*. 1985; 35: 510.

52. Patel IH, Venkataramanan R, Levy RH, Viswanathan CT, Ojemann LM. *Epilepsia*. 1982; 23: 283.

53. Bauer LA, Davis R, Wilensky A, Raisys V, Levy RH. *Clin Pharmacol Ther*. 1985; 37: 697.

54. Ando H, et al. *Chronobiol Int*. 2005; 22: 655.

55. Bruguerolle B, Prat M. *Life Sci*. 1990; 45: 2587.

56. Lemmer B, Nold G. *Br J Clin Pharmacol*. 1991; 32: 624.

57. Belanger PM. *Annu Rev Chronopharmacol*. 1988; 4: 1.

58. Feuers RJ, Scheving LE. *Annu Rev Chronopharmacol*. 1988; 4: 209.

59. Belanger PM, Labrecque G. In: Lemmer B, ed. *Chronopharmacology: Cellular and Biochemical Interactions*. Basel: Marcel Dekker; 1991: 15–34.

60. Nair V, Casper R. *Life Sci*. 1969; 8: 1291.

61. Ohno M, et al. *Eur J Clin Pharmacol*. 2000; 55: 861.

62. Shaw GL, et al. *J Nat Cancer Inst*. 1990; 82: 1573.

63. Tada H, et al. *J Clin Pharmacol*. 2003; 43: 859.

64. Cambar J, Cal JC, Tranchot J. In: Touitou Y, Haus E, eds. *Biological Rhythms in Clinical and Laboratory Medicine*. Paris: Springer-Verlag; 1992: 470–482.

65. Dettli L, Spring P. *Helv Med Acta*. 1966; 15: 134.

66. Beauchamp D, et al. *Antimicrob Agents Chemother*. 1997; 41: 1468.

67. Rebuelto M, Ambros L, Rubio M. *Biol Rhythm Res*. 2003; 34: 51.

68. Rebuelto M, Ambros L, Rubio M. *Antimicrob Agents Chemother*. 2003; 47: 809.

69. Rao V, Rambhau D, Srinivasu P. *Antimicrob Agents Chemother*. 1997; 41: 1802.

70. Lemmer B, Scheidel B, Blume H, Becker HJ. *Eur J Clin Pharmacol*. 1991; 40: 71.

71. Levi F, Zidani R. *Lancet*. 1997; 350: 681.

72. Ungerstedt U. *J Intern Med*. 1991; 230: 365.

73. Johansen MJ, Newman RA, Madden T. *Pharmacotherapy*. 1997; 17: 464.

74. Lehman JC, et al. *Acta Neurochir*. 1996; 67: 66.

75. Sheiner LB, Stanski DR, Vozeh S, Miller RD, Ham J. *Clin Pharmacol Ther*. 1979; 25: 358.

76. Hecquet B. *Annu Rev Chronopharmacol*. 1990; 6: 1.

77. Gries JM, Benowitz N, Verotta D. *Clin Pharmacol Ther*. 1996; 60: 385.

78. Aronson JK, Chappell MJ, Godfrey KR, Yew MK. *Eur J Clin Pharmacol*. 1993; 45: 357.

79. Koopmans R, Dingemanse J, Danhof M, Horsten GP, van Boxtel CJ. *Clin Pharmacol Ther*. 1991; 50: 16.

80. Shappell SA, et al. *J Clin Pharmacol*. 1996; 36: 1051.

81. Lemmer B. *Int J Clin Pharmacol Ther*. 1997; 35: 458.

82. Lemmer B, Portaluppi F. In: Redfern PH, Lemmer B, eds. *Physiology and Pharmacology of Biological Rhythms*. Heidelberg: Springer-Verlag; 1997: 251–298.

CHAPTER 4

CHEMICAL OSCILLATOR SYSTEMS FOR CHRONOTHERAPY

STEVEN A. GIANNOS

"If you don't find God in the next person you meet, it is a waste of time looking for him further."

— Mahatma Gandhi (1869–1948)

CONTENTS

4.1   INTRODUCTION

The goal of controlled release drug delivery is to optimize the pharmacological response by controlling the drug intake and directing the drug to the targeted biological receptors [1]. Transdermal delivery combines the advantages of conventional drug delivery methods, by delivering medications directly to the circulatory system using an external noninvasive device and circumventing the

Chronopharmaceutics: Science and Technology for Biological Rhythm-Guided Therapy and Prevention of Diseases, edited by Bi-Botti C. Youan
Copyright © 2009 John Wiley & Sons, Inc.

first-pass hepatic metabolism [2]. The transdermal system provides the user with a convenient and safe method of taking medication for a prolonged period, while reducing complications such as those associated with implantable systems [3, 4].

The original performance target for controlled drug delivery is to achieve a zero-order release rate of the drug, so that a constant efficacious drug concentration is maintained in the plasma. However, more than two decades of research in chronobiology and chronopharmacology have demonstrated the importance of biological rhythms to the dosing of medications [5–12]. Circadian rhythms, seasonal cycles, and fertility cycles should be considered a part of optimizing the therapeutic effect of a drug and its delivery system. Studies indicate that the onset of diseases, such as specific cancers, show strong seasonal dependency. Certain diseases, asthma and angina, for example, occur more frequently at particular times of the day: in the afternoon or evening for asthma and in the morning hours for angina [13]. The secretion of gastric acid has been found to increase in the afternoon, leading physicians to recommend that ulcer medications be taken in the afternoon for better efficacy. Moreover, Parkinson disease [14, 15], which is treated by L-dopa, and angina [16–20], which is treated by nitroglycerin, would be better managed with chronobiological therapy.

The continued interest in chronobiology, chronopharmacology, and chronotherapy demonstrates the importance of biological rhythms to the dosing of medications [21–23]. Research findings suggest that the onset and severity of many diseases are cyclic in nature, or follow circadian patterns. Drug tolerance adds to the need for modulation of drug dosing profiles. Additionally, skin irritation and sensitization caused by medications may require intervals during which no drug is administered. Smolensky and Labrecque [24] reviewed chronotherapeutics as well as chronopharmacokinetics. In *Body Clock Guide to Better Health: How to Use Your Body's Natural Clock to Fight Illness and Achieve Maximum Health*, Smolensky and Lamberg [25], discuss major health issues such as sleep, exercise, nutrition, medications, sexuality, and fertility in regard to chronobiology and chronotherapeutics.

There now seems to be a resurgence of interest in the development of pulsatile drug delivery systems due to their advantages of offering alternative ways for the delivery of drugs exhibiting chronopharmacological behavior, extensive first-pass metabolism, and the necessity of nighttime dosing [26–29]. Tolerance to various drugs and skin irritation and sensitization caused by transdermal and topical pharmaceuticals may also require intervals in which no drug is administered.

4.2   TRANSDERMAL DRUG DELIVERY

Traditionally, the most common form of drug delivery has been the oral route. While pills and tablets have the notable advantage of easy administration, they also have significant disadvantages such as poor bioavailability, due to hepatic metabolism (first pass) and the tendency to produce rapid blood level spikes (both high and low). Also, variations due to individual differences or food intake are additional concerns. This can lead to the need for high and/or frequent dosing, which can be both cost prohibitive and inconvenient.

During the last 30 years, transdermal drug delivery systems and topical pharmaceuticals have increasingly offered key advantages over the oral route. Transdermal patches have been useful in developing new applications for existing therapeutics and for reducing first-pass drug-degradation and metabolism effects. Transdermal patches can also reduce side effects; for example, the estradiol patch is used by more than a million patients annually and, in contrast to oral formulations, does not cause liver damage [30].

The 1970s saw the development and marketing of early transdermal therapeutic systems such as the scopolamine, nitroglycerin, and estradiol patches. Today there are transdermal systems available for drugs such as clonidine, fentanyl, lidocaine, nicotine, nitroglycerin, estradiol, oxybutynin, scopolamine, and testosterone. More recently, transdermal "patches" are now available for selegiline and methylphenidate. There are also combination patches for contraception, as well as hormone replacement [31]. Transdermal patches generally last from 1 to 7 days, depending on the drug formulation and system size. The annual U.S. market for transdermal patches is more than US $3 billion [32]. In the same way, transdermal nitroglycerin, fentanyl, and clonidine patches demonstrate fewer adverse effects than traditional oral dosage forms. Additionally, nicotine patches have helped people quit smoking and thereby increase lifespan [33].

4.2.1 Percutaneous Permeation

For conventional and pulsatile transdermal drug delivery systems to be effective, the drug must be able to penetrate the skin barrier and pass into the systemic circulation. The skin is one of the largest organs, representing about 16% of the body's weight. It is made up of four layers: the stratum corneum, the epidermis, the dermis, and subcutaneous tissues. It serves a multitude of functions including (1) protection from injury and desiccation, (2) participation in thermoregulation and maintenance of water balance, (3) reception of external stimuli from the environment, and (4) excretion of various substances. In general, these functions may be understood as protective, maintaining homeostasis, and sensing [34].

The barrier properties of skin are most attributable to its outermost layer, the stratum corneum. The stratum corneum is effectively a 10–20 μm thick matrix of dehydrated, dead keratinocytes (corneocytes) embedded in a lipid matrix. The penetration of topically applied solutes, shown in Figure 4.1, is generally considered to occur through or across the lipid component of the matrix [35, 36]. There are additional routes, however, most notably through sweat pores and hair follicles (see Figure 4.2).

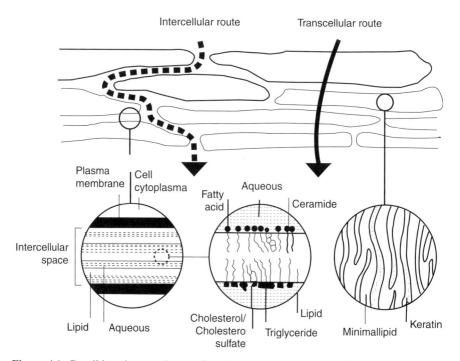

Figure 4.1. Possible micro pathways for drug penetration across human skin (intercellular and transcellular) [36].

Although transdermal delivery has been very successful as a controlled release technology platform, it has several limitations that prevent it from realizing its fullest potential.

1. Ionic drugs cannot be delivered.
2. High levels of medications cannot be achieved in blood/plasma.
3. Only limited applications to small molecular weight compounds (less than 500 Da) are possible.
4. Product components or dugs may cause irritation and/or sensitization.
5. Drugs cannot be delivered in a pulsatile fashion.

Therefore, in regard to these limitations, passive partitioning/diffusion has been traditionally limited to highly lipophilic drugs such as nicotine, hormones, and nitroglycerin. [37].

In order to address these restrictions, bold efforts and new technologies have been employed to overcome the skin barrier and allow for rapid skin permeation. Additionally, since 1997, transdermal drug delivery development has aligned with the life science and biopharmaceutical industries to deliver large molecules, peptides, and proteins (i.e. insulin, calcitonin, PTH(1–34)).

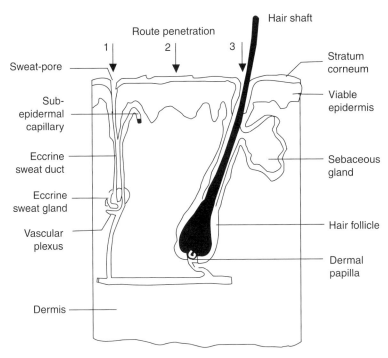

Figure 4.2. Possible macro routes for drug permeation across human skin via stratum corneum, hair follicles, or eccrine sweat glands [36].

The strategy has been to develop transdermal permeation enhancement techniques, either as pretreatments or continuous use devices, to increase the drug flux across the skin by either altering the skin barrier (primarily the stratum corneum) or increasing the energy of the drug molecules. These so-called active transdermal technologies include iontophoresis (which uses low voltage electrical current to drive charged drugs through the skin), electroporation (which uses short electrical pulses of high voltage to create transient aqueous pores in the skin), sonophoresis (which uses low frequency ultrasonic energy to disrupt the stratum corneum), thermal energy (which uses heat to make the skin more permeable and to increase the energy of drug molecules), photomechanical waves, microneedles, and jet-propelled particles. The current status of these emerging technologies, as solutions to the dilemma of how to make the skin more permeable and deliver a wider range of drugs transdermally, has recently been reviewed by Berner and Dinh [38], Mitragotri [39], and Cross and Roberts [40].

4.3 PULSATILE DRUG DELIVERY

Pulsatile delivery systems can be categorized as either externally modulated or self-regulated [41, 42]. Chronopharmaceutical drug delivery systems and programmed polymeric devices for pulsed drug delivery are self-regulated in the sense that they are governed by the inner mechanism of the device (i.e., hydrolysis, enzymatic degradation, osmotic pressure, and degradation with osmotic bursting of the device) [43]. The majority of these devices are designed for oral or subcutaneous application and are either in clinical development or are currently on the market. Reviews by Youan [44] and Stubbe et al. [43] outline the concepts that have been proposed to release medication in a pulsatile manner and describe currently marketed products. Additional pulsatile technologies for drug delivery have recently been reviewed by Stevens [45] and Giannos [46].

Pulsatile and temporally controlled transdermal and modulated topical drug delivery systems may be triggered using a variety of methods and can be classified as follows:

1. Systems exhibiting periodic changes due to external stimulation such as ultrasound, magnetism, or electrical current
2. Self-regulated systems releasing in response to chemical or enzymatic reactions
3. Self-regulated systems releasing in response to physical changes (pH, temperature, ionic strength)
4. Systems exhibiting periodic changes due to an internal timing mechanism such as solvent depletion or chemical oscillators [47–74]

4.3.1 Self-Regulated Systems Exhibiting Periodic Changes Due to an Internal Timing Mechanism

Internally regulated drug delivery modulation has been considered and investigated over the past 20 years. A number of transdermal methods such as solvent controlled, chemical oscillator controlled, and electromechanical-solvent controlled have shown feasibility in providing a temporally modulated delivery profile. In 1995, Siegel and Pitt [75] introduced a general scheme and simplified theory for open loop, sustained oscillatory drug release that does not require periodic external activation. The strategy was inspired by chemical oscillations and biochemical reactions such as the Belousov–Zhabotinsky (BZ) reaction [76] and the peroxidase–oxidase oscillator [77].

Burnette [78] investigated pharmacokinetic limits on the utility of sinusoidal drug delivery systems. In general, it was shown that the micro rate constants describing the drug's pharmacokinetics must be large (i.e., the system must be able to respond rapidly) for *sinusoidal* infusion to be of value. In other words, pharmacokinetic processes tend to smooth plasma drug concentration profiles, which may reduce the effectiveness of pulsatile delivery [78]. This pharmacokinetic restriction further limits the amount of possible drug candidates for temporal drug delivery. Nevertheless, by choosing a pharmacologically active agent with a relatively short half-life (less than 6 hours) and rapid clearance kinetics, pulsatile drug delivery can still be achieved [79].

4.4   APPLICATION OF CHEMICAL OSCILLATORS

Temporally controlled drug delivery systems, proposed by Giannos et al. [80] coupled pH oscillators with membrane diffusion in order to generate a periodic release of a drug or active ingredient transdermally, without external power sources and/or electronic controllers. The strategy was based on the observation that a drug may be rendered charged or uncharged relative to its pK_a value. Since only the uncharged form of a drug can permeate across lipophilic membranes, including the skin, a periodic delivery profile may be obtained (Figure 4.3) by oscillating the pH of the drug solution [80].

The approach originates from the nonlinear kinetics of chemical oscillators. Chemical oscillating reactions have been known for nearly a century, with the Belousov–Zhabotinsky (BZ) and the Landoldt reactions being the two best

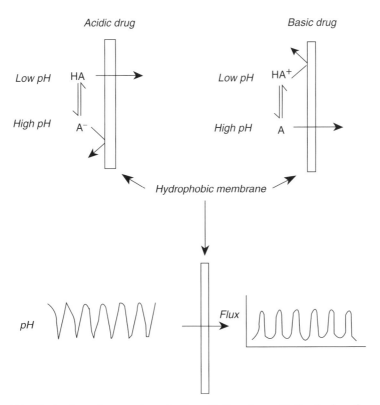

Figure 4.3. Illustration of conversion of pH oscillations to oscillation in drug flux across a lipophilic membrane [94].

Table 4.1. Examples of pH Oscillator Reactions

System	pH
Iodate–Sulfite–Thiourea	3.5–7.5
Iodate–Sulfite–Thiosulfate	4.1–6.5
Iodate–Sulfite–Ferrocyanide	2.5–8.0
Iodate–Hydroxylamine	2.8–5.5
Periodate–Hydroxylamine	
Periodate–Thiosulfate	4.0–6.0
Periodate–Manganese(II)	3.5–4.5
Hydrogen Peroxide–Ferrocyanide	5.0–7.0
Hydrogen Peroxide–Thiosulfate–Copper(II)	6.0–8.0
Hydrogen Peroxide–Bisulfite–Thiosulfate	
Peroxodisulfate–Thiosulfate–Copper(II)	2.3–3.0
Bromite–Iodide	
Bromate–Sulfite–Ferrocyanide	4.5–6.5
Bromate–Sulfite–Thiosulfate	

Source: Adapted from Reference [87].

characterized oscillators. The BZ systems, which are models for studying a wide variety of temporal and spatial instabilities in chemical systems, are generally accepted as the metal-ion-catalyzed oxidation and bromination of an organic substrate by acidic bromate. These colorful reactions illustrate the principles of chemical oscillators through cyclic changes in the color of the solutions [76].

The pH oscillators consist of those oscillating chemical reactions in which there is a large amplitude change in the pH, and in which the pH change is an important driving force rather than a consequence or an indicator of the oscillation [81–83]. The pH of a solution can be oscillated over a range of pH values from 2 to 10 by the reduction and oxidation (redox) reactions of salts, such as permanganates, iodates, sulfates, chlorates, or bromates (Table 4.1).

The first pH oscillator, the hydrogen peroxide–sulfide reaction, was discovered almost 30 years ago. The modified mixed Landoldt reaction (iodate–thiosulfate–sulfite) was used to generate the pH oscillations. With this oscillating system, the pH oscillates between 6.5 and 4, with a characteristic "spike" where the pH minimum is just above 4.0. If the pH falls below 4.0 for any length of time, the iodate–iodide (Dushman) reaction predominates and the solution turns brown. A proposed mechanism for this reaction is as follows:

$$A + B \rightarrow Y \tag{4.1a}$$

$$A + B + X \rightarrow P_1 \tag{4.1b}$$

$$A + Y + X \rightarrow 2X + P_2 \tag{4.1c}$$

where A corresponds to iodate, B to thiosulfate, Y to hydrogen sulfite, X to hydrogen ion, P_1 to tetrathionate, and P_2 to sulfate [84]. The basis for the

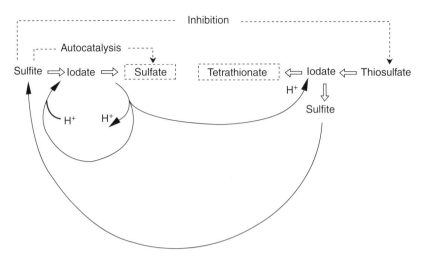

Figure 4.4. Diagram showing the modified mixed Landoldt pH oscillator reaction [89].

oscillatory behavior, as shown in Figure 4.4, is the *alternation* of the auto-catalysis of sulfite and the consumption of hydrogen ion and the formation of sulfite [85]. Furthermore, it was found that compounds with sulfonic acid groups such as poly 2-acrylamido-2-methyl-1-propane-sulfonic acid (PAMPS) or ion exchange resins such as Amberlite$^{®}$ or Nafion$^{®}$ can be substituted for sulfuric acid in the modified Landoldt oscillator [86].

4.4.1 Strategy for Temporal Drug Delivery

The key parameter for system design is the ratio of the characteristic time for permeation to the characteristic time of the oscillation of the driving force. This ratio must be small to produce a temporally controlled delivery profile. As an example, a periodic drug release profile can be obtained through the use of a pH chemical oscillation provided that the period of oscillation in the drug input is longer than the permeation of the drug across all diffusional barriers. In practice, the period of the pH oscillator must be longer than the pharma-cokinetic time lag, which is related to the sum of the characteristic times for obtaining steady-state flux through the membranes and steady-state plasma levels. The following analysis illustrates how this key parameter controls the delivery of a drug across a membrane.

Consider an ideal situation where a drug with a known pK_a is in an infinite reservoir in which the pH of the solution is periodically changed by a pH chemical oscillator. The instantaneous concentration of the uncharged form of the drug, $[C(t)]$, which can permeate across a hydrophobic membrane, is given by

$$C(t) = C_{\max}(1 + \sin \omega t)\, H(t) \qquad (4.2)$$

where C_{max} is the maximum concentration, t is time, ω is the frequency (or $2\pi/\omega$ is the period of oscillation), and $H(t)$ is the Heaviside function. The frequency, ω, is controlled by the kinetics of the pH oscillation and hence by the selection of the chemical oscillator. The flux of the drug across the membrane is then given by

$$\sum_{n=1}^{\infty} (-1)^{n+1} n^2 \left\{ \underbrace{\frac{1}{\left(n^4 + \lambda^2 \omega^2\right)^{1/2}} \sin\left[\omega t - \tan^{-1}\left(\frac{\lambda \omega}{n^2}\right)\right]}_{\text{forced oscillation}} + \underbrace{\frac{\lambda \omega}{\left(n^4 + \lambda^2 \omega^2\right)} e^{-n^2 t/\lambda}}_{\text{diffusion}} \right\}$$

$$(4.3)$$

The characteristic time for permeation, such as the lag time, is governed by the diffusivity and the thickness of the membrane. The first term of the above equation describes the contribution to the flux by the imposed periodic change of the driving force as modulated by the frequency-filtering effect of the membrane. The second term represents the transient permeation. Consequently, if the conditions are set up such that the second term dominates ($\lambda \omega \gg 1$), then the output flux decays to zero, the mean driving flux force for diffusion. However, if the conditions are set up such that the first term dominates ($\lambda \omega \ll 1$), then the flux of the drug across the membrane oscillates with a frequency distribution reflecting the oscillation of the driving force of the permeant and the filtering effect of the membrane. Defining the set of conditions, in which $\lambda \omega < 1$, is the underlying principle for the development of the temporally controlled delivery system [80].

This limit is exemplified by a single oscillation of the fluxes of benzoic acid and nicotine across an ethylene vinyl acetate copolymer membrane containing 28% vinyl acetate (Figure 4.5 and 4.6). The pK_a of benzoic acid is 4.2. As shown in Figure 4.5, the permeation of benzoic acid across the membrane responded to the change in pH during the addition of the iodate solution—increasing in flux when the pH of the solution decreased toward the pK_a of benzoic acid, and decreasing in flux when the pH of the solution increased above the pK_a of benzoic acid. In this experiment, the diffusional lag time of benzoic acid was found to be approximately 20 minutes.

The permeation of nicotine across this ethylene vinyl acetate copolymer membrane is shown in Figure 4.6. The pK_a values of nicotine are 3.4 and 7.9. In this illustration, nicotine freebase permeated across the membrane during the first 60 minutes, in the absence of the iodate oscillator. The diffusional lag time of nicotine across this membrane was approximately 30 minutes. Thereafter, the pH oscillatory reaction was initiated by the addition of the iodate solution. As shown in Figure 4.6, the flux of nicotine reached a maximum at approximately 90 minutes, and then it decreased in response to the lowering of the pH of the solution. The flux of nicotine increases again, responding to the increasing pH of the oscillator reaction [87].

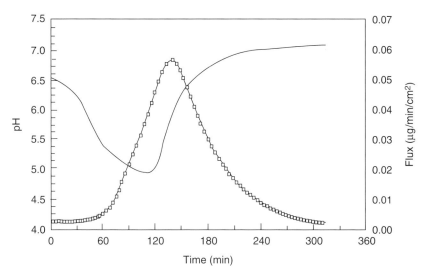

Figure 4.5. Permeation of benzoic acid across 28% vinyl acetate, ethylene vinyl acetate copolymer membrane. The pK_a of benzoic acid is 4.2. The flux of benzoic acid (dotted line) changes according to the change in the pH of the solution (solid line) [87].

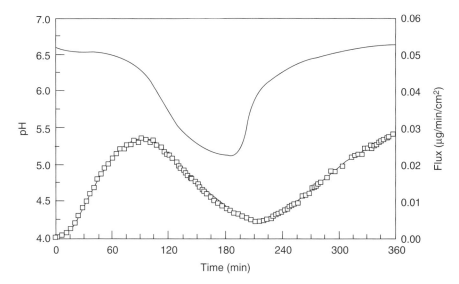

Figure 4.6. Permeation of nicotine across 28% vinyl acetate, ethylene vinyl acetate copolymer membrane. The pK_a values of nicotine are 3.4 and 7.9. The flux of nicotine (dotted line) changes according to the change in the pH of the solution (solid line) [87].

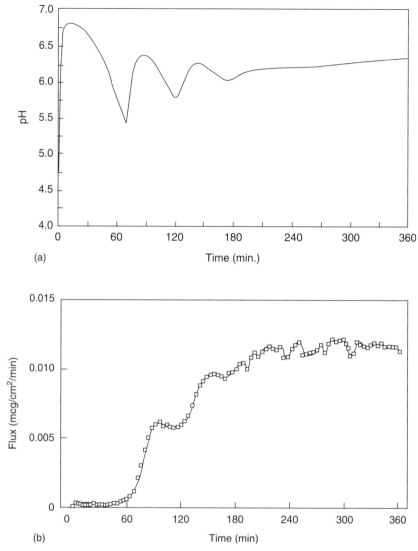

Figure 4.7. (a) pH oscillations observed using a semibatch configuration for benzoic acid permeation of benzoic acid across a 28% vinyl acetate, ethylene vinyl acetate copolymer membrane. (b) Permeation of benzoic acid across a 28% vinyl acetate, ethylene vinyl acetate copolymer membrane using a semibatch configuration. The pK_a of benzoic acid is 4.2. The flux of benzoic acid (dotted line) changes according to the change in the pH of the solution.

Figure 4.7a illustrates the change in the pH during the reaction with benzoic acid using a semibatch configuration, where the sulfoxide solution with the benzoic acid is added to an iodate solution. Figure 4.7b shows the resulting permeation of benzoic acid.

The implementation of this concept, shown in Figure 4.8, to a transdermal delivery system was described in U.S. Patent 6,068,853. As an example, a user-activated system [88] may be employed, where the reactants are initially separated in different compartments. The user-activated system is a two-chamber reservoir system, such that the compartments are separated by a weak seal during storage. The drug can be in either compartment, provided that the drug is stable in that environment. The user activates the system, prior to usage, by breaking the weak seal. The contents from the two compartments are mixed to form the pH-oscillating solution. The uncharged state of the drug then permeates across lipophilic barriers, such as the control membrane of the delivery system and skin. The use of a lipophilic control membrane ensures that the reactants, which are charged species, do not diffuse out of the drug delivery system thereby eliciting adverse biological responses [89].

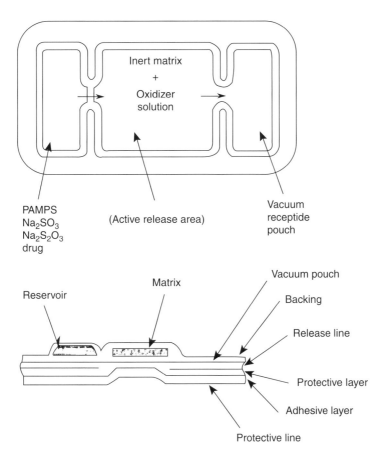

Figure 4.8. Illustration of a user-activated transdermal system for the temporal release of active compounds [89].

4.4.2 Limitations, Status, and Future for Oscillator Controlled Drug Delivery Systems

One limiting factor in the formulation of oscillator–diffusion systems, as described earlier, has been the need for a pH oscillating reaction that has a long enough periodic time, and a longer low pH state within a cycle, to allow diffusion across a membrane. Rábai and Hanazaki [90] described the bromate oscillator system, using marble as the acid accepting component. The basis for the oscillatory behavior is the autocatalysis of sulfite and the consumption of hydrogen ion by marble. The kinetics of the pH oscillations using bromate as the oxidizer and marble chips as the hydrogen acceptor are slower, thereby lengthening the oscillation periods to approximately an hour, as opposed to seconds in the modified Landoldt reaction [90]. Giannos and Dinh [91] obtained reproducible oscillations with nicotine sulfate and using the conditions described by Rábai and Hanazaki (Figure 4.9); however, they did not demonstrate modulated transport across a membrane.

Dolnik et al. [92] demonstrated a novel mechanism for controlling the frequency, amplitude, and existence of pH chemical oscillations. Using the mixed Landoldt (ferrocyanide–iodate–sulfite) pH oscillator, they showed that phosphate buffers could increase or decrease the frequency of oscillations. Furthermore, the same buffer can completely suppress or, conversely, induce oscillations when added to the appropriate composition [92]. Misra and Siegel [93] then followed by investigating the Rábai–Hanazaki pH oscillator with benzoic acid in order to obtain multipulse drug permeation across a membrane as well as study the buffering effects of the drug. Successful multiple, periodic pulses of drug flux across an ethylene vinyl acetate copolymer (EVAc) membrane, as shown in Figure 4.10, were achieved when the concentration

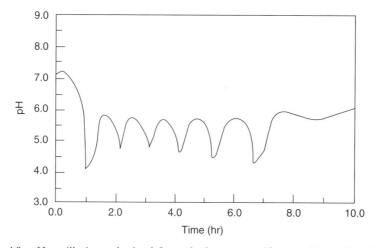

Figure 4.9. pH oscillations obtained from the bromate–sulfite–marble semibatch reaction (Rábai–anazaki pH oscillator reaction) containing nicotine hemisulfate [91].

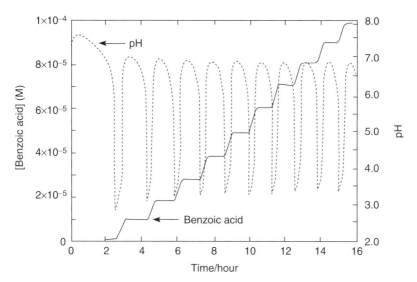

Figure 4.10. pH oscillations and corresponding drug flux of benzoic acid across 2-mm thick 28% vinyl acetate, ethylene vinyl acetate copolymer membrane [93].

of drug was sufficiently low. Additionally, Misra and Siegel [93] investigated the buffering effects of acidic drugs of varying concentration and acid dissociation constant, $pK(D)$, namely, benzoic acid, salicylic acid, and acetic acid with the Rábai–Hanazaki pH oscillator. Higher concentrations of drug had been shown to interfere with the ability of the chemical system to oscillate. Low concentrations of acidic drug can attenuate and ultimately quench chemical pH oscillators by a simple buffering mechanism [94].

The current limitations for the formulation of these coupled oscillator–diffusion systems are the following:

1. The ionized and nonionized forms of the drug have a finite buffer capacity that results in damping the pH oscillations. A concentration must be selected as a compromise between an acceptable amount of damping and the desired flux of the drug.
2. The oscillations are extremely sensitive to initial conditions. A regime where oscillations occur and which is relatively insensitive to these conditions must be determined empirically.
3. The desired frequency and amplitude are not always possible for a given oscillator. Time lags of 20 and 30 minutes for benzoic acid and nicotine, respectively, necessitate the use of a lower frequency than are typically observed with the iodate–thiosulfate oscillator. Membranes with time lags on the order of 5 minutes would exhibit multiple oscillations. Mathematical modeling and discovery of new oscillators should increase the predictability and adaptability of this technology [79].

4. In order to be effective, the active drug compound chosen must have a relatively short half-life, while at the same time drug distribution to the effect site, elimination, and receptor response must be shorter than the time period of periodic drug delivery [78].

4.5 CONCLUSION

The continued interest in chronopharmacology shows the ever-increasing need to develop technologies to control the temporal profile in drug delivery. Research findings suggest that the onset and severity of many diseases are cyclic in nature or follow circadian patterns. Drug tolerance, as well as irritation and sensitization issues, adds to the need for modulation of drug dosing profiles and the need for "off" periods. Moreover, side effects to various drugs may be circumvented through off periods during which no drug is administered as well as improved patient compliance through automated dosing.

Temporally controlled drug delivery systems and chemical oscillators can serve as models to inspire and direct innovative product concepts and new product development for chronotherapeutics. There are, however, pharmacokinetic limitations that cannot be overlooked. For one thing, in order to be able to use pulsatile drug delivery effectively, the body must be able to respond rapidly to the changes in delivery rate. For this to occur, the time frame for drug distribution to the effect site, elimination, and receptor response must be shorter than the time period of periodic drug delivery. Currently, drugs are not designed to have these characteristics [78].

A variety of physical and chemical concepts are now being explored to develop innovative technologies. Self-regulated transdermal systems are now being investigated. Thermoresponsive membranes, nanomaterials, and automated systems, such as Chrono Therapeutics' ChronoDose™ system, as well as intelligent materials for new dosage forms are being developed. The future success of chronotherapeutics and temporal drug delivery will depend not only on the successful integration of intelligent materials and the ease and cost effectiveness of manufacturing, but also on the pharmaceutical and medical community's acceptance of chronopharmacology, chronopharmaceutics and chronopharmacokinetics. Pharmaceutical companies could also benefit by taking advantage of these drug delivery technologies' ability to noninvasively deliver drugs with very short half-lives, multiple doses, and automated dosing while the patient is asleep or before the patient wakens in the morning. The hope is that accurate timing of drug delivery, synchronized with biological rhythms, will lead to more efficient and safer disease therapy.

REFERENCES

1. Berner B, Dinh SM. Fundamental concepts in controlled release. In: Kydonieus A, ed. *Treatise on Controlled Drug Delivery*. New York: Marcel Dekker; 1991.

2. Kydonieus A. Fundamentals of transdermal drug delivery. In: Kydonieus A, Berner B, eds. *Transdermal Delivery of Drugs*. Boca Raton, FL: CRC Press; 1987: 3–16.

3. Guy RH, Hadgraft J, Bucks DA. Transdermal drug delivery and cutaneous metabolism. *Xenobiotica*. 1987; 17(3): 325–343.

4. Ranade VV. Drug delivery systems. 6. Transdermal drug delivery. *J Clin Pharmacol*. 1991; 31: 401–418.

5. Reinnberg A, Halberg F. Circadian chronopharmacology. *Annu Rev Pharmacol*. 1971; 11: 455–492.

6. Smolensky MH, Reinberg A, Queng JT. The chronobiology and chronopharmacology of allergy. *Ann Allergy*. 1981; 47(4): 234–252.

7. Smolenskey MH, McGovern JP, Scott PH, Reinberg A. Chronobiology and asthma. II. Body-time dependent differences in the kinetics and effects of bronchodialator medications. *J Asthma*. 1987; 24: 91–134.

8. Hrushesky WJM. Temporally optimizable delivery systems: sine qua non for the next therapeutic revolution. *J Control Release*. 1992; 19: 363–368.

9. Hrushesky WJM. Timing is everything. *THE SCIENCES*. 1994; July/Aug: 33–37.

10. Lemmer B, Bruguerolle B. Chronopharmacokinetics. Are they clinically relevant? *Clin Pharmacokinet*. 1994; 26(6): 419–427.

11. Redfern P, Minors D, Waterhouse J. Circadian rhythms, jet lag, and chronobiotics: an overview. *Chronobiol Int*. 1994; 11(4): 253–265.

12. Halberg F, Cornelissen G, Wang Z, Wan C, Ulmer W, Katinas G, Singh R, Singh RK, Singh RK, Gupta BD, Singh RB, Kumar A, Kanabrocki E, Sothern RB, Rao G, Bhatt ML, Srivastava M, Rai G, Singh S, Pati AK, Nath P, Halberg F, Halberg J, Schwartzkopff O, Bakken E, Governor SVKS. Chronomics: circadian and circaseptan timing of radiotherapy, drugs, calories, perhaps nutriceuticals and beyond. *J Exp Ther Oncol*. 2003; 3(5): 223–260.

13. Lemmer B. Implications of chronopharmacokinetics for drug delivery: antiasthmatics, H2-blockers and cardiovascular active drugs. *Adv Drug Deliv Rev*. 1991; 6: 83–100.

14. Nutt JG. In: Penn RD, ed. *Neurological Applications of Implanted Drug Pumps*. New York: The New York Academy of Sciences. 1988: 194–199.

15. Altar CA, Berner B, Beall P, Carlsen SF, Boyar WC. Dopamine release and metabolism after chronic delivery of selective or nonselective dopamine autoreceptor agonists. *Mol Pharmacol*. 1988; 33(6): 690.

16. Yates FE, Benton LA. Characteristics of ultradian and circadian rhythms of selected cardiovasularvariables. In: Hrushesky WJM, Langer RS, Theeuwes F, eds. *Temporal Control of Drug Delivery*. New York: Annal NY Academy of Sciences; 1991: 38–56.

17. Wolff H-M, Bonn R. Principles of transdermal nitroglycerin administration. *Eur Heart J*. 1989; 10: 26–29.

18. Fujimura A, Ohashi K-I, Sugimoto K, Kumagai Y, Ebihara A. Chronopharmacological study of nitrendipine in healthy subjects. *J Clin Pharmacol*. 1989; 29: 909–915.

19. Krepp H-P, Turpe F. Antiischaemic effects of phasic release nitroglycerin system during acute and sustained therapy. *Eur Heart J*. 1989; 10: 36–42.

20. Wiegand A, Bauer KH, Bonn R, Trenk D, Jahnchen E. Pharmacodynamic and pharmacokinetic evaluation of a new transdermal delivery system with a time-dependent release of glyceryl trinitrate. *J Clin Pharmacol*. 1992; 32: 77–84.

21. Reinberg AE. Concepts of circadian chronopharmacology. In: Hrushesky WJM, Langer RS, Theeuwes F, eds. *Temporal Control of Drug Delivery*. New York: Annal NY Academy of Sciences; 1991: 102–115.

22. Lemmer B. The clinical relevance of chronopharmacology in therapeutics. *Pharmacol Res*. 1996; 33(2): 107–115.

23. Lemmer B. Clinical chronopharmacology: the importance of time in drug treatment. *Ciba Found Symp*. 1995; 183: 235–247; discussion 247–253 .

24. Smolensky MH, Labrecque G. Chronotherapeutics. *Pharm News*. 1997; 4(2): 10–16.

25. Smolensky MH, Lamberg L. *Body Clock Guide to Better Health: How to Use Your Body's Natural Clock to Fight Illness and Achieve Maximum Health*. New York: Henry Holt & Company; 2001.

26. Ohdo S. Changes in toxicity and effectiveness with timing of drug administration: implications for drug safety. *Drug Safety*. 2003; 26(14): 999–1010.

27. Bruguerolle B. Chronopharmacokinetics. Current status. *Clin Pharmacokinet*. 1998; 35(2): 83–94.

28. Gries JM, Benowitz N, Verotta D. Chronopharmacokinetics of nicotine. *Clin Pharmacol Ther*. 1996; 60(4): 385–395.

29. Gries JM, Benowitz N, Verotta D. Importance of chronopharmacokinetics in design and evaluation of transdermal drug delivery systems. *J Pharmacol Exp Ther*. 1998; 285(2): 457–463.

30. Cramer MP, Saks SR. Translating safety, efficacy and compliance into economic value for controlled release dosage forms. *Pharmacoeconomics*. 1994; 5: 482–504.

31. Cleary GW. Transdermal and transdermal-like delivery system opportunities. In: Boulton E, ed. *Business Briefing: Pharmatech 2004*. London: Business Briefings; 2004: 82–88.

32. Prausnitz MR, Mitragotri S, Langer R. Current status and future potential of transdermal drug delivery. *Nat Rev Drug Discov*. 2004; 3(2): 115–124.

33. Mucke HAM. *Transdermal and Transmucosal Therapeutics: New Developments in Drug Delivery*. Rockvile MD: Drug and Market Development Publishing; 2004: 36–37.

34. Fawcett DW, Bloom W. A Textbook of Histology, 10th edition, London: WB Saunders Company; 1975.

35. Roberts MS, Walters KA. The relationship between structure and barrier function of skin. In: Roberts MS, Walters KA, eds. *Dermal Absorption and Toxicity Assessment*. New York: Marcel Dekker; 1998: 1–42.

36. Williams AC, Barry BW. Skin absorption enhancers. *Crit Rev Ther Drug Carrier Syst*. 1992; 9(3–4): 305–353.

37. Panchagnula R. Transdermal delivery of drugs. *Indian J Pharmacol*. 1997; 29(3): 140–156.

38. Bret Berner B, Dinh SM, eds. *Electronically Controlled Drug Delivery*. Boca Raton, FL: CRC Press: 1998 .

39. Mitragotri S. Breaking the skin barrier. *Adv Drug Deliv Rev*. 2004; 56(5): X–X.

40. Cross SE, Roberts MS. Physical enhancement of transdermal drug application: is delivery technology keeping up with pharmaceutical development? *Curr Drug Del*. 2004; 1(1): 81–92.

41. Kost J, Langer RS. Responsive polymeric delivery systems. *Adv Drug Deliv Rev.* 2001; 46(1–3): 125–148.

42. Kost J. Intelligent drug delivery systems. In: Mathiowitz E, eds. *Encyclopedia of Controlled Drug Delivery.* Hoboken, NJ: Wiley; 1999: 445–459.

43. Stubbe BG, De Smedt SC, Demeester J. Programmed polymeric devices for pulsed drug delivery. *Pharm Res.* 2004; 21(10): 1732–1740.

44. Youan BB. Chronopharmaceutics: gimmick or clinically relevant approach to drug delivery? *J Control Release.* 2004; 98(3): 337–353.

45. Stevens NES. Chronopharmaceutical drug delivery. In: Redfern P, ed. *Chronotherapeutics.* London: Pharmaceutical Press; 2003: 283–307.

46. Giannos SA. Pulsatile delivery of drugs and topical actives. In: Wille JJ Jr, ed. *Skin Delivery Systems: Transdermals, Dermatologicals and Cosmetic Actives.* Oxford UK: Blackwell Publishing; 2006: 327–357.

47. Heller J. Modulated release from drug delivery devices. *Critical Rev Ther Drug Carrier Syst.* 1993; 10(3): 253–305.

48. Brucks R, Nanavaty M, Jung D, Siegel F. The effect of ultrasound on the in vitro penetration of ibuprofen through human epidermis. *Pharm Res.* 1989; 6(8): 697–701.

49. Asano J, Suisha F, Takada M, Kawasaki N, Miyazaki S. Effect of pulsed output ultrasound on the transdermal absorption of indomethacin from an ointment in rats. *Biol Pharm Bull.* 1997; 20(3): 288–291.

50. Lavon I, Kost J. Ultrasound and transdermal drug delivery. *Drug Discov Today.* 2004; 9(15): 670–676.

51. Mitragotri S, Kost J. Low-frequency sonophoresis: a review. *Adv Drug Deliv Rev.* 2004; 56(5): 589–601.

52. Edelman ER, Kost J, Bobech H, Langer RS. Regulation of drug release from polymer matrices by oscillating magnetic fields. *J Biomed Mater Res.* 1985; 19: 67–83.

53. Murthy SN, Hiremath SRR. Physical and chemical permeation enhancers in transdermal delivery of terbutaline sulphate. *AAPS PharmSciTech.* 2001; 2(1): X. Available at http://www.aapspharmscitech.org/view.asp?art=pt0201_tn1&pdf=yes. (Accessed December 15, 2004).

54. Murthy SN. Magnetophoresis: approach to enhance transdermal drug diffusion. *Die Pharm.* 1999; 54: 377–379.

55. Znaiden AP, Johnson AW, Bosko CA, Samaras S. Skin cosmetic care system and method. US Patent *6,761,896.* 2004.

56. Kalia YN, Naik A, Garrison J, Guy RH. Iontophoretic drug delivery. *Adv Drug Deliv Rev.* 2004; 56(5): 619–658.

57. Suzuki Y, Nagase Y, Iga K, Kawase M, Oka M, Yanai S, Matsumoto Y, Nakagawa S, Fukuda T, Adachi H, Higo N, Ogawa Y. Prevention of bone loss in ovariectomized rats by pulsatile transdermal iontophoretic administration of human PTH(1–34*).* *J Pharm Sci.* 2002; 91(2): 350–361.

58. Piggins HD, Cutler DJ, Rusak B. Ionophoretically applied substance P activates hamster suprachiasmatic nucleus neurons. *Brain Res Bull.* 1995; 37(5): 475–479.

59. Heller J. Modulated release from drug delivery devices. *Crit Rev Ther Drug Carrier Syst.* 1993; 10(3): 253–305.

60. Heller J. Chemically self-regulated drug delivery systems. *J Control Release*. 1988; 8(2): 111–125.

61. Siegel RA. pH-sensitive gels: swelling equilibria and applications for drug delivery. In: Kost J, ed. *Pulsed and Self-Regulated Drug Delivery*. Boca Raton, FL: CRC Press; 1990: 129–157.

62. Leroux JC, Siegel RA. Autonomous gel/enzyme oscillator fueled by glucose: preliminary evidence for oscillations. *Chaos*. 1999; (2): 267–275.

63. Heller J, Trescony PV. Controlled drug release by polymer dissolution. II: Enzyme-mediated delivery device. *J Pharm Sci*. 1979; (7): 919–921.

64. Siegel R. Modeling of self-regulating oscillatory drug delivery. In: Park K, ed. *Controlled Release: Challenges and Strategies*. Washington DC: American Chemical Society; 1997.

65. Zrínyi M, Szabó D, Filipcsei G, Fehér J. Electrical and magnetic field–sensitive smart polymer gels. In: Osada Y, Khokhlov AR, eds. *Polymer Gels and Networks*. New York: Marcel Dekker; 2001: 309–355.

66. Osada Y, Gong J. Stimuli-responsive polymer gels and their application to chemomechanical systems. *Prog Polym Sci*. 1993; 18: 187–226.

67. Yuk SH, Bae YH. Phase-transition polymers for drug delivery. *Crit Rev Ther Drug Carrier Syst*. 1999; 16(4): 385–423.

68. Peppas NA, Leobandung W. Stimuli-sensitive hydrogels: ideal carriers for chronobiology and chronotherapy. *J Biomater Sci Polym Ed*. 2004; 15(2): 125–144.

69. Kashyap N, Kumar N, Kumar R. Hydrogel applications: smart gels for drug delivery applications. *Drug Deliv Technol*. 2004; 4(7): 32–39.

70. Soppimath KS, Aminabhavi TM, Dave AM, Kumbar SG, Rudzinski WE. Stimulus-responsive "smart" hydrogels as novel drug delivery systems. *Drug Dev Ind Pharm*. 2002; (8): 957–974.

71. Lin S-Y. Chronotherapeutic approach to design a thermoresponsive membrane for transdermal drug delivery. *Curr Drug Deliv*. 2004; 1(3): 249–263.

72. Suzuki K, Yumura T, Tanaka Y, Akashi M. Thermo-responsive release from interpenetrating porous silica-poly(*N*-isopropylacrylamide) hybrid gels. *J Control Release*. 2001; 75(1–2): 183–189.

73. Jiang HL, Zhu KJ. Pulsatile protein release from a laminated device comprising polyanhydrides and pH-sensitive complexes. *Int J Pharm*. 2000; 194(1): 51–60.

74. Liu Y, Zhao M, Bergbreiter DE, Crooks RM. pH-switchable, ultrathin permselective membranes prepared from multilayer polymer composites. *J Am Chem Soc*. 1997; 119: 8720–8721.

75. Siegel RA, Pitt CG. A strategy for oscillatory drug release: general scheme and simplified theory. *J Control Release*. 1995; 33: 173–188.

76. Field RJ. Experimental and mechanistic characterization of bromate-ion-driven chemical oscillations and traveling waves in closed systems. In: Field RJ, Burger M, eds. *Oscillations and Traveling Waves in Chemical Systems*. Hoboken, NJ: Wiley-Interscience; 1983: 55–92.

77. Larter R, Olson DL, Scheeline A, Williksen EP, Horras GA, Klein ML. The peroxidase-oxidase oscillator and its constituent chemistries. *Chem Rev*. 1997; 97(3): 739–756.

78. Burnette RR. Fundamental pharmacokinetic limits on the utility of using a sinusoidal drug delivery system to enhance therapy. *J Pharmacokinet Biopharm.* 1992; 20(5): 477–500.

79. Burnette RR. Pharmacokinetics and dynamics of temporal delivery. In: Bret Berner B, Dinh SM, eds. *Electronically Controlled Drug Delivery.* Boca Raton, FL: CRC Press; 1998.

80. Giannos SA, Dinh SM, Berner B. Temporally controlled drug delivery systems: coupling of pH oscillators with membrane diffusion. *J Pharm Sci.* 1995; 84(5): 539–543.

81. Rábai G, Orban M, Epstein IR. Design of pH regulated oscillators. *Acc Chem Res.* 1990; 23: 258–263.

82. Luo Y, Epstein IR. A general model for pH oscillators. *J Am Chem Soc.* 1991; 113: 1518–1522.

83. Epstein IR, Orban M. Halogen-based oscillators in a flow reactor. In: Field RJ, Burger M, eds. *Oscillations and Traveling Waves in Chemical Systems.* Hoboken, NJ: Wiley-Interscience; 1983: 257–286.

84. Rábai G, Beck MT. Exotic kinetic phenomena and their chimical explanation in the iodate-thiosulfate-sulfite system. *J Phys Chem.* 1988; 92: 2804–2807.

85. Rábai G, Beck MT. High-amplitude hydrogen ion concentration oscillation in the iodate–thiosulfate–sulfite system under closed conditions. *J Phys Chem.* 1988; 92: 4831–4835.

86. Giannos SA, Dinh SM, Berner B. Polymeric substitution in a pH oscillator. *Macromol Rapid Commun.* 1995; 16: 527–531.

87. Giannos SA, Dinh SM. Novel Timing Systems for Transdermal Drug Delivery. *Polymer News.* 1996; 21: 118–124.

88. Dinh SM, Gargiulo P, Berner B. Nicotine transdermal delivery system. *Proc Int Symp Control Release Bioact Mater.* 1992; 19: 462.

89. Giannos SA, Dinh SM, Berner B. Temporally controlled drug delivery systems. US Patent *6,068,853.* 2000.

90. Rábai G, Hanazaki I. pH oscillations in the bromate–sulfite–marble semibatch and flow systems. *J Phys Chem.* 1996; 100: 10615–10619.

91. Giannos SA, Dinh SM. pH oscillation of a drug for temporal delivery. In: Dinh SM, DeNuzzio JD, Comfort AR, eds. *Intelligent Materials for Controlled Release.* Washington DC: American Chemical Society; 1999: 87–97.

92. Dolnik M, Gardner TS, Epstein IR, Collins JJ. Frequency control of an oscillatory reaction by reversible binding of an autocatalyst. *Phys Rev Lett.* 1999; 82(7): 1582–1585.

93. Misra GP, Siegel RA. Multipulse drug permeation across a membrane driven by a chemical pH-oscillator. *J Control Release.* 2002; 79(1–3): 293–297.

94. Misra GP, Siegel RA. Ionizable drugs and pH oscillators: buffering effects. *J Pharm Sci.* 2002; 91(9): 2003–2015.

CHAPTER 5

DIFFUCAPS® TECHNOLOGY FOR CONTROLLED RELEASE DRUG DELIVERY

GOPI VENKATESH

"I wasted time, and now doth time waste me; For now hath time made me his numbering clock; My thoughts are minutes."

— *William Shakespeare (1564–1616), Richard II*

CONTENTS

Chronopharmaceutics: Science and Technology for Biological Rhythm-Guided Therapy and Prevention of Diseases, edited by Bi-Botti C. Youan
Copyright © 2009 John Wiley & Sons, Inc.

5.1   INTRODUCTION

Most physiological, biochemical, and molecular processes in living organisms display predictable changes on a 24-hour schedule. Epidemiological studies have established that the symptoms of many chronic medical conditions and life-threatening events exhibit a circadian (24-hour) pattern related to the sleep–wake cycle [1, 2]. There is a high incidence of symptoms and events in a particular part of the day (e.g., cardiovascular events in the morning, gastroesophageal reflux disease at night) [3, 4]. Research in clinical drug delivery suggests that synchronizing drug therapies with circadian rhythms may provide a more efficacious treatment and/or minimize adverse side effects in many disease states [5]. However, much effort has been devoted to developing sophisticated drug delivery systems, such as osmotic devices for the oral route of administration, which remains the gold standard for drug delivery, exhibiting drug release at constant rates at or near the absorption sites. The absorption of therapeutic agents thus made available generally results in desired plasma concentrations leading to maximum efficacy and minimum toxic side effects. However, there are instances where maintaining a constant blood level of a drug is not desirable. In addition to a properly designed drug delivery system, the time of administration is equally important. For example, the novel Covera-HS™ (controlled onset, extended-release verapamil tablets based on Alza's OROS technology) has a delayed onset of approximately 4–5 hours after oral administration and has an extended release for approximately 18 hours. When taken at bedtime, this delivery system has been shown to provide an optimal plasma concentration of verapamil over a 24-hour period synchronized with the circadian rhythm variation of both blood pressure and heart rate. Thus drug delivery systems, which are tailored to deliver the drugs to the typical circadian rhythms of the disease states in patients in need of such treatments, need to be designed taking into account the time of administration, knowledge of the molecule, its pH-dependent solubility profile and absorption along the gastrointestinal tract, pharmacokinetic parameters, and elimination half-life. The unique pharmacokinetic profile needed for the target product can be calculated using computer simulation and modeling techniques, and the use of such methods results in reduced feasibility development time and enhances the probability of success of the program.

However, only a few such oral controlled-release systems [6–10] (e.g., drug delivery systems offered by Elan, Andrx, Alza, Penwest, Elite, Shire, Port Systems, and Eurand) are available due to potential limitations of the dosage form size and/or polymeric materials and their compositions used for producing such dosage forms. In this chapter, the concept of chronotherapeutic profiles, a process for developing and manufacturing controlled-release dosage forms comprising functionally coated drug-containing beads based on Diffucaps® technology, and results of clinical studies conducted in an attempt to validate the concept of chronotherapy are discussed.

5.2   **EURAND'S DIFFUCAPS TECHNOLOGY**

Eurand's Diffucaps technology (see Figure 5.1 for the structure) involves the preparation of (1) (immediate release IR) beads (i.e., drug-containing cores such as beads, pellets, and micro tablets, typically provided with a protective seal-coat), (2) barrier-coated beads by providing a (sustained-release SR) or an enteric-coating membrane on IR beads, (3) (timed, pulsatile release TPR) beads by providing a lag-time coating on IR or barrier-coated beads, and (4) finished dosage forms, hard gelatin capsules, conventional or orally disintegrating tablets, comprising one or more coated spherical bead populations (IR beads, barrier-coated (SR or enteric) beads, and/or TPR beads). Such a dosage form exhibits a composite drug-release profile mimicking the target profile calculated by deconvoluting a simulated target pharmacokinetic (PK) profile. The active core of the novel dosage form may comprise an inert particle such as a sugar sphere or a cellulose sphere with a desired particle size range. Alternatively, drug-containing cores (microgranules, pellets, or microtablets) may be prepared by granulation, rotogranulation, or granulation followed by extrusion-spheronization or by compression into microtablets (about 1–2 mm in diameter), consisting of the drug, a polymeric binder, and optionally fillers/diluents. The drug load in the cores could be as high as 60% by weight in drug-layered beads and as high as 95% in pellets and microtablets. These IR beads provide a bolus dose of the active ingredient. The IR beads coated with a water-insoluble polymer (e.g., ethylcellulose) alone or in combination with a water-soluble polymer such as polyvinylpyrrolidone (PVP) provide an extended or sustained-release profile of the active ingredient contained in the core by a diffusion mechanism. If an enteric polymer (e.g., hypromellose phthalate—HPMCP) is used to apply a membrane on IR beads, the drug is released in the form of a delayed pulse. If the IR or barrier-coated beads are provided with a molecularly dispersed membrane of a blend of a water-insoluble polymer and an enteric polymer, the resulting beads—TPR (timed, pulsatile release)

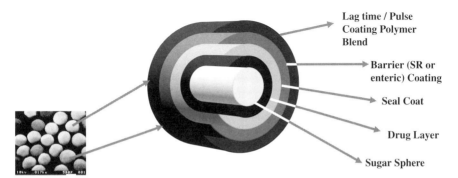

Figure 5.1. Scanning electron micrographs and schematic of Diffucaps beads. (*See color insert.*)

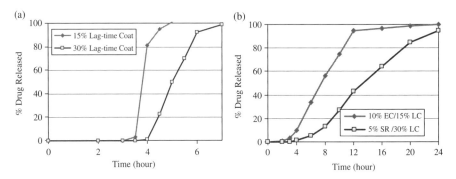

Figure 5.2. Conceptual drug release profiles for Diffucaps beads: (a) a rapid release "Pulse" and (b) sustained-release (SR) profile.

beads—exhibit a release profile as a rapid pulse or a sustained-release profile over a period of up to 20 hours after a delayed onset of drug release (i.e., following a predetermined lagtime of up to about 10 hours) (see Figure 5.2 for conceptual profiles). Generally, the individual polymeric coating can be applied on the active cores from a solution or an aqueous suspension for a weight gain of up to 60% (about 1.5–15% for the barrier coating and about 10–60% for the lag-time coating). The achievable duration of the drug release following the lagtime depends on the nature of the active ingredient as well as the composition and thickness of the barrier-coating and lag-time coating membranes.

The Diffucaps approach has enabled Eurand to develop finished dosage forms comprising one or more coated spherical bead populations (IR beads, barrier-coated (SR or enteric) beads, TPR beads) providing target plasma concentrations to synchronize drug therapies with circadian rhythms of the disease state. For example, Innopran® XL, a new chronotherapeutic formulation of propranolol hydrochloride comprising TPR beads (i.e., IR beads coated with combinations of patented functional polymers), exhibits a time-delayed release synchronizing with the circadian rhythm variation of blood pressure when dosed at bed time (at about 10:00 PM).

5.3 ADVANTAGES OF DIFFUCAPS

Diffucaps beads (typically < 1.5 mm in diameter) including Orbexa®, extruded-spheronized pellets (also < 1.5 mm in diameter), and Microtabs™ (typically about 1.5 mm in diameter) are small in size and therefore have an advantage over nondisintegrating monolithic tablets. Particles or tablets that are 2–3 mm or larger are known to exhibit greater variability in residence times in the stomach and in the small intestine compared to multiparticulate formulations, especially in the presence of food [11, 12]. Consequently, the in vivo release profiles and the extent of absorption of drugs with pH-dependent solubility are often less variable with multiparticulate products. In addition, two or more Diffucaps bead populations can readily be combined into a dosage form, permitting easier adjustment of pharmacokinetic profile and/or creation of multiple strengths of a drug product.

5.4 MANUFACTURING PROCESS FOR DIFFUCAPS-BASED PRODUCTS

The manufacturing process for Diffucaps-based capsules is shown in Figure 5.3. The process consists of aqueous druglayering, SR coating, and lag-time coating to produce TPR beads in fluid-bed equipment, Glatt GPCG 120 or FluidAir FA0300, and encapsulation of TPR beads alone and/or IR or SR beads (barrier coated) into hard gelatin capsules using a commercial capsule-filling equipment, MG Futura. If the intended dosage form is a conventional tablet, the required bead populations are blended with pharmaceutically acceptable excipients, such as microcrystalline cellulose Starch 1500, and/or lactose, and magnesium stearate (lubricant), and are compressed into tablets on a commercial rotary tablet press such as Fette TP2200. Alternatively, if the finished dosage form is an orally disintegrating tablet (ODT), the required bead populations are blended with AdvaTab® base granulation, a flavor, a sweetener, and a disintegrant and are compressed into tablets using a Hata tablet press TP 2000, equipped with a Matsui Ex-Lube system. The base granulation is manufactured by granulating mannitol and Crospovidone with water in

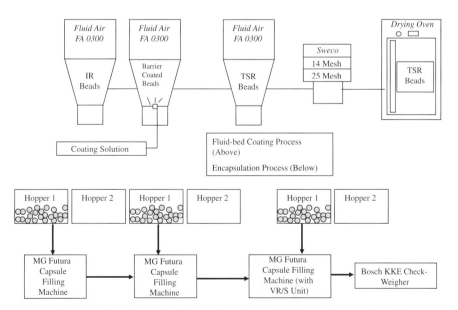

Figure 5.3. Manufacturing of Diffucaps-based capsule dosage forms—flow diagrams.

accordance with the disclosure in EP 0914818 B1. The ODT thus produced rapidly disintegrates on contact with the saliva in the oral cavity, forming a viscous, smooth ready-to-swallow suspension containing the coated beads.

Formulation development in accordance with the Diffucaps technology consists of developing processes to produce the following beads:

- Drug-containing cores (drug-layered beads, pellets, or microtablets, here-after referred to as IR beads for simplicity)
- Barrier-coated beads (SR beads or enteric-coated beads comprising IR beads coated with a water-insoluble polymer (e.g., ethylcellulose) alone or in combination with a water-soluble polymer such as polyethylene glycol or polyvinylpyrrolidone or IR beads coated with an enteric polymer (e.g., hypromellose phthalate)
- TPR beads comprising IR, SR, or enteric-coated beads provided with a molecularly dispersed membrane consisting of a combination of water-insoluble and enteric polymers at a predetermined ratio

5.4.1 Immediate Release (IR) Beads

Immediate-release beads comprising drug-containing cores are prepared by (1) drug-layering and seal coating in fluid-bed equipment; (2) granulation using Granulex or Rotogranulator; (3) granulation–extrusion–spheronization; and (4) high–shear granulation-compression.

IR Beads by Drug Layering IR beads are prepared by layering onto inert particles such as sugar spheres (also called nonpareil seeds) or cellulose spheres from a solution or suspension in water or an aqueous-solvent mixture of the drug using fluid-bed equipment such as Glatt GPCG 3 or GPCG 5 (pilot-scale), Glatt GPCG 120, or Fluid Air FA 0300 (scale-up or commercial scale) equipped with 18-in. or 32-in. bottom-spray Wurster insert. During the preliminary investigations to determine the suitable binder, solution or suspension, optimum binder concentration, and solid content depending on the viscosity of the ensuing solution/suspension, the required drug load is fixed so as to keep the size of the finished dosage form (e.g., capsule or tablet) for the highest strength (dose) as small as possible.

During the initial runs, some of the operating variables, which might have a significant impact on the product quality (i.e., a higher product yield with a minimum of agglomeration and/or spray drying with reproducible release profiles) are identified, optimized, and monitored. These are the drug-to-binder ratio, inlet air temperature setting, spray/flow rate, atomization pressure, product temperature, and the fluidization air volume. The outlet air tempera-ture/exiting humidity in turn is a function of and controlled by these process variables. These parameters should be monitored/controlled throughout the process to develop a robust process. Examples provided in later sections include drug layering of (1) propranolol hydrochloride from an aqueous solution, (2) nizatidine from an aqueous suspension, and (3) cyclobenzaprine hydrochloride from a solution in a 50:50 acetone–water solvent mixture.

Preparation of IR Beads The Glatt GPCG-5 equipped with a 9-in. bottom spray Wurster insert (10-in. partition height) with the setup parameters shown in Table 5.1 is used for the preparation of IR beads. The equipment is charged with sugar spheres (e.g., 25–30 mesh) and fluidization is begun at a product temperature of 45–50 °C. The spray rate applied initially is approximately 8 mL/min and gradually increased to 80 mL/min while increasing the inlet air volume to maintain proper fluidization. Immediately following drug layering, the beads are provided with a protective seal coat of Opadry® Clear. The beads are dried in the fluid-bed coater at the same temperature setting for approximately 5 minutes, as a precautionary measure to drive off excessive surface moisture. The IR beads are then sieved by passing through suitable screens (e.g., 16/25 mesh) to discard oversized beads (>16 mesh screen, i.e., retained on the screen) and fines (<25 mesh, i.e., passing through the screen).

Case Study: Propranolol Hydrochloride IR Beads To produce a 5-kg batch of IR beads, 2800 g of propranolol hydrochloride USP was dissolved in 9816 g of purified water USP with 145 g of povidone (PVP-K29/32) USP as a binder at a solids content of 30% by weight. Glatt GPCG 5 was charged with 1955 g of 25–30 mesh sugar spheres and coated with the drug-layering solution. Also, a seal coat was provided by spraying an aqueous solution of 100 g of Opadry Clear premix in 1250 g of water (approximately 8% solids). The beads

Table 5.1. Setup Parameters for Drug Layering

Equipment Parameters	Purpose
Distribution plate, B	Proper fluidization pattern
Screen, 100-mesh Dutch weave	Prevent beads from falling into bottom chamber
Partition gap, 1 inch	Proper, adequate fluidization pattern
Exhaust flap setting, 38–39% (~ 150 cfm)	
Nozzle tip, 1.0 mm	Proper atomization of coating solution
Atomization air pressure, 1.5 bar	
Flow rate, 8–80 mL/min	Proper coating and to avoid agglomeration
Product temperature, 44–49 °C	

were dried in the unit for approximately 5 minutes to drive off excessive surface moisture.

Case Study: Preparation of Nizatidine IR Beads Micronized Nizatidine (168 kg), a histamine H_2-receptor antagonist indicated for the treatment of peptic ulcer and gastroesophageal reflux disease (GERD), was slowly added to an aqueous solution of 18.6 kg of hydroxypropylcellulose (Klucel LF) and mixed well. Glatt GPCG 60 equipped with a 32-in. bottom-spray Wurster insert was charged with 107.4 kg of 25–30 mesh sugar spheres, which were sprayed with the drug-layering suspension. The drug-layered beads were coated with a protective seal coat of Opadry Clear at 2% by weight and dried in the Glatt unit to drive off excessive surface moisture. The IR beads with a desired sieve cut were further processed for creating Nizatidine Circadian Rhythm Release (CRR) Capsules, 150 mg (75 mg IR and 75 mg TPR beads).

Case Study: Preparation of Cyclobenzaprine Hydrochloride IR Beads Cyclobenzaprine hydrochloride (2.5 kg), a centrally acting skeletal muscle relaxant, was dissolved in 50:50 acetone–water at 25% solids. Glatt GPCG 5 equipped with a 9-in. bottom-spray Wurster insert was charged with 7.3 kg of 20–25 mesh sugar spheres and coated with the drug-layering solution. Upon completion of drug layering, the beads were provided with a protective seal coat of Opadry Clear at 2% by weight and dried for 5 minutes to drive off surface moisture.

IR Beads by Granulation Granurex is an integrated unit for granulation and drying. The trapezoid rotor generates dynamic particle movement during granulation and improves productivity. Granulex has a built-in drying mechanism, which is designed to blow dry air onto the granules. Granurex GX-40 was charged with 3 kg of 350–500 μm sugar spheres and 6 kg of pancrelipase and granulated by spraying a solution of 2.5% povidone (PVP K-30) in 50:50 ethanol–water (nozzle; 0.7 mm in diameter; spray rate; about 20 mL/min; rotor speed; 300 rpm; air volume; 0.3 3 m/min; product temperature; 20 °C). The granulation process was repeated twice using 3 kg of 500–710-μm granules of the first batch or using 3 kg of 700–1000-μm granules of the second batch to produce 710–1400-μm granules with a usual yield of 88%. These granules (almost spherical) may be provided with a seal coat prior to processing into SR or TPR beads.

Alternatively, a fluid-bed granulator such as Glatt GPCG 1, equipped with a rotating disk, tangential spraying nozzle, and a powder feeder, allows both layering of fine powder on inert particles such as sugar spheres or on fine particles of the active agent and direct spheronization of a wetted or melted mass. For example, GPCG 1 was charged with 990 g of milled pancrelipase (<500 μm) and 10 g of Aerosil V200 and granulation is carried out while spraying water at a rate of 10 g/min (process parameters: rotor speed; 1000 rpm; atomization pressure; 1.5 bar; product temperature; 29 °C; air volume;

35% flap; disk; smooth). About 50% spherical granules were in the particle size range of 600–1080 μm.

IR Beads by Granulation–Extrusion–Spheronization   Extruded–spheronized beads can also be prepared by first granulating the active agent with a filler such as lactose and binder (the binder may be dissolved in the granulating fluid for better consistency) in a planetary or high shear mixer; the wet mass is fed into an extruder such as a Nica extruder and the resulting extrudate is spheronized in a Nica spheronizer and finally dried in a fluid-bed drier or in a tray drying oven.

IR Beads by Granulation–Microtabletting   An active agent is blended with other excipients such as lactose and microcrystalline cellulose and granulated using a binder solution in a planetary or high shear mixer or in a fluid-bed granulator and dried. The dried granulation is milled to pass through preferably a 40 mesh sieve, blended with a disintegrant and a lubricant in a blender, and compressed into microtablets on a tablet press equipped with specially fabricated micropunches and dies. A rotary tablet press equipped with 29 stations, with each station being equipped with 16 microtooling, can produce about 14,000 tablets per hour when operated at about 30 rpm. The primary requirement for the success in producing microtablets meeting the USP content uniformity criterion is that the particles should be small ($< 400\,\mu m$, preferably $< 300\,\mu m$) and free flowing. Resulting microtablets (about 1.5 mm in diameter and weighing about 4–6 mg) may be seal coated prior to further coating with functional polymers.

5.4.2 Barrier-Coated (SR or Enteric) Beads

Barrier-coated beads are produced by coating IR beads with a plasticized solution or aqueous dispersion of a water-insoluble polymer such as ethylcellulose alone or in combination with a water-soluble polymer such as polyvinylpyrrolidone or with a plasticized solution or aqueous dispersion of an enteric polymer such as hypromellose phthalate. The purpose of this barrier coating is to sustain the drug release over several hours or to provide a delayed pulse when tested by a two-stage dissolution methodology.

Case Study: Propranolol HCl EC-10 Coated Beads   In these GPCG 5 batches ($\sim 5.0\,kg$), the equipment was charged with 4910 g of IR beads and fluidization was begun at a product temperature of $27.5 \pm 2.5\,°C$. The barrier coating solution was prepared by dissolving 81.75 g ethylcellulose (Ethocel Premium 10 cps—EC-10 for short) and 8.2 g diethyl phthalate in 900 mL of 98/2 acetone/water. The spray rate was initially set at 5 mL/min and then gradually increased to 30 mL/min during the coating operation at an air volume of around 150–160 cfm (exhaust flap set at 38–39% to achieve adequate fluidization). These conditions resulted in a product temperature in the range of 28–30 °C. Following completion of spraying, the beads were dried for 5 minutes as a precautionary measure to ensure low residual acetone levels. The beads were sieved to discard oversized (>16 mesh) and fines (undersized) (<25 mesh) beads. The resulting barrier-coated beads with a coating of 1.8% by weight sustain the drug release over a period of about 16 hours.

5.4.3 Lag-Time Coated (TPR) Beads

Timed, pulsatile-release (TPR) or timed, sustained-release (TSR) beads are produced by spraying a lag-time coating (also called pulse coating) solution of a mixture of a water-insoluble polymer and an enteric polymer at a ratio of from about 90:10 to 50:50 directly onto IR or barrier-coated beads for a weight gain of up to 50% by weight. The purpose of this lag-time coating is to provide a lag time of up to 10 hours (i.e., a period of no appreciable (not more than 10%) release), followed by a rapid pulsatile release or a sustained-release over several hours when tested by a two-stage dissolution methodology.

Case Study: Propranolol HCl TPR Beads In these GPCG 5 batches (∼5.0 kg), the equipment was charged with 4250 g of EC-10 coated beads and fluidization was begun at a product temperature of 27.5 ± 2.5 °C. A pulse coating solution was prepared by dissolving 227.5 g of EC-10, 200 g of HPMCP (HP-55), and 72.5 g of diethyl phthalate in 3750 g of 98:2 acetone–water. The spray rate was initially set at 5 mL/min and then gradually increased to 30 mL/min during the coating operation at an air volume of around 150–160 cfm (exhaust flap set at 38–39% to achieve adequate fluidization). These conditions resulted in a product temperature in the range of 28–30 °C. Following completion of spraying, the beads were dried for 5 minutes as a precautionary measure to ensure low residual acetone levels. The beads were also heat treated at 60 °C for 4 hours in a conventional oven and subsequently sieved to discard oversized (>14 mesh) and fines (undersized) (<25 mesh) beads. The resulting barrier-coated beads with a drug load of about 46.7% by weight sustain the drug release over a period of about 20 hours.

5.4.4 Encapsulation Process

The encapsulation process consists of filling hard gelatin capsules with one or more bead populations using a commercial capsule filling equipment, MG Futura, equipped with two bead-filling hoppers. MG Futura consists of 32 dosing segments and can produce 96,000 capsules per hour. When three or more bead populations need to be filled, two or more bead populations are blended together in a V-blender and tested for blend homogeneity. To manufacture capsule dosage forms, the shell hopper on the Futura is filled with empty capsules while one or both bead-dosing hoppers are filled with the test beads, and the valve on hopper 1 is opened to deliver the amount of beads required to fill each capsule based on the potency of the beads. After verifying that 20 capsules are filled to the target weight in the manual operation, the first hopper valve is closed and the second hopper valve is opened and the weight of the beads filled is adjusted. After verifying that the fill weights of 20 capsules filled with beads from both hoppers are within predetermined specifications, the machine is set up to run in the auto mode. During the encapsulation process, the MG Futura check weighs one capsule approximately every 10 seconds to verify compliance with the predetermined weight specification tolerances. In-process visual and weight checks are executed by the operator throughout the run. The filled capsules are subsequently passed through a Bosch KKE2500 check-weighing machine that weighs and confirms that every individual capsule is within predetermined weight limits.

5.5   DISSOLUTION TESTING

Dissolution testing of Diffucaps beads comprising methylphenidate is conducted using a USP Apparatus 2 (paddles at 50 rpm) in 500 mL of purified water USP at 37 °C and cumulative drug release with time is determined by HPLC on samples pulled at selected time intervals. Dissolution testing of Diffucaps beads comprising propranolol hydrochloride or nizatidine is conducted using a USP Apparatus 1 (baskets at 100 rpm) and a two-stage dissolution medium at 37 °C (first 2 hours in 700 mL of 0.1 N hydrochloric acid) followed by dissolution testing at pH 6.8 obtained by the addition of 200 mL of pH modifier. Cumulative drug release with time is determined by HPLC on samples pulled at selected time intervals.

5.6   MECHANISM OF DRUG RELEASE FROM TPR/TSR BEADS

The water-insoluble and enteric polymers are molecularly dispersed in the lag-time coating membrane applied on the drug cores. During dissolution testing in the two-stage dissolution medium, little water is imbibed into the core as the polymeric system is least permeable in the acidic medium. When the pH of the medium is changed to 6.8, the penetrating dissolution medium selectively dissolves the enteric polymer molecule starting from the outermost membrane layer and moving toward the core, thereby creating tortuous micropore channels (see Figure 5.4). The tortuosity increases with increasing coating thickness and/or at ratios of water-insoluble polymer to enteric polymer greater than 1:1, and consequently, the drug release from the TPR beads having no barrier coat may not be rapid-release "pulses" but tends to be increasingly sustained (see Figure 5.5). In conclusion, the use of uncoated or suitably barrier-coated IR beads enables the development of time-delayed pulsatile release or time-delayed sustained release of the active pharmaceutical agent for absorption along the gastrointestinal tract.

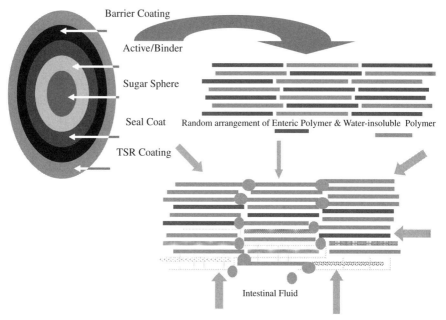

Figure 5.4. Mechanism of drug release from Diffucaps-based TPR beads. (*See color insert.*)

Assumptions/Rationale The pH in the small intestine region [13] varies from about 6.0 to about 7.5 depending on the gastric conditions (fasted or fed, fat content, house waves timing, etc.). Typical resident times [14] in the stomach, duodenum, jejunum, and ileum are, respectively, 0.5 h (0–2.0 h), 0.5 h (0–1.0 hr), 1.25 h (0.5–2.0 h), and 1.5 h (0.5–2.5 h). As discussed earlier, Diffucaps beads with a diameter of 2 mm or less are supposed to have a

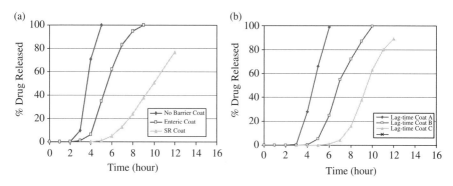

Figure 5.5. Drug release profiles following a predetermined lag-time: (a) rapid release/ SR profiles from TPR beads with an inner barrier coating (none, enteric, or SR) and (b) SR profiles from TPR beads with no inner barrier coating.

predictable transit time through the duodenum region, namely, in about an hour (0–3.0 h). During the in vitro drug-release testing of TPR beads that are <2 mm, the resident time in the acidic dissolution media was deliberately chosen to be 2 h to address this scenario. If the drug has a significant food effect, the time of dosage administration needs to be specified accordingly to take advantage of chronotherapy.

5.7 APPLICATIONS OF DIFFUCAPS TECHNOLOGY FOR CHRONOTHERAPY

A major objective of chronotherapy is to synchronize drug delivery with circadian rhythm in order to optimize efficacy and/or minimize side effects, that is, to deliver the drug in higher concentrations during the time of greatest need and in lower concentrations when the need is less. Eurand has developed circadian rhythm release (CRR) dosage forms for the treatment of school-going children with ADHD (attention deficit hyperactivity disorder), morning protection against target organ damage from hypertension and angina, and healing of GERD (gastro esophageal reflux disorder).

5.8 DIFFUCAPS EXAMPLE: METADATE® CD (METHYLPHENIDATE MR)

Stimulant therapy with pharmacologically active agents such as methylphenidate hydrochloride (MPH) is the mainstay of treatment for children, adolescents, and adults with attention deficit hyperactivity disorder (ADHD). The pharmacodynamic (PD) effects of IR MPH match the pharmacokinetic (PK) profile of a given dose, with a maximum effect ∼1.5–2.0 h after dosing and a half-life of about 2–3 h [15], requiring frequent dosing to maintain effectiveness across the day. It is important to maintain adequate plasma levels so as to avoid the need for midday dosing of a scheduled drug product in the school and to have the plasma levels decrease after school hours so that sideeffects of appetite suppression and insomnia are not manifested. The initially marketed SR formulations, including Ritalin® SR to be administered at breakfast, were not well accepted in clinical practice. Eurand developed a once-daily dosage form comprising 20 mg MPH, Metadate® CD for Celltech Pharmaceuticals, Inc. (now part of UCB Pharma, Inc.), as a bimodal, multiparticulate capsule formulation comprising both 30% IR and 70% SR beads of MPH. The formulation has been designed to deliver a portion of the dose for rapid onset of action and the remainder of the dose in a controlled manner for approximately 12 hours. See Figure 5.6 for the in vitro drug-release profiles from MR capsules, 20 mg (30% IR/70% ER) (i.e., initial stability and stability when stored at accelerated stability conditions—40 °C/75% RH–up to 6 months).

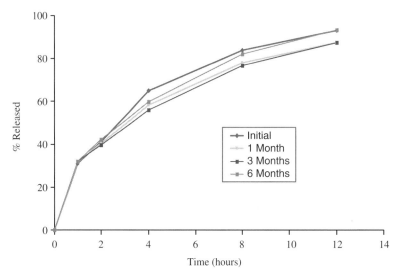

Figure 5.6. Drug release profiles from methylphenidate hydrochloride MR capsules (Metadate CD): accelerated stability data.

PK Study of MPH A randomized six-way crossover study in 24 healthy subjects (Protocol MAI 1001-01) was performed, and the six ways included the following dosings: (1) 1×10 mg Ritalin IR, (2) 1×10 mg Ritalin IR at 0 and 4 h, (3) 1×20 mg Ritalin SR, (4) 1×25 mg MR capsules (20% IR/80% SR beads, also referred to as ER beads), (5) 1×25 mg MR capsules (30% IR/70% SR beads), and (6) 1×25 mg MR capsules (40% IR/60% SR beads). Pharmacokinetics assessments demonstrated that unique, slower methylphenidate elimination rate processes following the administration of the Diffucaps formulations are limited by the release rates from the respective formulations. Based on the pharmacokinetics data, it was decided to reduce the dose to 20 mg, use ER beads with a faster drug release profile, and choose two ratios of IR beads to ER beads, namely, 30/70 and 40/60 for further investigation. Per Protocol MAI 1001-02, the plasma profiles were obtained in a randomized, two-double-blind, crossover comparison of IR bid and placebo in stage 1 and two doses of two MR capsules in stage 2 in 24 healthy children [16]. Children received MR capsules (30% IR/70% ER and 40% IR/60% ER beads, single and double doses) and one dosing regimen of Ritalin IR tablets (10 mg bid). MPH plasma concentrations versus time profiles are presented in Figure 5.7. A level "A correlation" was established between the in vitro release and in vivo absorption with a correlation coefficient of $r^2 = 0.98$ and a slope of almost 1, as per the U.S. _Food and Drug Administration_ (FDA) guidelines, _Guidance for Industry: Extended Release Oral Dosage Forms._ Food has no effect on early exposure and the pharmacokinetic profiles up to 8 h after dosing [16].

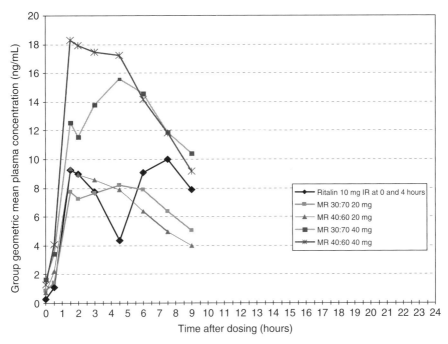

Figure 5.7. Mean plasma concentration–time profiles for MPH MR capsules (30/70 and 60/40 IR/SR beads) versus Ritalin 10 mg bid.

***Performance Comparison Between Metadate CD and Concerta*®**   Metadate CD, 20 mg and Concerta® comprising 18 mg (4 mg IR and 14 mg SR portion) were compared in a crossover clinical study in patients at 10 centers across the United States [17, 18]. Eligible patients were assigned to a dose level according to their preexisting dosing requirements for MPH and remained at this level for the study duration (level 1 dosing, one unit dose of Metadate vs. Concerta vs. Placebo; level 2 dosing; 2 unit doses of Metadate vs. Concerta vs. Placebo; level 3 dosing; 3 unit doses of Metadate vs. Concerta vs. Placebo). Each of the three treatments was administered for 7 days (in the assigned sequence) without an intervening washout period. The patients were assessed in the laboratory school on days 7, 14, and 21. Despite the similarity in overall and maximum exposure to MPH, the differences in early and late exposure to MPH with these two once-daily MPH formulations resulted in detectable and potentially important differences in clinical efficacy during the day. The early and late phase higher exposures of MPH (see Figure 5.8) with Metadate (6 mg IR and faster SR profile) and Concerta (4 mg IR and slower SR profile) appear to have resulted in superior performance of Metadate and Concerta in the early and late phases, respectively [17, 18].

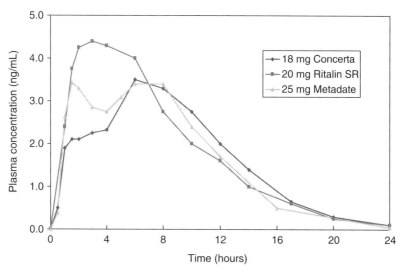

Figure 5.8. Mean plasma concentration–time profiles for 25 mg Metadate CD, 18 mg Concerta versus 20 mg Ritalin SR.

Single Versus Multiple Dose Administrations   The study in children of age 6–12 years confirmed that Metadate CD and Concerta that were compared in this study meet the published FDA criteria for single-dose bioequivalence of a modified release oral dosage form; however, the results of this study suggest that the PD effects of these two formulations are not equivalent. The study suggests that single-dose bioequivalence comparisons that are based only on AUC and C_{max} may be insensitive to clinically important differences in PD effects for this class of agents in this patient population [17, 18].

5.9   DIFFUCAPS EXAMPLE: INNOPRAN XL (PROPRANOLOL CRR)

Propranolol hydrochloride USP, a novel, nonselective beta-adrenergic receptor-blocking agent is indicated for the management of hypertension [15]. Propranolol is rapidly and almost completely absorbed from the gastrointestinal tract. Its biological half-life is approximately 4 hours. There is a well-established circadian variation in frequency of onset of cardiovascular events including ventricular arrhythmias, stroke, angina, and myocardial infarction; they are more common during the period each day when people rise from sleep and in the morning hours. The peak frequency of such events is exhibited in the morning hours, theoretically in conjunction with the morning surge in systolic blood pressure and heart rate. Blood pressure peaks in late morning, then falls during afternoon and evening. Blood pressure is generally lowest between 8 PM and 2 AM. This rise in blood pressure corresponds to increased secretion of catecholamines (adrenal hormones) and rennin. This early morning blood pressure rise may be accentuated in patients with hypertension, and hence there is an excess risk of cardiovascular events: about 40% higher risk of heart attack, about 30% risk of sudden cardiac death, and about 50% increased risk of stroke [19, 20]. There is also some evidence of a secondary peak in frequency of such events in the late afternoon or evening hours [21].

The BHAT (Beta blocker Heart Attack Trial) study demonstrated the therapeutic role of beta blockers in decreasing morbidity and mortality from morning cardiovascular events. For example, propranolol is associated with an approximately 25% decrease in the morning peak incidence of sudden cardiac death compared to placebo [22, 23]. The marketed sustained release products of propranolol hydrochloride, Inderal® LA 80, 120, and 160 mg (Wyeth), which release the active agent at a near-constant rate with a T_{max} of approximately 6 h, do not provide chronotherapy for hypertension. Thus it would be physiologically advantageous to tailor plasma concentrations of propranolol to the typical circadian patterns of blood pressure and heart rate.

Pilot PK Supplies   In 2000 Eurand began the development of a circadian rhythm release dosage form of propranolol hydrochloride. In order to assess the type of in vitro release profiles as well as the ratio of IR to TSR beads needed to achieve a circadian rhythm effect under in vivo conditions, a modeling exercise was performed using the pharmacokinetic parameters available in the literature [24, 25]. The mean serum concentrations achieved in healthy volunteers on oral dosing of 160 mg immediate release and extended release propranolol HCl were fitted to a linear one-compartment model [24].

Ka: $0.7\,h^{-1}$
Ke: $0.18\,h^{-1}$
Vd/F: 837.1 L

where F was given a value of 1.0 and 0.7 for IR and extended release dosage forms, respectively.

Using these parameters and a three-stage dissolution medium (i.e., dissolution testing in 0.1 N HCl for the first 2 h, at pH of 4.0 for the next 2 h, and at pH 6.8 for the remainder), the 20 mg IR bead portion was estimated to provide the desired in vivo profile when combined with 140 mg TSR with a lag time of approximately 6 h when tested using the three-stage dissolution methodology. The IR bead portion was kept the same for the other two strengths, namely, 80 and 120 mg. A randomized, double blind, double-dummy, single dose, two-way crossover PK safety study was performed by Omnicare Clinical Research per Clinical Protocol No. RelPro 3000 by doing the above pilot clinical supplies (80- and 160-mg MR capsules) in 12 healthy volunteers after dinner at 7–7:30 PM. The main measurements included plasma-free propranolol levels, C_{max}, T_{max}, AUC $_{(0-72\,h)}$, and $T_{1/2}$. The study results indicated that under in vivo conditions, the lag time achieved was of the order of approximately 4 h instead of about 6 h anticipated based on the three-stage dissolution procedure. Furthermore, the anticipated bimodal plasma profile was not observed even in the 80-mg dose. A comparison of the actual plasma level obtained for 160-mg MR capsules in Study RelPro 3000 with the simulated in vivo plasma levels of 160-mg MR capsules (using the three-stage dissolution method) and 160-mg Inderal LA suggested that administration of CRR capsules containing only the TSR beads at bedtime (at about 10:00 PM) would provide therapeutically better plasma concentration profiles in the early morning hours and that the two-stage dissolution methodology better corresponds to the drug release under in vivo conditions. Accordingly, the capsules comprising TSR beads were tested using the two-stage dissolution methodology since then.

Pivotal Clinical Study and NDA Approval   Eurand has subsequently developed a CRR capsule formulation (Innopran XL) comprising only TSR beads with a delayed onset of approximately 4 h to afford morning protection against target organ damage from hypertension and angina (see Figure 5.9).

A randomized, open-label, active-controlled, two-period crossover clinical study was conducted comparing the pharmacokinetics of Innopran XL and long-acting propranolol (Inderal LA) per preapproved study design: $n = 35$ healthy male nonsmoking subjects between the ages of 18 and 45 years with a

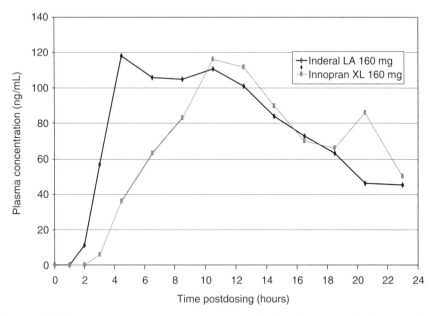

Figure 5.9. Mean plasma concentration–time profiles for Innopran XL (propranolol CRR) 160 mg versus Inderal LA 160 mg in Pilot Clinical Protocol No. RelPro 3007.

body weight within $+20\%$ of the ideal for height; first drug; 1–3 days (single dose), 4–9 days (multiple dose); 9–15 days (washout); second drug, 16–18 days (single dose), 19–23 days (multipledose). For the single-dose study, subjects fasted for 4 hours received a single dose of Innopran or Inderal LA between 9:30 and 10:30 PM and the multiple-dose phase of the study began on day 4. Plasma samples were analyzed for total propranolol (conjugated and unconjugated) using a validated HPLC method. The mean plasma concentration–time profiles of propranolol following administration of the single and multiple doses of Innopran XL and Inderal LA are presented in Figures 5.10 and 5.11. Propranolol is released after the initial delay of about 4 hours such that maximum plasma level occurs in the early morning hours when the hypertensive patient is most at risk [26]. In contrast, the commercially available SR product, Inderal LA, delivers an appreciable fraction of the dose within 3 hours postdosing with a potential for hypotension.

A randomized, multicenter, double-blind, placebo-controlled, parallel group pivotal efficacy study had 420 patients enrolled at 42 centers in the United States who were dosed placebo and 80, 120, 160, and 640 mg at bedtime during 12 weeks/patient study. The results demonstrated statistically significant differences versus placebo in controlling morning and evening blood pressure (6). The Innopran XL products, 80 and 120 mg, were launched in the first quarter of 2003 following the approval of NDA 021-438.

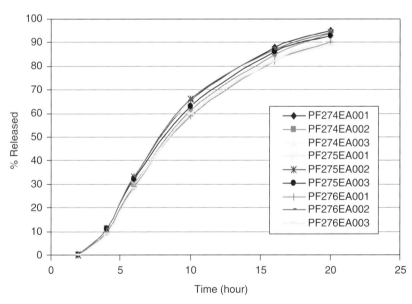

Figure 5.10. Release profiles for propranolol hydrochloride CRR capsules, 80, 120, and 160 mg of registration batches.

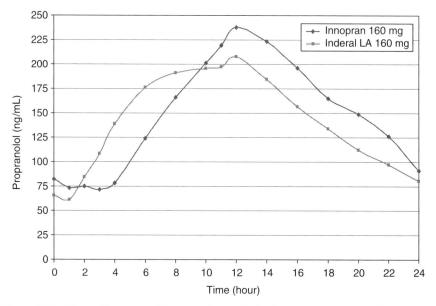

Figure 5.11. Mean Innopran 24-hour clock single-dose concentration–time profile compared with Inderal LA 160 mg.

5.10 DIFFUCAPS EXAMPLE: AXID XL (NIZATIDINE CRR)

During the 24-hour cycle, there are typically four peaks of gastric acid secretion: one peak following each meal and the overnight (nocturnal) peak after bedtime. Gastroesophageal reflux disease (GERD) involves regurgitation of gastric acid into the esophagus, which produces heartburn. Chronotherapy is important in the GI area, treatment of ulcers and heartburn throughout the day and GERD episodes can be improved by timing drug availability before meals and before midnight [4].

Nizatidine, a histamine H_2-receptor antagonist, has a short elimination half-life (1–2 h) and hence an IR dose delivers a single peak with rapid decline in drug concentration, thus necessitating a twice-a-day (bid) dosing regimen [15]. The MR capsules (Axid XL) comprising both IR and TPR beads with a delayed onset of approximately 2–3 h are designed to provide therapeutic levels of nizatidine for morning and afternoon heartburn (AM dose) or provide therapeutic levels for evening and nocturnal heartburn (PM dose). Both twice-daily (bid) and once-daily (qd) regimens were studied in the clinical trial program. Two identical multicenter, randomized, double-blind, placebo-controlled, parallel group studies with 312 patients per study were enrolled at 100 centers in the United States to evaluate efficacy of healing of endoscopically proven GERD. Doses taken include placebo, Axid XL 150 mg twice daily (AM and PM) before meals versus Axid 2×150 mg taken before

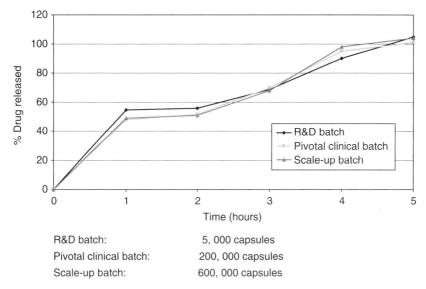

R&D batch:	5, 000 capsules
Pivotal clinical batch:	200, 000 capsules
Scale-up batch:	600, 000 capsules

Figure 5.12. Drug release profiles for 150 mg Nizatidine CRR capsules manufactured at pilot, pivotal and commercial scales (batch size: 5 kg vs. 80 kg vs. 300 kg).

dinner (study duration was 8 weeks per patient). Figure 5.12 shows the in vitro profiles from CRR capsules (150 mg) produced at a R&D/pilot scale (batch size 5–10 kg), semicommercial scale (batch size 80–100 kg), and pivotal/commercial scale (batch size 300 kg). Figure 5.13 shows the mean plasma

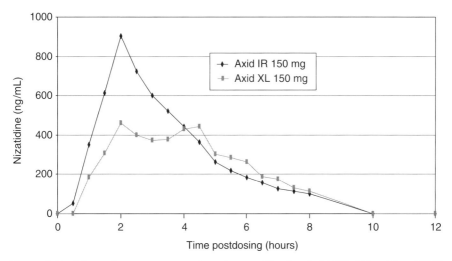

Figure 5.13. Mean plasma concentration–time profiles for Axid XL (Nizatidine CRR) capsules 150 mg versus Axid 150 mg.

concentration–time levels obtained in the pivotal clinical study [27]. Bioavailability of Axid XL was 92% of that of Axid (IR capsules) with an acid suppression at 430 ng/mL. The results showed statistically significant healing of GERD for both the twice-daily and once-daily dosing regimens with Axid XL.

5.11 TECHNICAL AND REGULATORY CHALLENGES

There are several technical challenges to be overcome to develop chronotherapeutic delivery systems. These include low potency and poor solubility in GI fluids, lack of adequate absorption in the lower GI tract, hepatic elimination, undesired conversion/metabolism into inactive metabolites, and significant food effect. From a regulatory perspective, proving that treatment efficacy is improved by timing the oral administration of the chronotherapeutic dosage form is difficult and it is expensive to get the required label approved by the regulatory agency.

5.12 CONCLUSION

In spite of several technical challenges in the development of chronotherapeutic dosage forms and timing of the dosing, significant progress has been made not only in the development of technologies such as Diffucaps, OROS® and TIMERx® technologies but also in determining the timing for dosing of the medication.

ACKNOWLEDGMENTS

The author thanks Reliant Pharmaceuticals, LLC (Liberty Corner, NJ), and, in particular, Mr. Joseph Krivulka, Dr. Keith Rotenberg, Dr. Neil Manowitz (all formerly of Reliant), and Dr. George Bobotas for sponsoring CRR projects at Eurand, Inc. The author also thanks UCB Pharma, Inc. (formerly Celltech/Medeva Pharma) for the clinical data on Metadate CD. He is thankful to John Fraher and the past and present colleagues of Eurand, Inc. who made significant contributions for the successful completion of projects.

REFERENCES

1. Waterdouse J. *Drug Deliv Syst.* 2000; 1: 45–51.
2. Redfern PH. *Drug Deliv Syst.* 2002; 2: 21–23.
3. Anwar YA, White WB. *Chronotherapeutics Cardiovasc Dis Drugs.* 1998; 55: 631–643.

4. Amidon GL. Optimizing oral delivery: PK/PD and controlled release, Presented at the Formulation Optimization and Clinical Pharmacology, A Capsugel Sponsored Conference at Tokyo, April 23, 1999, p. 16.

5. Youan BC. *Control Release*. 2004; 98: 337–353.

6. (a) Jao F, Wong PSL, Huyuh HT, McChesney K, Wat PK, inventors; Alza Corporation, assignee. Verapamil therapy. US Patent 5,160, 744. November 3, 1992. (b) Jao F, Wong PSL, Huyuh HT, McChesney K, Wat PK, inventors; Alza Corporation, assignee. Therapy delayed. US Patent 5,190,765. March 2, 1993. (c) Jao F, Wong PSL, Huyuh HT, McChesney K, Wat PK, inventors; Alza Corporation, assignee. Therapy delayed. US Patent 5,252,338. October 12, 1993.

7. Panoz DE, Geoghegan EJ, inventors; Elan Corporation, assignee. Controlled absorption of pharmaceutical compositions. US Patent 4,863,742. September 5, 1989.

8. Fuisz R, inventor; Fuisz Technology Ltd. (now part of Biovail Corporation), assignee. Recipient-dosage delivery system. US Patent 4,963,742. October 12, 1999.

9. (a) Bettman MJ, Percel PJ, Hensley DL, Vishnupad KS, Venkatesh GM, inventors; Eurand, Inc., assignee. Methylphenidate modified release formulations. US Patent 6,344,215. February 5, 2002. (b) Percel PJ, Vishnupad KS, Venkatesh GM, inventors; Eurand Pharmaceuticals Ltd, assignee. Timed, sustained release systems for propranolol. US Patent 6,500,454. December 31, 2002. (c) Percel PJ, Vishnupad KS, Venkatesh GM, inventors; Eurand Pharmaceuticals Ltd, assignee. Timed, pulsatile drug delivery systems. US Patent 6,627,223. September 30, 2003; and (d) Percel PJ, Vyas NH, Vishnupad KS, Venkatesh GM, inventors; Eurand Pharmaceuticals Ltd, assignee. Pulsatile release histamine H_2 antagonist dosage forms. US Patent 6,663,888. December 16, 2003.

10. Penwest Pharmaceutical Company's TIMERx® proprietary oral controlled release technology and related Geminex® and ChronoDose™ systems.

11. Khosla R, Feely LC, Davis SS. *Int J Pharm*. 1989; 53: 107–117.

12. Rhie JK, Hayashi Y, Welage LS, Frens J, Wald RJ, Barnett JL, Amidon GE, Putcha L, Amidon GL. *Pharm Res*. 1998; 15: 233–238.

13. Rao KA, Yazaki E, Evans DF, Carbon R. *Br J Sports Med*. 2004, 38: 482–487.

14. Prior DV, Wilding IR, Davis SS, Pharmaceutical Visions: *Absorption*. 2002.

15. Physicians Desk Reference, 54–59th editions, 2000–2005.

16. Greenhill LL, Findling RL, Swanson JM. ADHD Study Group. A double-blind, placebo-controlled study of modified-release methylphenidate in children with attention-deficit/hyperactivity disorder. *Pediatrics*. 2002; 109: 107–111.

17. Swanson JM, et al. Development of a new once-daily formulation of methylphenidate for the treatment of ADHD: proof of product studies. *Arch Gen Psychiatry*. 2003; 60: 204–211.

18. Swanson JM, et al. A comparison of once-daily extended-release methylphenidate formulations in children with attention-deficit/hyperactivity disorder in the laboratory school (The Comacs Study). *Pediatrics*. 2004; 114: 1132–1151.

19. Muller JE, et al. Circadian variation in the frequency of onset of acute myocardial infarction. *N Eng J Med*. 1985; 313(21): 1315–1322.

20. Smolensky MH, Portaluppi F. Chronopharmacology and chronotherapy of cardio-vascular medications: relevance to prevention and treatment of coronary heart disease. *Am Heart J.* 1999; 137: S14–S24.

21. Aronow WS, Chul A, Mercando AD, Epstein S. Effect of propranolol on circadian variation of myocardial ischemia in elderly patients with heart diseases and complex ventricular arrhythmias. *Am J Cardiol.* 1995; 75: 837–839.

22. Douglas-Jones AP. Comparison of a once daily long-acting formulation of propranolol with conventional propranolol given twice daily in patients with mild to moderate hypertension. *J Intern Med Res.* 1979; 7(3): 221–223.

23. Lalonde RL, Pieper JA, Straka RJ, Bottorff MB, Mirvis DM. Propranolol pharmacokinetics and pharmacodynamics after single doses and at steady state. *Eur J Clin Pharmacol.* 1987; 33(3): 315–318.

24. Estimation Program Winnonlin™ Nonlinear, Version 1.5, Scientific Consulting, Inc. and Stella, Version 5.5.1, High Performance Systems, Inc.

25. Rekhi GS, Jambhekar SS. Bioavailability and in-vitro/in-vivo correlation for propranolol hydrochloride extended release bead products prepared using aqueous polymeric dispersions. *J Pharm Pharmacol.* 1996; 34: 1276–1284.

26. Sica D, Frishman WH, Manowitz N. Pharmacokinetics of propranolol after single and multiple dosing with sustained-release proporanolol or propranolol CR (Innopran XL), a new chronotherapeutic formulation. *Heart Dis.* 2003; 5: 176–181.

27. Clinical data available at Reliant Pharmaceuticals, LLC.

CHAPTER 6

CHRONOTOPIC™ TECHNOLOGY

M. E. SANGALLI, A. MARONI, L. ZEMA, M. CEREA, and
A. GAZZANIGA

"Fall seven times, stand up eight."

— *Japanese Proverb*

CONTENTS

6.1   SCOPE AND DESIGN CONCEPT

The Chronotopic technology relates to an oral delivery system designed for time-based pulsatile release, which is generally referred to as the liberation of drugs after a predetermined lag phase starting at the time of administration [1]. In contrast to triggered pulsatile delivery, in which release is initiated by external chemical, thermal, electrical, magnetic, ultrasonic, or enzymatic stimuli, in the case of time-based devices only inherent mechanisms are exploited to control the onset of release, irrespective of environment variables such as pH, ionic strength, and temperature [2]. The primary rationale behind time-based oral pulsatile delivery is to enable the chronotherapy of pathologies with symptoms mainly recurring in the night or on awakening, such as ischemic heart disease, bronchial asthma, and rheumatoid arthritis [3–5]. In fact, provided that release is programmed to take place at that particular time, higher drug levels after evening dosing could be achieved when they are especially required. This would expectably improve both the efficacy and tolerability of the pharmacological treatment without impairing patient

Chronopharmaceutics: Science and Technology for Biological Rhythm-Guided Therapy and Prevention of Diseases, edited by Bi-Botti C. Youan
Copyright © 2009 John Wiley & Sons, Inc.

compliance [1, 6–9]. As a further application, colon delivery, which is regarded as potentially beneficial to the treatment of inflammatory bowel disease (IBD) and the enhancement of oral peptide bioavailability, is pursued relying on the time-dependent approach [10–14]. Such a strategy envisages the exploitation of the relative reproducibility in small intestinel transit time (SITT), that has been shown to last 3–5 hours practically independent of characteristics of the dosage forms as well as fasting or fed state of the subjects [15].

The Chronotopic system, which was first presented in the early 1990s, is basically composed of a drug-containing core provided with an outer release-controlling coating (Figure 6.1) [16–29]. Both single- and multiple-unit dosage forms, such as tablets and capsules or minitablets and pellets, have been employed as the inner drug formulation. Cores meant for either an immediate or a prolonged liberation of the active ingredient have been proposed. However, the main focus has so far been on the accomplishment of a rapid and transient delayed release, which is generally considered as the most challenging and also appealing pulsatile delivery mode. The outer barrier has been obtained through the application of swellable hydrophilic polymers of different viscosity grade, typically hydroxypropyl methylcellulose (HPMC), by exploiting a variety of methods. When exposed to the aqueous fluids, these polymers undergo a glassy–rubbery transition. In the hydrated state, they are subject to permeability increase, dissolution, and/or mechanical erosion phe-nomena, which delay the delivery of drugs from the core (Figures 6.2 and 6.3). The system has been shown to provide the pursued pulsatile release behavior

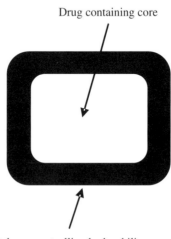

Figure 6.1. Scheme of the Chronotopic system for pulsatile release (cross-sectional view).

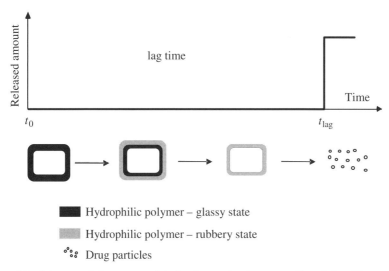

Figure 6.2. Scheme of the expected behavior and release profile of the Chronotopic system. (Adapted from Ref. 16.)

in vitro and in vivo, with programmable lag phases followed by drug release according to the core characteristics. It has turned out possible to finely modulate the lag time by relying on differing coating materials and coating thickness values. Moreover, depending on such variables, diverse mechanisms have been hypothesized and, in some instances, demonstrated to be involved in the control of release [28]. When proper modifications have been introduced into the system design, the Chronotopic technology has shown to yield oral time-dependent colon delivery as well [20, 29]. In particular, the application of an outer enteric film has easily allowed the highly variable and unpredictable

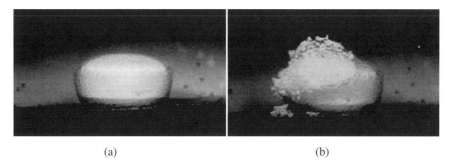

Figure 6.3. Morphological changes undergone by the release-controlling HPMC coating in aqueous medium: (a) formation of a gel layer and (b) disruption of said layer along with disintegration of the tablet core. (*See color insert.*)

gastric emptying time to be overcome. As a result, it has been possible to exploit the relative consistent SITT by purposely selecting the physical–chemical characteristics and amount of the hydrophilic polymer to be employed as the release-delaying agent. Accordingly, the system in its two-layer configuration is expected to keep intact as long as it is located in the stomach. After gastric emptying, the pH-induced dissolution of the enteric coating enables the interaction of the underlying swellable polymer with the aqueous intestinal fluid. This works as a triggering signal for the lag phase, which is programmed to protect the core for a period roughly corresponding to the average SITT. Hence, at the end of the delay time, the device is assumed to be positioned in the colon, where drug delivery may take place.

6.2 FORMULATION DEVELOPMENT AND IN VITRO PERFORMANCE

Throughout the evolution of the Chronotopic technology, much effort has been spent on the preparation and characterization of the polymeric layer responsible for the control of release. Since early developmental stages, hydrophilic cellulose ethers have been identified as potentially interesting coating agents. In particular, HPMC candidates were selected in view of their special suitability for meeting the technology requirements due to a number of advantageous features. Indeed, they are well known to present swelling properties in a range of modes and degrees, consolidated safety profile, ease of handling, general availability in several grades, and reasonable costs as well. However, the coating operations turned out a challenging step that involved the solution of a number of practical drawbacks. These were chiefly connected with the need for obtaining layers provided with thickness values on the order of a few hundred microns. Only a limited experience had until then been gained on HPMC coating, which was essentially confined to the application onto solid dosage forms of rather thin films intended for taste masking or cosmetic purposes. The choice of a suitable coating technique was then the first issue to deal with. Both press- and spray-coating appeared worth exploring. In principle, press-coating seemed more attractive because of its relative simplicity and immediate availability [16]. Moreover, a skill background previously acquired in tableting procedures, including the preparation of multilayered tablets, could advantageously be exploited. However, double compression was soon discarded due to some inherent problems, such as primarily the difficulties encountered in having the core correctly positioned in the die center, which might impact on the homogeneity of the coat thickness and, in turn, on the lag time reproducibility. By way of example, the cross-section of a press-coated system is shown in Figure 6.4. Furthermore, special equipment and time-consuming multiple-step processes, likely associated with poor scale-up prospects, would have been necessary. Finally, the remarkable polymer amount required by such a technique would have not only hindered the achievement of rather short lag phases, but also the preparation of the system in multiple-unit

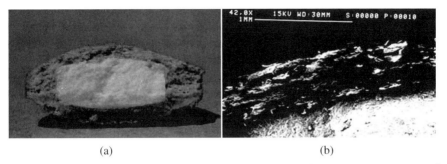

(a)   (b)

Figure 6.4. (a) Photograph of a cross-sectioned Methocel K100 LV press-coated system and (b) SEM photomicrograph (magnification 42.0X) of a coating detail. (*See color insert.*)

form as well as in single units from relatively large starting cores (e.g., because of high drug doses). These appeared as potential limitations to the technology versatility, which should represent a primary goal for any delivery platform. The in vitro performances displayed by press-coated systems were shown not to fully match the pursued pulsatile release patterns (Figure 6.5). Prior to quantitative delivery, in fact, a diffusion phase was observed, during which a

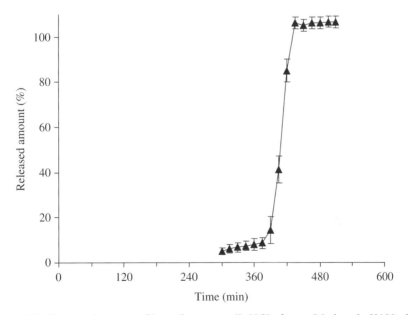

Figure 6.5. Mean release profiles of verapamil·HCl from Methocel K100 LV (177.6 mg/cm^2) press-coated systems based on tablet (60 mg weight, 4.5 mm diameter) cores (paddle apparatus, 900 mL distilled water, 37±0.5 °C, 50 rpm, 278 nm UV detection, 6 replicates, standard deviation indicated by bars). (Adapted from Ref. 16.)

relatively high percentage of model drug was slowly released. Again, this was attributed to the large quantity of polymer necessarily applied.

Spray-coating was then attempted on tablet cores in fluid bed and rotating pan [16–18, 21]. Initially, high-viscosity HPMC grades (Methocel K4 M and K15 M) were taken into consideration as they were assumed to be more effective in ensuring a long-lasting protection of the drug core from the gastrointestinal fluids (i.e. in deferring the onset of release) [16, 17]. However, owing to their viscosity properties, water solutions of these polymers could hardly be used for film-coating operations. In order to reduce the viscosity of such solutions, thus improving their chances of being sprayed, hydro-alcoholic vehicles were employed. In particular, ethanol was utilized in order to prevent the coating formulations from excessively thickening as a consequence of polymer dissolution. On the other hand, following solvent evaporation, the coalescence of polymeric particles adhering to the substrate surface was dependent on an adequate hydration degree of the particles themselves. Hence a vehicle composition was sought that could provide an acceptable balance between the overall feasibility of the coating process and the ability of the suspended polymer to ultimately form a continuous coat. The obtained spray-coated systems exhibited highly satisfactory physical–pharmaceutical requisites and release performance with lag phases increasing in length as a function of the coating level (Figures 6.6 and 6.7). Hydro-alcoholic film-coating was therefore demonstrated to be a potentially suitable and hypothetically scalable technique for the application of HPMC release-delaying layers onto solid dosage forms. Still, the use of organic solvents, which is well known to raise major environmental, safety-related, and consequent regulatory problems, remained an open issue. In order to overcome it, the feasibility of HPMC-based aqueous spray-coating procedures was subsequently explored by comparing the outcome of different polymer viscosity

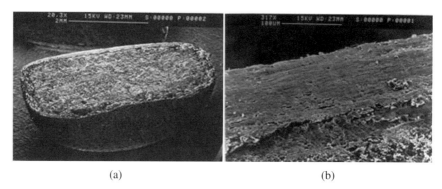

(a)   (b)

Figure 6.6. (a) SEM photomicrograph (magnification 20.3X) of a cross-sectioned system based on tablet (20 mg weight, 4 mm diameter) core and (b) SEM photomicrograph (magnification 317X) of a coating detail (coating agent: Methocel K15M 5% w/w in 95.6:4.4 v/v ethanol/water mixture).

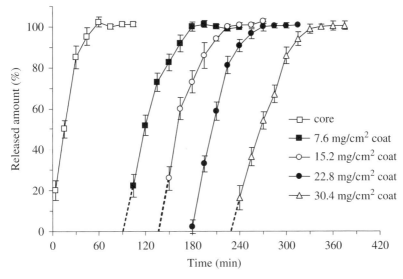

Figure 6.7. Mean release profiles of indomethacin from tablet cores (20 mg weight, 4.5 mm diameter) and systems with increasing coating level (coating agent: Methocel K15M 5% w/w in 95.6:4.4 v/v ethanol/water mixture; test: paddle apparatus, 900 mL simulated intestinal fluid, 37 ± 0.5 °C, 50 rpm, 318 nm UV detection, 6 replicates, standard deviation indicated by bars). (Adapted from Ref. 16.)

grades applied up to 20% weight gain with respect to the original tablet mass, approximately corresponding to 32 mg/cm² coating level [21]. The investigation focused on Methocel E5, E50, and K4 M, the 2% w/v aqueous solutions of which at 20 °C have viscosity of 5, 50, and 4000 mPa s, respectively. The coating process in fluid bed apparatus involved a preliminary set up of the operating conditions. Particular attention was directed to the polymer content and spray rate of the coating solutions, which turned out to be especially critical. As expected, higher polymer viscosity was related to longer process times, mainly due to the need for lowering the HPMC content in the coating solution. The operating parameters finally adopted for 1-kg batches are reported in Table 6.1.

Table 6.1. Operating Parameters for Methocel E5, E50, and K4M (16%, 8%, and 2% w/v) Aqueous Spray-Coating Agents (Fluid Bed Equipment)

Parameter	Methocel E5	Methocel E50	Methocel K4M
Inlet air temperature (°C)	62	60	62
Outlet air temperature (°C)	41	40	39
Nebulizing air pressure (bar)	3.5	3.5	3.5
Nozzle port size (mm)	1.2	1.2	1.2
Spray rate (g/min)	4.8	5.7	8.8

Source: Adapted from Ref. 21.

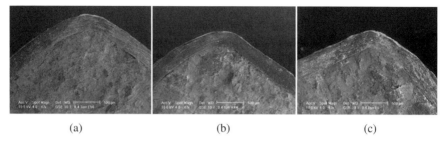

(a)   (b)   (c)

Figure 6.8. ESEM photomicrographs (magnification 47X) of cross-sectioned (a) Methocel E5-, (b) E50-, and (c) K4M-coated systems based on tablet (204 mg weight, 6.8 mm diameter) cores (coating agents: Methocel E5 16%, E50 8%, and K4M 2% w/v water solutions; coating level: 32 mg/cm^2). (Adapted from Ref. 21.)

With all polymers under examination it was possible to obtain yields $>70\%$ and coat layers exhibiting homogeneous thickness as well as smooth surface (Figure 6.8). Release tests were performed in an adapted disintegration apparatus in order to limit adhesion phenomena of the gelled units, which might impair data reliability when using a conventional dissolution testing procedure. The functional coatings were proved capable of delaying the drug liberation (Figure 6.9). Their effectiveness in the control of release increased as a function of the polymer viscosity characteristics. Release patterns showing the typical lag phase followed by a prompt and complete delivery of the model

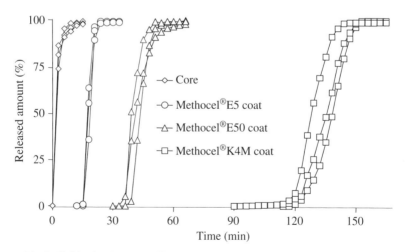

Figure 6.9. Individual release profiles of acetaminophen from tablet (204 mg weight, 6.8 mm diameter) cores and systems coated with different HPMC grades (coating agents: Methocel E5 16%, E50 8%, and K4M 2% w/v water solutions; test: modified disintegration apparatus, 900 mL distilled water, $37 \pm 0.5\,°C$, 31 cycles/min, 248 nm UV detection). (Adapted from Ref. 21.)

drug were attained. Only in the case of Methocel K4M-coated systems a limited percentage ($< 5\%$) of the drug content leached out prior to quantitative release. In this respect, it was hypothesized that Methocel K4M may form a sufficiently resistant gel layer still capable of withstanding extensive erosion after complete hydration, meanwhile allowing drug molecules to diffuse outward. Hence the overall results seemingly pointed out process and performance benefits for low- and high-viscosity polymer grades, respectively. In order to evaluate the coating agents taking account of both these aspects, special parameters were introduced, that is, the time equivalent process parameter (TEPP), given by the ratio between process time (min) and in vitro lag time (min), and the time equivalent thickness parameter (TETP), given by the ratio between coat thickness (μm) and in vitro lag time (min). TEPP and TETP thus represent the process time and coat thickness needed to attain a lag time unit, respectively. Favorable TEPP and TETP results were shown by Methocel K4M (Table 6.2). However, as a consequence of its highly effective control on drug release, possible difficulties were anticipated in a fine modulation of lag time relying on the selection of this polymer coating level. On the other hand, Methocel E50 yielded reasonable process time and feasible manufacturing both in fluid bed and rotating pan [18, 21]. These benefits were coupled with a satisfactory capability of deferring drug delivery without markedly impacting on the relevant rate, and with an appreciable flexibility in the modulation of lag time without entailing excessive coat thickness values (Figure 6.10). In particular, a linear correlation was found between lag time and Methocel E50 coating level. Further advantages were the robustness of its coating formulations and the intra- as well as inter batch performance reproducibility of the coated systems. Moreover, when the batch size was raised from 1 to 15 kg, consistent physical–pharmaceutical characteristics and in vitro release behavior were obtained, thus suggesting the potential viability of a large-scale production. The consistency of in vitro performance was assessed for Methocel E50-based systems under differing physiological pH and ionic strength conditions as well (Figures 6.11 and 6.12). In the case of ionic strength, a marked influence on the delay duration was only noticed at values not included in the physiological 0.01–0.166 range described for the gastrointestinal fluids [30]. pH and ionic strength independency is regarded as an important feature for time-controlled oral pulsatile delivery systems, as their release outcome might otherwise be affected by the considerable variations to which such parameters

Table 6.2. TEPP and TETP Values for Methocel E5, E50, and K4M Aqueous Spray-Coating Agents (Fluid Bed Equipment)

Parameter	Methocel E5	Methocel E50	Methocel K4M
TEPP	34.6	23.0	18.0
TETP (μm/min)	21.8	7.2	2.0

Source: Adapted from Ref. [21].

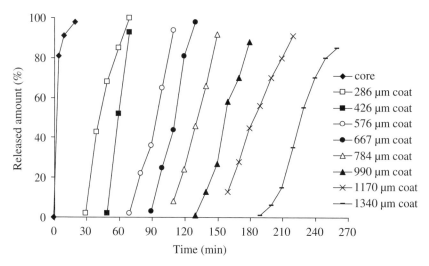

Figure 6.10. Mean release profiles of methyl 4-hydroxybenzoate sodium salt from tablet (180 mg weight, 6.7 mm diameter) cores and systems with increasing coat thickness (coating agent: Methocel E50 7.5% w/v water solution; test: paddle apparatus, 900 mL distilled water, $37 \pm 0.5\,°C$, 100 rpm, 6 replicates, 257 nm UV detection). (Adapted from Ref. 18.)

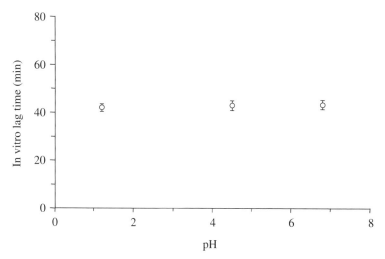

Figure 6.11. In vitro lag time as a function of the medium pH for systems with Methocel E50 ($32\,mg/cm^2$) coating (modified disintegration apparatus, 900 mL simulated gastric fluid, phosphate buffer or simulated intestinal fluid, $37 \pm 0.5\,°C$, 31 cycles/min, 248 nm UV detection). (Adapted from Ref. 21.)

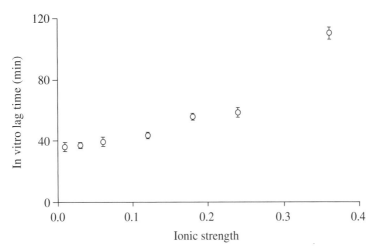

Figure 6.12. In vitro lag time as a function of the medium ionic strength for systems with Methocel E50 ($32\,mg/cm^2$) coating (modified disintegration apparatus, 900 mL distilled water or NaCl solutions, $37 \pm 0.5\,°C$, 31 cycles/min, 248 nm UV detection). (Adapted from Ref. 21.)

are susceptible. According to the above findings, Methocel E50 was subsequently relied on for any further development study.

The possibility of applying the Chronotopic technology to hard- and soft-gelatin capsule cores was also investigated [22–24]. Much interest is focused on this line extension, which could enable a time-controlled liberation of solid multiparticulate (e.g., microspheres, solid-lipid nanospheres, self-microemulsifying drug delivery systems), semisolid, and liquid preparations incorporated within the capsule shells. As it has recently been suggested that stability and gastrointestinal absorption chances of peptides and proteins would benefit from conveyance in dispersed formulations [31–33], capsule-based pulsatile delivery systems might be advantageous for the purpose of enhancing the oral bioavailability of said drugs, particularly through time-dependent colon targeting. Following a progressive adjustment of the operating parameters, chiefly aimed at preventing sticking and shrinking phenomena of the gelatin shells, the previous Methocel E50 aqueous spray-coating procedure was successfully adapted to capsule substrates with no need for the application of any protective subcoating. Coated units with good physical–pharmaceutical requisites were obtained from both hard- and soft-gelatin capsules (Figure 6.13), which provided programmable delays prior to a prompt release of the model drug.

More recent studies were undertaken with the aim of further improving the overall time and yield of Methocel E50 coating processes [26, 27]. In this respect, the feasibility of tangential spray-coating in rotary fluid bed and powder layering was preliminarily assessed with core tablets. Notably, the

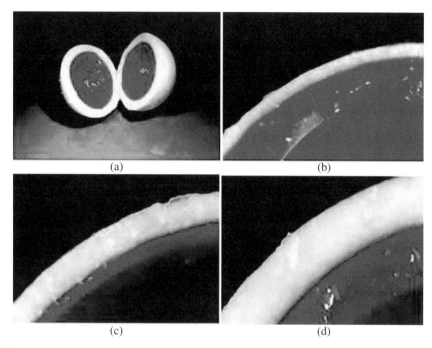

(a)   (b)

(c)   (d)

Figure 6.13. (a) Cross-sectioned Methocel E50-coated system based on soft-gelatin capsule (size 2 round C) core and (b–d) details of coatings with increasing thickness. (*See color insert.*)

process time necessary to reach a coating level of approximately 50 mg/cm^2 was shown to decrease from the 13 hours required by top-spray coating in fluid bed to 6 and 2 hours when operating by film-coating in rotary tangential-spray fluid bed or by powder layering, respectively. Currently, in-depth investigations are ongoing into the application of the latter technique, which involves no solvent vehicle for the coating polymer and might therefore prove highly advantageous in the manufacturing of the Chronotopic system.

6.3   IN VIVO STUDIES

A number of preliminary human in vivo studies have been undertaken on prototypes of promising Chronotopic formulations at different stages of the technology evolution. Various aspects have been evaluated, such as the achievement of a lag time preceding the model drug appearance in the sampled biological fluid and of a subsequent rapid increase in its concentration, the possibility of modulating said lag time by varying the coating level, and, finally, the reproducibility of performance. In addition, even though no in vitro–in vivo correlation has purposely been sought, the overall in vivo results have been compared with the corresponding in vitro data.

Pharmacokinetic, γ-scintigraphic, and pharmacoscintigraphic analyses have been carried out with spray-coated systems based on tablets of differing sizes or on hard-gelatin capsules with increasing low-viscosity HPMC (Methocel E50) coating level. For each study, a limited number of healthy volunteers in the fasting and/or fed state have been enrolled. Acetaminophen and antipyrine have been selected as model drugs for the pharmacokinetic investigations as, in addition to a well-established safety profile, they present the advantageous feature of reaching saliva concentrations comparable with the corresponding plasma levels. Accordingly, they allow non invasive biological sampling to be effected. Both drugs have been assayed in saliva by a high-performance liquid chromatography (HPLC) method. Imaging investigations have been carried out with labeled *placebo* units or else with a preparation containing 5-aminosalicylic acid (5-ASA, mesalazine), which is a major therapeutic tool in the management of IBD [34].

The first in vivo investigation was performed with fasting male volunteers, who were administered a single dose of the antipyrine-containing formulations under examination [20]. These included immediate-release tableted cores and systems coated up to increasing coat thicknesses. The obtained concentration profiles highlighted a delayed appearance of antipyrine in saliva (Figure 6.14).

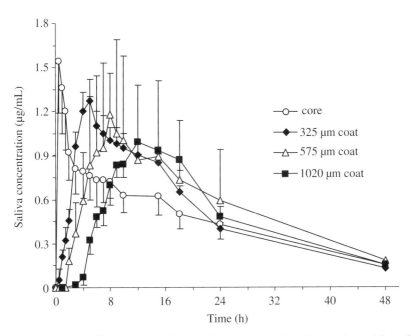

Figure 6.14. Mean saliva concentration profiles of antipyrine after oral administration of tablet (155 mg weight, 6 mm diameter) cores and systems with increasing Methocel E50 coat thickness (4 fasting volunteers, standard deviation indicated by bars). (Adapted from ref. 20.)

Table 6.3. Mean Pharmacokinetic Data After Oral Administration of Tablet Cores and Systems with Increasing Methocel E50 Coat Thickness[a]

Formulation	t_{lag} (h)	C_{max} (µg/mL)	t_{max} (h)	$AUC_{o-\infty}$ (µg. h/mL)
Core	—	1.54 ($\pm$0.35)	0.74 ($\pm$0.41)	23.21 ($\pm$3.70)
325 µm Coat	0.52 ($\pm$0.40)	1.27 ($\pm$0.15)	5.03 ($\pm$1.11)	24.30 ($\pm$4.72)
575 µm Coat	1.80 ($\pm$0.71)	1.18 ($\pm$0.28)	7.42 ($\pm$1.20)	22.04 ($\pm$4.51)
1020 µm Coat	3.94 ($\pm$1.53)	0.99 ($\pm$0.08)	11.69 ($\pm$1.54)	20.82 ($\pm$3.22)

Source: Adapted from Ref. [20].
[a] Four fasting volunteers, standard deviation in parentheses.

Lag times were shown to lengthen as a function of the applied amount of hydrophilic polymer, that is, of the thickness of the release-controlling layer. Mean AUC values turned out quite similar, whereas the peak concentration (C_{max}) displayed a diminishing trend with rising coating levels (Table 6.3). A linear correlation was found between thickness of the applied HPMC layer and lag time, thus pointing out the possibility of timing in vivo drug release (Figure 6.15). In addition, it is interesting to underscore that, for each coating level, in vitro and in vivo delays of the same rank order were obtained. Although not expressly sought, this preliminary result might represent an encouraging premise for the future development of in vitro–in vivo

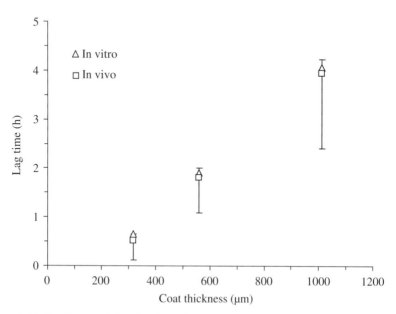

Figure 6.15. In vitro and in vivo lag time as a function of the coat thickness for Methocel E50-coated systems based on tablet (155 mg weight, 6 mm diameter) cores. (Adapted from Ref. 20.)

correlations. Moreover, it indicated the potential reliability of the adopted release testing procedure. With a view to time-dependent colon delivery, the above protocol was repeated on the same formulations, each provided with an outer gastric-resistant film. The relevant saliva concentration curves appeared very similar to those yielded by the corresponding preparations with the HPMC coating only. As expected, longer lag times were observed owing to the presence of the external enteric coating that prevents the interaction between hydrophilic polymer and aqueous biological fluids during the whole gastric residence of the units.

Pharmacokinetic analyses were also focused on hard-gelatin capsule-based Chronotopic systems. Acetaminophen plasma levels clearly delayed as a function of the coat thickness were attained in fasting subjects. Again, in vivo lag times turned out consistent with the in vitro lag phases (Figure 6.16) [24].

The above-described pharmacokinetic results were supported by a γ-scintigraphic evaluation performed with fasting subjects on a *placebo* formulation analogous for composition and preparation procedures to the previously tested antipyrine-containing gastric-resistant tablet system [20]. As indicated by data presented in Table 6.4, all units were shown to disintegrate in the large bowel. In some volunteers, they started to break up in the cecum. The disintegration time after gastric emptying results confirmed the ability of the system to delay drug release throughout the intestine for a programmable period of time. Furthermore, the relatively low variability of such values seemed to point out reproducible in vivo performances.

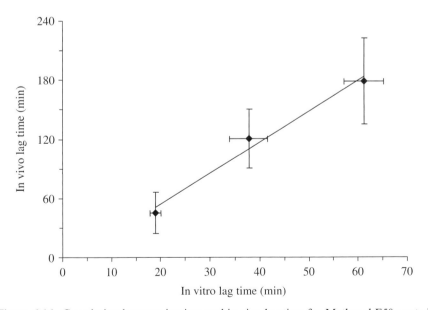

Figure 6.16. Correlation between in vitro and in vivo lag time for Methocel E50-coated systems based on hard-gelatin capsule (DBcaps® size B) cores.

Table 6.4. Individual and Mean γ-Scintigraphic Data After Oral Administration (Fasting Condition) of Gastric-Resistant Methocel E50 (≅1000 μm)-Coated Systems Based on *Placebo* Tablet (155 mg weight, 6 mm diameter) Cores

Parameter	Subject						Mean (SD)
	1	2	3	4	5	6	
Gastric residence (h)	1.0	2.0	0.5	0.5	1.0	0.5	0.9 (±0.5)
SITT (h)	7.0	5.0	3.5	4.5	4.5	5.5	5.0 (±1.1)
Colon arrival (h)	8.0	7.0	4.0	5.0	5.5	6.0	5.9 (±1.3)
Disintegration time after gastric emptying (h)	7.0	6.0	4.5	5.5	5.0	6.0	5.7 (±0.8)
Disintegration site	Cecum/ ascending colon	Ascending colon	Cecum/ ascending colon	Ascending colon	Cecum/ ascending colon	Ascending colon	

Source: Adapted from Ref. 20.

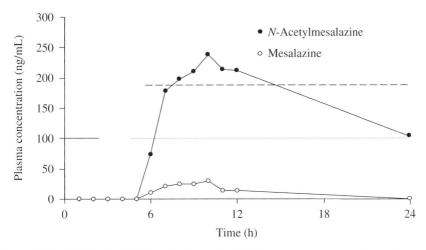

Figure 6.17. Individual 5-ASA and *N*-acetyl 5-ASA concentration profiles after oral administration (fed condition) of a Methocel E50 ($\cong 900\,\mu m$)-coated system based on tablet (550 mg weight, 11 mm diameter) core. Gastric residence and colon transit are represented as a solid and a dotted line, respectively, whereas the dashed line indicates disintegration.

A pharmacoscintigraphic investigation was subsequently carried out into the in vivo behavior of 5-ASA-containing enteric-coated Chronotopic systems administered to fasted and fed volunteers [29]. Combined imaging and pharmacokinetic techniques were employed to acquire information about the actual sites of release and absorption by relating the gastrointestinal performance of the dosage form to the corresponding plasma levels of 5-ASA or its *N*-acetyl metabolite. Scintigraphic results showed that, according to the pulsatile release characteristics of the system, disintegration always occurred in the colon under fasting and fed conditions. By comparing imaging findings with plasma concentration profiles of 5-ASA and its metabolite, the drug was assessed to reach the bloodstream as soon as disintegration started (Figure 6.17). Hence it was not detected in the plasma before the dosage form had reached the colon, thus demonstrating that release and absorption were consistently delayed throughout the intestinal tract.

The overall in vivo results have therefore highlighted the suitability of the Chronotopic technology for delaying delivery after oral administration of the systems to both fasting and fed volunteers. Moreover, the possibility of opportunely timing the onset of drug plasma levels by selecting an adequate thickness for the HPMC coating layer has been established.

6.4 CONCLUSION

The described oral pulsatile delivery system is the mainstay of the Chronotopic technology. Basically, the underlying working mechanism relies on a hydrophilic swellable polymeric coating, which delays drug release from an inner core for a programmable period of time. Hence, through the use of conventional pharmaceutical equipment and standard materials, a versatile delivery platform has been obtained, suited for delivering drugs with different physical–chemical properties as well as pharmacological indications. In particular, because of its special ability to yield lag phases on the order of a few hours, the system could prove a useful means of accomplishing the chronotherapy of illness states with mainly night or early-morning symptoms, such as ischemic heart disease, bronchial asthma, and rheumatoid arthritis. Although the possible chronopharmaceutical application embodies the primary rationale behind the Chronotopic technology, it is noteworthy that the attainable delay times are also consistent with those involved by the time-dependent formulation approach to colon delivery. This is being extensively investigated for the local treatment of large bowel pathologies and a potential bioavailability enhancement for orally administered peptide drugs. As regards both pulsatile and colon delivery modes, proof-of-concept has been achieved through preliminary human studies. In this respect, future research steps envisage more in-depth in vivo investigations, possibly based on active ingredients with a specific chronotherapeutic indication in their recommended dose range. Further development efforts will be directed toward an easy production scale-up.

In conclusion, the inherent advantages of the Chronotopic technology can be summarized in the relative simplicity of design, working principle and manufacturing, general availability of the equipment and materials to be employed, versatility in terms of starting core formulations as well as drugs to be delivered, and, finally, remarkable flexibility in the modulation of delay.

REFERENCES

1. Maroni A, Zema L, Cerea M, Sangalli ME. *Expert Opin Drug Deliv*. 2005; 2(5): 856.
2. Stubbe BG, De Smedt SC, Demeester J. *Pharm Res*. 2004; 21(10): 1732.
3. Lemmer B. *J Control Release*. 1991; 16(1–2): 63.
4. Hrushesky WJM. *Sciences*. 1994; 34(4): 32.
5. Smolensky MH, Reinberg AE, Martin RJ, Haus E. *Chronobiol Int*. 1999; 16(5): 539.
6. Youan BBC. *J Control Release*. 2004; 98(3): 337.
7. Bussemer T, Otto I, Bodmeier R. *Crit Rev Ther Drug Carrier Syst*. 2001; 18(5): 433.
8. Gothoskar AV, Joshi AM, Joshi NH. *Drug Deliv Technol*. 2004; 4(5).
9. Vyas SP, Sood A, Venugopalan P, Mysore N. *Pharmazie*. 1997; 52(11): 815.
10. Gazzaniga A, Maroni A, Sangalli ME, Zema L. *Expert Opin Drug Deliv*. 2006; 3(5): 583.
11. Gazzaniga A, Giordano F, Sangalli ME, Zema L. *STP Pharma Prat*. 1994; 4(5): 336.
12. Leopold CS. *Pharm Sci Technol Today*. 1999; 2(5): 197.

13. Rubinstein A et al. *J Control Release*. 1997; 46(1–2): 59.

14. Friend DR. *Adv Drug Deliv Rev*. 2005; 57(2): 247.

15. Davis SS. *J Control Release*. 1985; 2: 27.

16. Gazzaniga A, Sangalli ME, Giordano F. *Eur J Pharm Biopharm*. 1994; 40(4): 246.

17. Gazzaniga A, Iamartino P, Maffione G, Sangalli ME. *Int J Pharm*. 1994; 108(1): 77.

18. Gazzaniga A, Busetti C, Moro L, Sangalli ME, Giordano F. *STP Pharma Sci*. 1995; 5(1): 83.

19. Busetti C, Crimella T. WO9832425 (1998).

20. Sangalli ME et al. *J Control Release*. 2001; 73(1): 103.

21. Sangalli ME et al. *Eur J Pharm Sci*. 2004; 22(5): 469.

22. Maroni A et al. *Proc Int Symp Control Release Bioact Mater*. 1999; 26: 885.

23. Busetti C, Crimella T. US6190692 (2001).

24. Maroni A et al. *AAPS Pharm Sci*. 2001; 3(3): T3120.

25. Maroni A et al. *Proc Int Symp Control Release Bioact Mater*. 2005; 32: 745.

26. Pirulli V et al. *Proc Int Symp Control Release Bioact Mater*. 2004; 31: 391.

27. Cerea M et al. *Proc Int Symp Control Release Bioact Mater*. 2006; 33: 882.

28. Zema L et al. *J Pharm Sci*. 2007; 96(6): 1527.

29. Sangalli ME et al. *Proc Int Meet Pharm Biopharm Pharm Tech*. 2004; 1: 815.

30. Johnson JL, Holinej J, Williams MD. *Int J Pharm*. 1993; 90(2): 151.

31. Carino GP, Mathiowitz E. *Adv Drug Deliv Rev*. 1999; 35(2–3): 249.

32. Jung T et al. *Eur J Pharm Biopharm*. 2000; 50(1): 147.

33. Barratt G. *Cell Mol Life Sci*. 2003; 60(1): 21.

34. Klotz U, Schwab M. *Adv Drug Deliv Rev*. 2005; 57(2): 267.

CHAPTER 7

CHRONOTHERAPY USING EGALET® TECHNOLOGY

DANIEL BAR-SHALOM, CLIVE G. WILSON, and NEENA WASHINGTON

"The difference between what we do and what we are capable of doing would suffice to solve most of the world's problems."

— *Mahatma Gandhi (1869–1948)*

CONTENTS

7.1 INTRODUCTION

Egalet is a novel erosion-based oral controlled-delivery dosage form that offers two distinct systems, the *constant release* (2K) system or the *delayed release* (3K) system. The constant release system consists of two components: an impermeable coat and a matrix. The drug is distributed evenly throughout the matrix which is eroded by gut movements and gastrointestinal fluids as it travels through the gut. The delayed release form consists of an impermeable shell with two lag plugs, enclosing a plug of active drug in the middle of the unit. After the inert plugs have eroded, the drug is released, thus a lag time occurs. Time of release can then be modulated by the length and composition of

Chronopharmaceutics: Science and Technology for Biological Rhythm-Guided Therapy and Prevention of Diseases, edited by Bi-Botti C. Youan
Copyright © 2009 John Wiley & Sons, Inc.

the plugs. It is the delayed release system that lends itself neatly to the field of chronobiology as the drug release can be timed to match the peak in the disease rhythm.

7.2 OVERVIEW

The realization that the disease state of a body displays a periodicity has led to the development of a relatively new branch of therapy, chronotherapeutics. Chronotherapeutics aims to take advantage of the disease's chronobiology to provide optimum plasma levels of drug, resulting in maximum efficacy and minimum side effects to the patient. This can be achieved by both accurately timing the dosing of the patient and the release of the drug from the delivery system. As more evidence is being obtained that improvement of efficacy of a medication can be achieved if its administration is coordinated with day-night patterns and biological rhythms, it brings into question the traditional practice of prescribing medication at evenly spaced time intervals throughout the day in an attempt to maintain constant drug levels throughout a 24-hour period.

Many disease types display chronobiological patterns (e.g., neoplastic, respiratory, and gastrointestinal diseases). For example, the likelihood of myocardial infarction, stroke, ventricular ectopy, and sudden cardiac death occurring between 6 AM and noon is greater than at other times of the day [1]. The risk of myocardial infarction is 40% higher, the risk of cardiac death is 29% higher, and the risk of stroke is 49% higher than would be expected to occur by chance alone. This could be caused by numerous factors but the main one is higher levels of circulating catecholamines, which increase vasoconstriction, blood pressure, and heart rate. Thus increased shear forces in blood vessels, along with myocardial oxygen consumption, create the opportunity for plaque rupture.

Another disease with demonstrable chronobiologic patterns is rheumatoid arthritis. Patients often suffer their worst symptoms when they wake up in the morning but taking medication once awake leads to a significant delay before these are alleviated. Taking the medication the night before seems an obvious solution; however, drugs such as ibuprofen need to be administered 4–6 hours before achieving their maximum benefit, so their peak effectiveness will occur prior to the patient waking and the effect will be in decline as the patient gets up.

Asthma could also be considered a prime candidate for chronotherapy as normal lung function undergoes circadian changes, reaching a low point in the early morning hours, a dip that is particularly pronounced in asthmatics. It has been estimated that symptoms of asthma occur 50–100 times more often at night than during the day. One method to treat the symptoms in the early hours is to use a long-acting bronchodilator; however, this produces sustained high doses of drug even when none is required, thus increasing the risk of unwanted side effects.

Rather than maintaining high levels of medication throughout the night with the associated risk of producing side effects, a better method of delivering drugs for such types of diseases is to use a time-delayed delivery method. The timing between administration of the formulation and release of the drug has to be carefully controlled to achieve release at the required time. To perform this operation successfully and reproducibly, many factors have to be taken into consideration before the release characteristics of a dose form can be specified for each disease state. For oral drug delivery, it is important to understand not only how the gastrointestinal tract handles the dose form in both fasted and fed modes, but also the effect of chronobiology on gut motility. In the majority of cases, drugs must leave the stomach before they are absorbed. However, the gastric residence time of an oral formulation is highly dependent on the presence or absence of food, and if food is present, the calorific value of the meal. Gastric emptying rates of the drug and its associated dose form present the most variable part of the whole gastrointestinal transit process [2].

Gastric emptying demonstrates a circadian rhythm as identical meals empty significantly more slowly at 8 PM than at 8 AM [3]. This factor needs to be taken into account for dose forms, as are the currently available chronothera-pies for hypertension, which are designed to be taken upon retiring for drug release in the early hours of the morning. Enteric coating of the dose form can ensure that the time delay starts after the dosage form leaves the stomach, but the ultimate release from time of ingestion is now unpredictable. Once past the stomach, the small intestine transit time of dosage forms is relatively constant at around 4 hours [4]. However, the velocity of the migrating myoelectric complex (MMC), which controls transit through the small intestine of large, single units, also displays a circadian rhythm as its speed of migration during the day is more than double that observed at night [5]. The advantage here is that units removed from the stomach by the MMC at night will have a longer time within the small intestine for drug absorption to occur.

Currently, the commercially successful solid oral controlled release technolo-gies are almost exclusively based on diffusion of water either directly into a matrix or through a membrane to release drug. These systems work well for water-soluble drugs, but not for poorly soluble or non-water-soluble drugs.

Egalet technology [6, 7] (Egalet a/s, Denmark) is relatively new to the market, but offers distinct advantages over more conventional controlled release dose forms. The primary one is its ability to deliver water-insoluble compounds in a controlled manner as drug release involves the process of erosion rather than diffusion. An added advantage is that active compounds entrapped in the matrix are also protected from oxygen and humidity and therefore Egalet technology appears suited for chemically unstable substances and thus may increase shelf life. Egalet technology also allows burst or delayed-release of drugs and allows combinations of different drugs to be delivered in one unit.

7.3 EGALET TECHNOLOGY

Egalet Technology offers two distinct systems, the constant release (Figure 7.1) system or the delayed release system (Figure 7.2). The constant release system consists of two components: an impermeable coat and a matrix. The drug is distributed evenly throughout the matrix, which is eroded by gut movements and gastrointestinal fluids as it travels through the gut. The delayed release form consists of an impermeable shell with two lag plugs, enclosing a plug of active drug in the middle of the unit. After the inert plugs have eroded, the drug is released; thus a lag time occurs. Time of release can then be modulated by the length and composition of the plugs. The shells are made of (slowly) biodegradable polymers (such as ethylcellulose) and including plasticizers (such as cetostearyl alcohol), while the matrix of the plugs comprises a mixture of pharmaceutical excipients including polymers like polyethylene oxide (PEO).

7.4 EGALET MATRIX EROSION

The drug release mechanism is achieved by surface erosion, effected through water diffusion, polymer hydration, disentanglement, and dissolution. The matrix is designed to erode when in contact with available water but, at the same time, it is desirable that water does not diffuse into the matrix until the point of release, thus avoiding hydrolysis and diffusion of the drug. It has the added benefit of reducing the effects of luminal enzymatic activity. A balance is required where the erosion is as fast as the diffusion of water into the matrix. The diffusion of water into the edges of the matrix produces only a thin hydrating/dissolving thin layer and leaving a dry core even after 4 hours [8]. The rate of drug release from Egalet can be altered by adjusting the composition of the matrix.

As Egalet is a matrix enclosed in a tube open at both ends, the area available for erosion will be the same at all times; thus the matrix gives a zero-order release profile of drugs in vitro independent of pH but directly dependent on rate of agitation [5]. Altering the diameter and length of the shell can easily be achieved to modify the release accordingly. The tube can be non erodible and

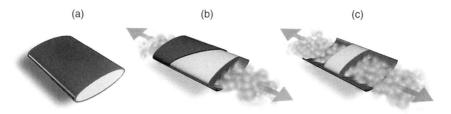

(a)   (b)   (c)

Figure 7.1. Egalet constant release (2K): (a) intact unit, (b) onset or erosion, and (c) further erosion showing the unit retaining the surface area for erosion. (*See color insert.*)

(a) (b) (c)

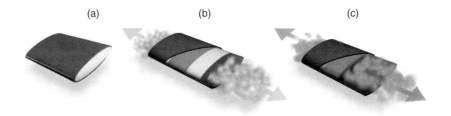

Figure 7.2. Delayed release (3K) form of Egalet: (a) intact unit (b) erosion of the time delay inert plugs, and (c) drug release. (*See color insert.*)

non degradable but degradability obviates the concern about residues in feces and an erodible shell affords yet another element of control of the rate of release.

7.5 MANUFACTURE

Egalet manufacturing can consist of a conventional two-component, injection molding process [9]. This design provides an efficient manufacturing process coupled with high accuracy in dimensions, weight, and content. It also allows the dosage form to be easily tailored to meet a variety of requirements.

Different materials added to the matrix will have profound effects on the erosion rates and, in addition, the processability of the matrix in production. This is also true for the active compounds, since very water-soluble ones will speed the erosion, whereas water-insoluble ones will slow it; for example, testosterone base will stop release altogether even at low concentrations. The pK_a of the active compounds will therefore also have a significant effect on the erosion. This is also true for excipients: for example, cellulose derivatives add plasticity, whereas starch, lactose, sucrose, and mannitol, which are convenient fillers, normally have little impact on the release, other than the solubility effect mentioned earlier. These can be used to compensate for water-soluble or water-insoluble drugs or to adjust the rate of erosion. Other additives may modify the crystallinity of the matrix or other parameters. Generally, the active drug should not exceed 50% of the matrix.

7.6 CLINICAL EXPERIENCE

Initial clinical studies with Egalet have been carried out using the 2K system containing an antihypertensive drug. The studies were performed to assess the suitability of Egalet to replace twice daily dosing with a once-daily therapy for carvedilol. Two pharmacokinetic studies were carried out; the first to compare the pharmacokinetics of Egalet carvedilol and an immediate release (IR) tablet

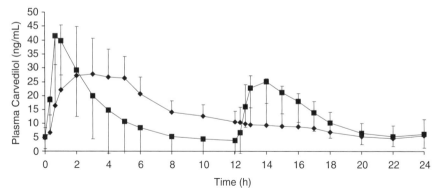

Figure 7.3. The $AUC_{(0-24)}$ for the single 25-mg dose of carvedilol delivered in Egalet carvedilol and twice daily 12.5-mg doses of carvedilol delivered in the IR formulation were 312.5 ± 185.7 and 303.4 ± 195.4 ng mL/h, respectively (mean $\pm$ SD). The $AUC_{(0-24)}$ for Egalet carvedilol was tested and found to be equivalent to the IR tablets with 90% CI.

formulation each containing 25 mg of carvedilol [10]. In the second study, Egalet carvedilol 25 mg was compared to twice-daily dosing of 12.5-mg IR tablets [10].

For the first study, the areas under the plasma–concentration time curve (AUC) were equivalent with a 90% confidence interval for Egalet carvedilol and IR formulation. The C_{max} for carvedilol was statistically lower with Egalet carvedilol than the IR formulation ($p < 0.001$). The T_{max} was delayed from 60 min with the IR formulation to 180 min with Egalet carvedilol.

The steady-state plasma concentration time curve for study 2 is shown in Figure 7.3. Hence it can be concluded that a once-daily 25-mg dose of carvedilol delivered in an Egalet drug delivery system in healthy volunteers provides the same total daily systemic exposure of drug as when administered with twice-daily dosing in a 12.5-mg IR tablet.

Drug release from Egalet 3 K formulation has been demonstrated in vivo also using the technique of γ-scintigraphy. The radiolabeled core was released when the unit entered the ascending colon. The released radioactivity gives a close approximation to the release and spread of the drug prior to absorption from the large bowel. The radiolabel can be seen to disperse as it passes through the ascending and transverse sections of the colon. Drug absorption usually ceases past the transverse colon due to the lack of water available. Preliminary work using quinine as a model drug demonstrates that the in vivo release of drug from Egalet 3K formulation is consistently slower than the in vitro prediction. This is almost certainly due to the reduced motility and water availability in the distal regions of the gastrointestinal tract. The data from these studies confirm the need for more sophisticated in vitro testing methods that can more closely mimic the in vivo conditions and thus be better predictors of in vivo behavior.

7.7 FUTURE WORK

As mentioned previously, blood pressure also displays chronobiology, with the peak occurring between 6 AM and noon and it generally being at it lowest between midnight and 6 AM. These changes in blood pressure parallel the morning activation in catecholamines, renin, and angiotensin. Activity and sleep influence the level of blood pressure throughout the day.

As an example, an extension to the clinical studies already performed with Egalet could be to manufacture a 3K system loaded with an antihypertensive such as carvedilol. As Egalet has proved that it can successfully deliver a drug for 24 hours, the 3K system could be used to tailor the drug release to target the elevation in blood pressure by having a higher concentration of drug in the center plug, which is released at 6 AM. A lower payload of drug can be administered between taking the drug at bedtime and 6 AM, thus providing 24-hour protection against hypertension and tailoring its release profile to match the peaks and troughs in the blood pressure cycle.

Currently, there are four antihypertensive products that are chronotherapeutic medications. These are verapamil (Covera HS) [11], Verelan PM [12], diltiazem (Cardizem LA) [13], and propranolol (Innopran XL) [14].

Covera HS incorporates ALZA's controlled onset, extended release delivery system, COER-24. The COER tablet comprises three layers. The outermost layer is a semi permeable membrane that regulates penetration of water into the tablet; the second layer continues to absorb water from the gut and allows penetration to the third layer. The third layer consists of osmogen, which osmotically expands, delivering drug through laser-drilled holes at the outer layer at a constant rate for approximately 24 hours. The second layer between the active drug core and the semi permeable membrane enables release to be delayed. The medication is designed to be taken at bedtime. The delivery system releases in two stages. First, it provides for a 4–5-hour delay in drug release after bedtime administration. At approximately 3 hours before awakening, drug release occurs so that peak levels of medication coincide with waking and the first hours of activity. Second, the extended release of drug in the gastrointestinal tract provides control of blood pressure for the remainder of the day.

Verelan PM uses the CODAS Chronotherapeutic Oral Drug Absorption System (Elan) and is also designed for bedtime dosing. It too is designed to release its drug after a 4–5-hour delay. The dose form uses pellet-filled capsules, which are coated with a non enteric release-controlling polymer. The polymer consists of both water-soluble and water-insoluble polymers. Water from the gastrointestinal tract dissolves the soluble polymer leaving a porous insoluble matrix through which the drug can escape. The water-insoluble polymer coat continues to act as a barrier, maintaining the controlled release of the drug [15]. Rate of release is essentially independent of pH, posture, and food.

Cardizem LA employs a graded extended release tablet delivery system. The diltiazem graded-response system consists of polymer-coated beads compressed into a tablet. This creates a lag time in tablet dissolution, allowing for detectable plasma concentrations within 3–4 hours and maximal concentrations within 11–18 hours post dose. The system consists of nonpareil seeds powder-layered with the drug, coated with a mixture of Eudragit S100 and L100 polymers (enteropolymers). The dissolution profile of the system shows an initial lag period followed by rapid release of the drug above pH 6.8 in the colon.

The chronotherapeutic formulation of propranolol, Innopran XL, consists of a capsule containing encapsulated beads. The beads have a central core granule, then a drug layer. This is surrounded by a dual-membrane coating, the outer one is a delayed membrane, while the inner one provides the controlled release of the drug.

Now that antihypertensive classes that have been formulated as chronotherapeutics are beginning to establish a track record in the treatment of hypertension, even though further studies are needed to examine the efficacy of chronotherapies for reducing the incidence of cardiovascular events [16], it seems likely that Egalet, with its unique ability to easily tailor drug release characteristics, will find a niche in the sector too.

7.8 CONCLUSION

One of the key factors to successfully utilizing Egalet technology for chronotherapeutics, prior to customizing Egalet release characteristics, is to map the window of absorption, in terms of both time of absorption after oral ingestion and position within the gut at which the drug needs to be released. The chronobiology of the gut's motility needs to be understood and factored in. However, it does appear that Egalet technology is adaptable enough to offer the field of chronotherapeutics a versatile and powerful tool, particularly for delivering poorly soluble or labile drugs.

REFERENCES

1. http://www.touchcardiology.com/ chronobiology-chronotherapeutics-possible-strategy-a409-1.html.
2. Washington N, Washington C, Wilson CG. In: *Physiological Pharmaceutics: Barriers to Drug Absorption*, 2nd edition. London: Taylor and Francis; 2001: 75–108.
3. Goo RH, Moore JG, Greenberg E, Alazraki NP. *Gastroenterology*. 1987; 93: 515.
4. Davis SS, Hardy JG, Fara JW. *Gut*. 1986; 27: 886.
5. Kumar D, Wingate D, Ruckebusch Y. *Gastroenterology*. 1986; 91: 926.
6. Bar-Shalom D, Bukh N, Kindt-Larsen T. *Ann NY Acad Sci*. 1991; 618: 578.
7. Bar-Shalom D, Kindt-Larsen T. US Patent 5 213: 8081993.

8. Metz H, Bar-Shalom D, Hemmingsen P, Fischer G, Mäder K. Presented at the Controlled Release Society, Vienna, Austria, 2006.

9. Cuff G, Raouf F. *Pharm Tech Eur*. 1999; 4: 18.

10. Data on File. Egalet 2004.

11. Verapamil CODAS (Verelan PM) product information. New York: G D Searle & Co.

12. Verapamil (Veralan PM) product information. Mequon, WI: Schwarz Pharma, Inc.

13. Diltiazem (Cardizem LA) product information. Morrisville, NC: Biovail Pharmaceuticals, Inc.

14. Propranolol (Innopran XL) product information. Liberty Corners, NJ: Reliant Pharmaceuticals.

15. Smith DHG, Neutel JM, Weber MA. *Am J Hypertens*. 2001; 14: 14.

16. Prisant LM. *Clinl Cornerstone*. 2004; 6: 17.

CHAPTER 8

CHRONSET™: AN OROS® DELIVERY SYSTEM FOR CHRONOTHERAPY

LIANG C. DONG, CRYSTAL POLLOCK-DOVE, and
PATRICK S.L. WONG

"Progress isn't made by early risers. It's made by lazy men trying to find easier ways to do something."

— *Robert A. Heinlein (1907–1988)*

CONTENTS

8.1 INTRODUCTION

Chronobiology is concerned with the circadian rhythm of biological functions, which has been realized to play a pivotal role in the exacerbation of many diseases. Chronotherapeutical delivery systems, also referred to as time-controlled delivery systems, were developed for treatment of cardiovascular diseases [1–5], asthma [6–8], and osteoarthritis [9, 10].

Covera HS® (verapamil hydrochloride) is a commercial product developed by ALZA utilizing controlled-onset extended-release (COER) technology,

Chronopharmaceutics: Science and Technology for Biological Rhythm-Guided Therapy and Prevention of Diseases, edited by Bi-Botti C. Youan

which is one of the well-known OROS® delivery systems [11–13]. Several time-controlled delivery systems have been reported, either for chronotherapy, site-specific delivery, or avoiding development of drug tolerance [14–21].

CHRONSET™ is another proprietary OROS delivery system that reproducibly delivers a bolus drug dose (>80% drug release within 15 minutes) in a time- or site-specific manner to the gastrointestinal tract (GIT) [22–24]. Using the CHRONSET technology, the drug formulation is completely protected from chemical and enzymatic degradation in the GIT before release, and the timing of release is unaffected by GIT contents. By specifically balancing the osmotic engine, the semipermeable membrane, and the other attributes of the system configuration, drug release onset times varying from 1 to 20 hours can be achieved. The design of CHRONSET, its operation mechanism, the control features, and in vivo performance in human volunteers are described.

8.2 SYSTEM DESIGN AND CONTROL FEATURES

Figure 8.1 shows the configuration of the CHRONSET delivery system. The system is composed of two compartments—the drug vessel and the osmotic engine cap. These two compartments are telescopically engaged. When the system is exposed to an aqueous medium, water permeates into the osmotic engine cap via a rate-controlling membrane. Hydration of the osmotic engine leads to its expansion, which exerts a driving force via a piston against the ridge of the drug vessel. The two compartments separate from each other by sliding apart. After disengaging, the open mouth of the drug vessel is exposed to the fluid environment. The ejecting layer is quickly swollen by the easily accessible fluid and expels the formulation out of the drug vessel. Therefore the

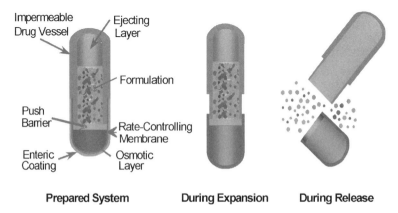

Figure 8.1. Cross section of CHRONSET system before and after operation. (*See color insert.*)

CHRONSET can deliver essentially the entire dose and minimizes the drug residue in the drug vessel after the operation.

8.3 SYSTEM MANUFACTURING

A flow diagram of the CHRONSET manufacturing steps is shown in Figure 8.2. The wall of the vessel and the rate-controlling membrane of the cap are both fabricated by an injection molding process. The vessel is made of water-impermeable ethylene-co-vinyl acetate copolymer (EVA), while the cap is made of proprietary water-permeable blends of polycaprolactone (TONE) and flux enhancers. After mixing, cooling, and pelletizing the blends, two membrane shapes were prepared from the pellets using a cold runner injection-molding machine. Disks were produced for permeability experiments and caps were made for the CHRONSET systems.

The osmotic granulation and barrier layer granulation were prepared on a fluid bed granulator using standard granulation techniques. Using standard tableting procedures and equipment, the osmotic engine was compressed as a bilayer tablet with an osmotic polymer blend on the concave side and an inert barrier layer on the flat side. An osmotic/barrier bilayer tablet was placed firmly inside the CHRONSET cap. The CHRONSET vessel was assembled with a Jr. Tylenol® tablet on top of the ejecting layer tablet inside the EVA vessel.

8.4 MEASUREMENT OF MEMBRANE PERMEABILITY

Membrane permeability was measured using side-by-side diffusion cells made by Crown Glass. Membranes were cut into 1-in. diameter circles. The thickness was measured at the center of the dry membrane. A ring of stopcock grease was placed around the outer wall of the diffusion cell on either side of the tight seal "sandwich." The membrane was clamped firmly into place. The cells were maintained at 37 °C by a water bath. Saturated potassium chloride solution was

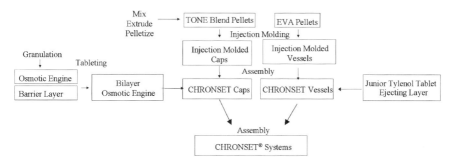

Figure 8.2. Flow diagram for manufacturing CHRONSET systems.

added to the donor reservoir and allowed to equilibrate to 37 °C. A water flow detector was placed into the donor reservoir. Deionized water was added to the receptor reservoir, and the volume of water diffusing from the receptor to the donor reservoir was recorded as a function of time. Stir bars were used to prevent a stagnant boundary layer from forming on either side of the membrane. The slope (dV/dt) of the volume transported through the membrane due to osmotic pressure was used to calculate the permeability (K) according to the equation

$$K = \frac{dV}{dt}\left(\frac{l}{A\Pi}\right) \tag{8.1}$$

where A is the permeation area, Π is the osmotic pressure of saturated KCl, and l is the thickness of the membrane tested. Permeability was expressed in units of $cm^2/h \cdot atm$. Figure 8.3 plots the effects of flux enhancement on the permeability of polycaprolactone membranes.

8.5 MEASUREMENT OF SYSTEM EXPANSION

For the mathematical modeling experiment, injection-molded CHRONSET caps with the composition of TONE/flux enhancers were used. The osmotic engine was composed of NaCl/Na carboxylmethylcellulose and the barrier layer was 50 mg of an inert material. Three osmotic engine weights were tested: 150, 200, and 250 mg. For each osmotic engine weight, three CHRONSET

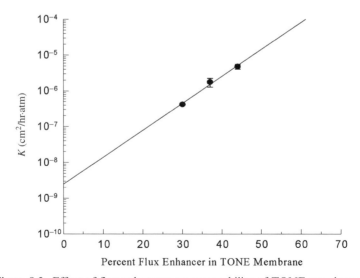

Figure 8.3. Effect of flux enhancers on permeability of TONE membranes.

systems were prepared. After measuring the initial length of the dry CHRON-SET systems, the systems were placed in simulated intestinal fluid (SIF) at 37 °C. At each time point, the expansion of the system was measured by the increase in system length using a pair of digital calipers. Care was taken not to compress or disturb the system during measurement. The actual progression of the osmotic engine and a mathematical model of the progression were compared.

8.6 MATHEMATICAL MODELING OF THE CHRONSET ONSET TIME

Water permeation rate through the injection-molded cap membrane (dV/dt) can be expressed by Eq. 8.2:

$$\frac{dV}{dt} = \frac{KA\Pi}{l} \tag{8.2}$$

where K is the osmotic membrane permeability, A is the permeation area, Π is the osmotic pressure of the osmotic engine, and l is the membrane thickness. Water permeation rate can also be expressed by Eq. 8.3:

$$\frac{dV}{dt} = \frac{d(\pi R_i^2 h)}{dt} = \frac{\pi R_i^2 dh}{dt} \tag{8.3}$$

where R_i is the inner radius of the cap and dh is the increase of the osmotic engine height during operation.

Therefore

$$\frac{dh}{dt} = \frac{KA\Pi}{\pi R_i^2 l} \tag{8.4}$$

Since $(R_o - R_i)/R_i$ is small for the configuration of the osmotic engine cap, the overall permeation area, A, can be reduced to the following simple expression:

$$A = A_d + 2\pi R_i(h_0 + h) \tag{8.5}$$

A_d is the permeation area of the dome part of the cap, which is constant with time; and h_0 and h are, respectively, the initial height of the cylindrical part of the osmotic engine and the increase of the osmotic engine height at time t.

Replacing A in Eq. 8.4 with Eq. 8.5 leads to

$$\frac{dh}{dt} = \frac{K\Pi[A_d + 2\pi R_i(h_0 + h)]}{\pi R_i^2 l} \tag{8.6}$$

Integration of Eq. 8.6 and rearrangement result in

$$\ln\left[\frac{A_d + 2\pi R_i(h_0 + h)}{A_d + 2\pi R_i h_0}\right] = \frac{2K\Pi}{R_i l}t \qquad (8.7)$$

The onset time (t_d) of the system, defined as the time at which the vessel and the cap are disengaged, can be estimated by Eq. 8.8:

$$t_d = \frac{R_i l}{2K\Pi}\ln\left[\frac{A_d + 2\pi R_i(h_0 + h_\infty)}{A_d + 2\pi R_i h_0}\right] \qquad (8.8)$$

where h_∞ is the increase of the osmotic engine height at time infinity, that is, at the time when the drug vessel and the osmotic engine cap are disengaged.

The parameters of this CHRONSET configuration are listed in Table 8.1. These parameters were used for mathematic modeling to evaluate the osmotic pressure of the osmotic engine, to estimate the onset time of the system, and to simulate the impact of the height of the osmotic engine on the onset time.

Figure 8.4 is the plot of $\ln\{[A_d + 2\pi R_i(h_0 + h)]/(A_d + 2\pi R_i h_0)\}$ versus time for various weights of the osmotic engine. The solid line is the regression of all the experimental data. From the slope of this regression line, we estimated the osmotic pressure of the osmotic engine to be 462 atm.

Figure 8.5 displays the onset time of the CHRONSET as a function of the osmotic engine height (h_{osm}). The experimental data agree reasonably well with the data estimated by Eq. 8.8.

Table 8.1. Parameters of CHRONSET Configuration for Mathematic Modeling

Parameter	Symbol	Value[a]
Permeation area of the dome part of the osmotic engine	A_d	0.511 (cm^2)
Height of the dome part of the osmotic engine	h_d	0.229 (cm)
Inner radius of the cap	R_i	0.357 (cm)
Osmotic membrane permeability of TONE/Polyox/ PEG 63/27/10 CHRONSET Caps	K	1.76×10^{-6} (cm^2/h · atm)
Thickness of the injection-molded cap membrane	l	0.0381 (cm)
Initial height of the cylindrical part of the osmotic engine	h_0	$h_0 = h_{osm} - h_c - h_b$

[a] h_{osm} and h_b are the heights of the osmotic engine tablet and the barrier layer (the piston of the osmotic engine), respectively. The length of the osmotic engine cap is 1.156 cm.

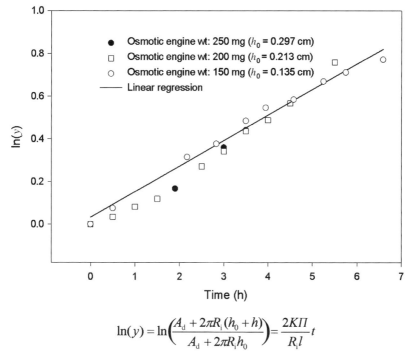

$$\ln(y) = \ln\!\left(\frac{A_d + 2\pi R_i(h_0 + h)}{A_d + 2\pi R_i h_0}\right) = \frac{2K\varPi}{R_i l}t$$

Figure 8.4. Regression of CHRONSET expansion.

8.7   IN VITRO AND IN VIVO FUNCTION

A clinical trial in humans was performed with 12 volunteers using 2-hour and 6-hour CHRONSET systems filled with a Jr. Tylenol tablet. The objective of this study was to evaluate the in vivo function of CHRONSET with different onset times and to find the in vitro and in vivo correlation in terms of its onset time.

The release profiles of these CHRONSET systems were measured in SIF using the United States Pharmacopeia (USP) Type VII method with 15-minute time intervals. The time interval at which the CHRONSET cap disengaged with its body was designated the system onset time. The acetaminophen concentration in SIF was analyzed to determine the release profile of these two CHRONSET systems along with the Jr. Tylenol tablet. Figure 8.6 also shows the in vitro release profiles from the clinical batches in SIF. Within 5 minutes, the Jr. Tylenol tablet was completely dissolved in SIF. The release profile also clearly indicates rapid bolus delivery of acetaminophen for both CHRONSET systems after their respective onsets.

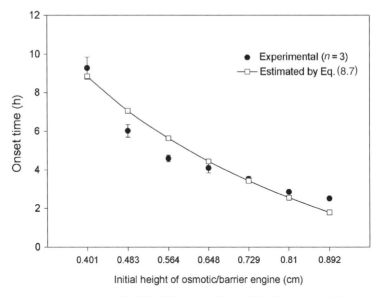

Osmotic engine : NaCl/Na CMC; Barrier: 50 mg with its thickness of 0.122 cm;
The error bars represent the standard deviations of $n = 3$.

Figure 8.5. Onset time of the CHRONSET as a function of the initial osmotic engine height.

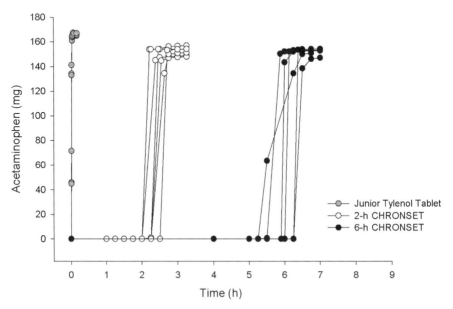

Figure 8.6. In vitro release profiles of IR Jr. Tylenol tablets for 2- and 6-hour CHRONSET systems, $n = 6$.

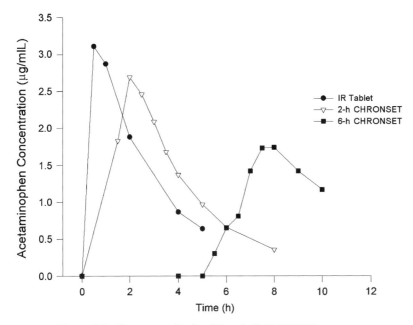

Figure 8.7. Plasma profile for IR and CHRONSET systems.

8.8 CLINICAL RESULTS

Figure 8.7 shows representative plasma profiles for the immediate release Jr. Tylenol tablet, 2-hour CHRONSET, and 6-hour CHRONSET. The bioavailability (BA) of the 2–hour CHRONSET was the same as the immediate release tablet, while the 6-hour CHRONSET had a BA of 84% relative to the immediate release tablet (Table 8.2). The compromised BA can be attributed to either the slow drug absorption in the colon or incomplete delivery of the drug. Incomplete delivery of a drug is a concern for all delayed bolus delivery systems, especially for the long-onset delivery systems, since these systems are unlikely to release their entire payloads at the distal intestine, where the intestinal fluid is lacking. To overcome this obstacle, an ejecting layer was incorporated into the drug vessel of CHRONSET to facilitate the rapid release of the drug tablet. The drug residues measured on the recovered, spent systems were low at $<0.4\%$

Table 8.2. CHRONSET Clinical Results: Average Bioavailability and Residuals

CHRONSET System	BA (%)		Residual (%)	
	2 h	6 h	2 h	6 h
Average	105	84	0.08	0.37
SD	18	21	0.12	0.37
CV	17%	25%	143%	99%

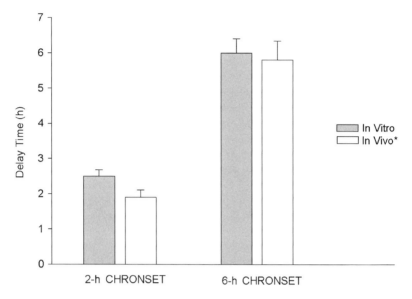

* Based on deconvolution of plasma acetaminophen data

Figure 8.8. In vitro–in vivo correlation of delay times for 2- and 6-hour CHRONSET systems.

(Table 8.2), indicating that the ejecting layer functioned effectively in vivo. Therefore the compromised BA for the 6-hour system can be attributed to the slow absorption of acetaminophen in the colon. As shown in Figure 8.8, the in vivo onset times, estimated by deconvolution of the plasma acetaminophen data, are correlated well with the in vitro data for both the 2- and 6-hour CHRONSET systems. The 2-hour CHRONSET systems are very successful in vivo. The 6-hour CHRONSET systems performed well overall but have an incomplete absorption due to slower acetaminophen absorption in the colon.

8.9 CONCLUSION

CHRONSET, an ALZA proprietary delivery system, is a pulsatile delivery dosage form capable of releasing the drug formulation at a predetermined time for chronotherapy. Clinical study has demonstrated that the system functions well in vivo as designed.

ACKNOWLEDGMENT

Our colleagues at ALZA Corporation are greatly appreciated for their contribution to developing the CHRONSET system.

REFERENCES

1. White WB. A chronotherapeutic approach to the management of hypertension. *Am J Hypertension*. 1996; 9(4 Pt 3): 29S–33S.

2. White WB, et al. Effects of controlled-onset extended-release verapamil on nocturnal blood pressure (dippers Versus nondippers). *Am J Cardiol*. 1997; 80(4): 469–474.

3. Glasser SP. Circadian variations and chronotherapeutic implications for cardiovascular management: a focus on COER verapamil. *Heart Dis*. 1999; 1(4): 226–232.

4. Sica D, Frishman WH, Manowitz N. Pharmacokinetics of propranolol after single and multiple dosing with sustained release propranolol or propranolol CR (Innopran XL), a new chronotherapeutic formulation. *Heart Dis*. 2003; 5(3): 176–181.

5. Claas Steven A, Glasser Stephen P. Long-acting diltiazem HCL for the chronotherapeutic treatment of hypertension and chronic stable angina pectoris. *Expert Opin Pharmacother*. 2005; 6(5): 765–776.

6. Goldenheim PD, Conrad EA, Schein LK. Treatment of asthma by a controlled-release theophylline tablet formulation: a review of the North American experience with nocturnal dosing. *Chronobiol Int*. 1987; 4(3): 397–408.

7. Burioka N, et al. Theophylline chronotherapy of nocturnal asthma using bathyphase of circadian rhythm in peak expiratory flow rate. *Biomed Pharmacother*. 2001; 55(suppl 1): 142S–146S.

8. Middle MV, et al. Double-blind randomized cross-over trial of nocturnal elixir theophylline supplementation of a twice-daily sustained-release theophylline tablet formulation in asthmatic patients. *Chronobiol Int*. 1993; 10(4): 277–289.

9. Levi F, Le Louarn C, Reinberg A. Timing optimizes sustained-release indomethacin treatment of osteoarthritis. *Clin Pharmacol Ther*. 1985; 37(1): 77–84.

10. Reinberg A, Levi F. Clinical chronopharmacology with special reference to NSAIDs. *Scand J Rheumatol Suppl*. 1987; 65, 118–122.

11. Theeuwes F. Elementary osmotic pump. *J Pharm Sci*. 1975; 64, 1987–1991.

12. Swanson DR, et al. Nifedipine gastrointestinal therapeutic system. *Am J Med*. 1987; 83(suppl 6B): 3–9.

13. Wong PSL, Gupta SK, Stewart BE. Osmotically controlled tablets. *Modified-Release Drug Deliv Technol* 2003; 126, 101.

14. Crison JR, et al. Programmable oral release technology, Port System: a novel dosage form for time and site specific oral drug delivery. *Proc Int Symp Control Release Bioact Mater*. 1995; 22, 278–279.

15. McNeill ME, Rashid A. Stevens HNE, inventors. *Dispensing device*. US patent 5,342,624. 1994.

16. Krogel I, Bodmeier R. Evaluation of an enzyme-containing capsular shaped pulsatile drug delivery system. *Pharm Res*. 1999; 16(9): 1424–1429.

17. Ishino R, et al. Design and preparation of pulsatile release tablet as a new oral drug delivery system. *Chem Pharm Bull*. 1992; 40(11): 3036–3041.

18. Niwa K, et al. Preparation and evaluation of a time-controlled release capsule made of ethyl cellulose for colon delivery of drugs. *J Drug Targeting*. 1995; 3(2): 83–89.

19. Peppas Nicholas A, Leobandung W. Stimuli-sensitive hydrogels: ideal carriers for chronobiology and chronotherapy. *J Biomater Sci Polym Ed*. 2004; 15(2): 125–144.

20. Pozzi F, Furlani P, inventors. Programmed release oral solid pharmaceutical dosage form. US patent 5,310,558. 1994.

21. Friend DR, Fedorak RN, inventors; SRI International USA, assigner. Pharmaceutical compositions and methods for colonic delivery of corticosteroids. Patent Application WO9322334. 1993.

22. Fix JA, et al. Chronset oral osmotic system capabilities and applications. Book of Abstracts, 213th ACS National Meeting, San Francisco, April 13–17, 1997: PMSE-233.

23. Dong LC, et al, inventors. Drug delivery device with minimal residual drug retention. US patent 5,902,605. 1999.

24. Wong PSL, et al. inventors. Device for administering active agent to biological environment. US patent 5,312,388. 1995.

CHAPTER 9

CONTROLLED RELEASE MICROCHIPS

KAREN DANIEL, HONG LINH HO DUC, MICHAEL CIMA, and ROBERT LANGER

> "Our brains are seventy-year clocks. The Angel of Life winds them up once for all, then closes the case, and gives the key into the hand of the Angel of the Resurrection."
>
> — *Häfez (1315–1390)*

CONTENTS

9.1 INTRODUCTION

This chapter focuses on two types of microchip drug delivery devices that have been developed: a solid-state silicon microchip (active device) and a resorbable

Chronopharmaceutics: Science and Technology for Biological Rhythm-Guided Therapy and Prevention of Diseases, edited by Bi-Botti C. Youan
Copyright © 2009 John Wiley & Sons, Inc.

polymeric microchip (passive device). These devices contain small reservoirs that are loaded with a drug and separated from the outside environment by a thin membrane (Figure 9.1). The active silicon-based microchip membranes are thin layers of gold. When a drug needs to be released from a reservoir in the active device, a voltage is applied, which causes electrochemical dissolution of the gold anode membrane. The passive polymeric device contains biodegradable polymer membranes. The composition, molecular weight, and thickness of the membrane determine when the drug depot is released from reservoirs in the passive polymeric device. Both the active and the passive microchip have demonstrated in vitro and in vivo pulsatile release of multiple compounds [1–4]. The ultimate goal for the active device is an autonomous device that can either be remotely activated or include sensors to activate the release of drugs when needed. MicroChips, Inc. is currently developing implantable drug delivery and biosensing devices based on technology similar to the active microchip device described in this chapter (go to www.mchips.com for more information).

These microreservoir devices are well suited for applications in chronotherapy due to their ability to achieve repeated pulsatile release of drug depots. Another benefit of these microchip devices, compared to micropumps, is that they contain no moving parts and are capable of delivering drugs in the solid, liquid, or gel state. The microchip design also protects the drug depot from the outside environment before release. This protection might decrease the amount of drug required to see a therapeutic effect or increase the time period over which delivery of active drug can occur.

The first therapeutic application investigated with these microchips was delivery of carmustine, also known as BCNU, a potent anti cancer drug used in chemotherapy. This drug has serious side effects when delivered systemically at the level required for efficacious therapy in the brain. Local drug delivery would therefore be a welcome alternative, to maintain efficacy while decreasing or even eliminating serious side effects. The following sections describe the device fabrication process, results from in vivo biocompatibility studies, and results from in vitro and in vivo release studies using both types of microchip devices, culminating in delivery of BCNU to a 9L glioma rat tumor model. The studies described here could easily be extended to investigate therapeutic delivery of a chronotherapeutic compound. Controlled release microchips are uniquely suited for applications where the timing of delivery is crucial. The delivery of hormones or other molecules that actuate a cascade of subsequent regulatory molecules in the body would allow these devices to replace or augment certain systems in the body that are not functioning properly. Adenohypophyseal hormones such as gonadotropin, growth hormone, and thyrotropin, for example, are important in the reproduction, growth, and regulation of other body systems such as the cardiovascular system.

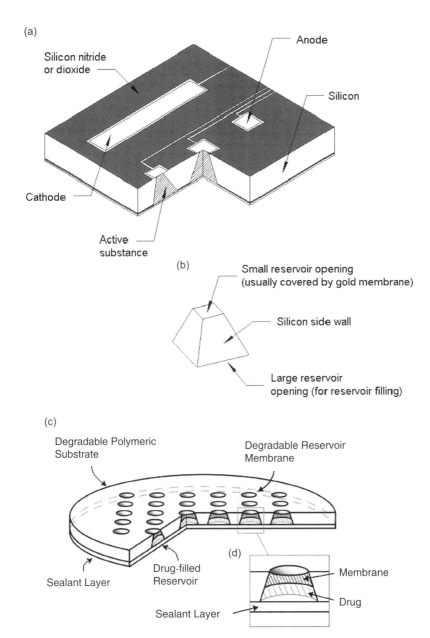

Figure 9.1. Schematic of two types of controlled release microchip devices: (a) active, silicon device, (b) close-up of single reservoir in active device [4], (c) passive, polymeric device, and (d) close-up of single reservoir in passive device [1]. (Parts (a) and (b) reproduced from *Nature* © 1999 and parts (c) and (d) reproduced from *Nature Materials* ©2003, with permission from Nature Publishing Group.)

9.2 ACTIVE SILICON MICROCHIP

9.2.1 Fabrication

The active device is fabricated using standard microfabrication techniques, which have been detailed previously [4]. Arrays of square pyramidal wells (Figure 9.1b) are etched into a silicon wafer using silicon nitride as an etch stop. Each reservoir has a volume of 25 nL and is approximately 50 μm × 50 μm on the small square end. Gold is sputtered onto the wafer surface and etched to form the anodes and cathodes. Gold is an ideal membrane material because it is resistant to spontaneous corrosion in many solutions and has a low reactivity with other substances. It has also been shown to be biocompatible. Portions of the gold circuits that must not be corroded are protected by an adherent, non porous silicon dioxide (SiO_2) coating deposited by plasma-enhanced chemical vapor deposition.

9.2.2 Activation

Gold resists spontaneous corrosion in vivo, but the presence of a small amount of chloride ions creates an electric potential region that favors the formation of soluble gold chloride complexes. Reproducible gold dissolution can be achieved by holding the anode potential in this corrosion region. Potentials above this region cause a passivating gold oxide layer to form, which slows the gold corrosion. Difficulty in holding the anode potential in the corrosion region can be overcome by using a square wave potential that cycles between a passivating potential and a lower potential that removes the passivated layer. Continuous cycling eventually leads to opening of the membrane, which has been observed to be a combination of electrochemical and mechanical failure, due to the difference in density of the gold and its oxide formed at the surface of the membrane.

  A bulge test apparatus was constructed to measure the mechanical integrity of the gold membranes, since capillary forces from the liquid material in a filled membrane can exert a stress on the gold membrane anode. The apparatus was pressurized, and the resulting deflection of the membranes was measured using interferometry. Calculations and subsequent measurements indicate that these capillary forces are three orders of magnitude smaller than that required to rupture a 0.3-μm thick gold membrane, which can withstand pressures up to 60 lb/in.^{2} [5]. Prototype devices have been shown to operate reliably even after being stored for over a year [4].

9.2.3 In Situ Monitoring of Drug Delivery

The ability to monitor the release of drugs in situ is an important part of a drug delivery device. It provides an alternative to the use of radiolabeled compounds to measure the amount of released drug in vivo, since these compounds can partition in different parts of the body and in body fluids. Some of these partition coefficients are known, but are also subject to experimental variation, which can be particularly large in biological systems. An in situ monitoring system would therefore bypass this variation by measuring directly the amount of drug remaining in the device.

The active microchip was modified to include an impedance-based sensor that allows noninvasive, real-time monitoring of drug release [6]. The sensor consists of two gold electrodes, deposited by electron beam evaporation, on opposite sides of the reservoir. The impedance signal between the sensor electrodes changes as the release medium penetrates into the reservoir and the drug dissolves. Figure 9.2 is a schematic of a reservoir with the sensing electrodes and depicts an idealized representation of drug release from a reservoir. An equivalent circuit was formulated to interpret the impedance measurements on reservoirs filled with phosphate-buffered saline solutions of varying concentrations. The sensor was used to monitor in vitro release of mannitol from the active device, and the equivalent circuit model correlated solution resistance and double layer capacitance with the drug release rate. The release rates measured with the impedance sensor were comparable to those measured by radioactivity counting during in vitro release of radiolabeled mannitol (Figure 9.3) [7]. This sensor was shown to work both in vitro and in vivo, as a proof-of-concept, but needs further development to fully integrate it with our current package [6].

9.2.4 Biocompatibility

One of the most important features of any implantable drug delivery device is its biocompatibility. The most intelligent design will not be acceptable if it

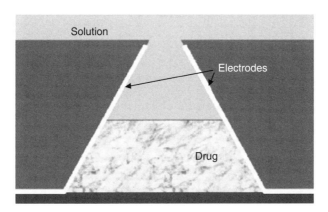

Figure 9.2. Idealized representation of drug release from a reservoir [6]. (Reproduced from *Journal of the Electrochemical Society.* © 2005, with permission from The Electrochemical Society.)

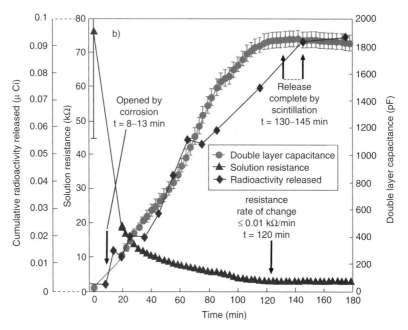

Figure 9.3. Comparison of cumulative radioactivity released with solution resistance and double layer capacitance during in vitro release of ^{14}C-mannitol [7]. (Reproduced with permission from MIT © 2004.)

triggers an adverse reaction in the body because of its materials or function. Biofouling is also a factor in the viability of the device. Biofouling is the adherence of cells onto the device, which can lead to reduced functionality if the device depends on exposed surfaces to function properly. Biocompatibility of the materials and activation process, as well as biofouling of the electrodes, was studied in a series of experiments, which are described next.

Materials The biocompatibility and biofouling of the materials used in our silicon device—metallic gold, silicon nitride, silicon dioxide, and silicon—were evaluated using a cage implant system in a rodent model [8]. Material samples were placed in stainless steel cages and implanted subcutaneously. Inflammatory exudate samples from inside the cage were collected on days 4, 7, 14, and 21 and analyzed to determine leukocyte concentration. The only sample with a significantly higher ($p < 0.05$) leukocyte concentration than the empty cage controls was silicon (days 7 and 14). By day 21, none of the materials had a leukocyte concentration that differed significantly from the empty cage controls. Biofouling was analyzed by calculating the cell density of macrophages or foreign body giant cells (FBGCs) on the surface of each sample. Cages were explanted on days 4, 7, 14, and 21, and the samples were removed and rinsed in a sterile isotonic phosphate buffered saline (PBS) solution. Scanning electron microscopy (SEM) image analysis was used to quantify the surface cell density. The number of macrophages and FBGCs decreased with time for all materials, but at day 21 the surface cell density of the silicon sample was significantly higher than the other three materials tested. These results identify the active device materials (gold, silicon nitride, silicon dioxide, and silicon) as biocompatible, with gold, silicon nitride, and silicon dioxide showing reduced biofouling [8].

Activation and Biofouling   The next step in our biocompatibility study was to investigate the effects of activating our devices in vivo, as well as potential effects of biofouling on device functionality. The first experiment was conducted on macroelectrodes approximately 5000 times larger than the anodes on our device, to investigate the role of the applied voltage and gold electrolysis products in modulating the inflammatory response, and the temporal adhesion of cellular populations onto the electrodes. This experiment was conducted in either stainless steel cages or direct implants against two controls—devices to which voltage was not applied (uncorroded), and inert platinum electrodes to which voltage was applied (electrical controls)—in order to separate the effects of applied voltage and gold electrolysis products [9].

Voltammetry was applied to the directly implanted gold surfaces and the inert platinum electrodes on days 4, 7, 14, 21, 28, 35, 42, and 49 after implantation. Cage-implanted electrodes were activated on days 3, 7, or 13 after implantation. Total leukocyte concentrations were calculated for exudate samples taken at various points before and after activation. The inflammatory response rapidly decreased to control levels 72 hours after voltage was applied with no significant cell concentration difference between the corroded devices and electrical controls. Histological evaluation of the direct implant samples quantified the thickness of the fibrous capsule that formed around the devices. The samples with voltage applied and the uncorroded controls all showed an increase in fibrous capsule thickness until a plateau was reached between 14 and 28 days. The magnitude of the inflammatory response from the uncorroded controls was smaller than from the applied electricity devices. This suggests that the inflammatory response to the corrosion of gold membranes is a combination of the response both to the applied voltage and to the gold decomposition products. Voltammetry analysis of the direct implants showed no change in the gold corrosion peak current with time, which suggests that the fibrous capsule does not interfere with dissolution of the gold membrane [9].

The last step in our biocompatibility studies was to examine the biological effects of repeated electrochemical activation of active devices [10]. Controls were microchips with no applied voltage and microchips with voltage applied on inert platinum electrodes. Devices were implanted subcutaneously both with and without stainless steel mesh cages for 4, 7, 14, 21, or 28 days before activation. They were then activated every other day for five activations. Exudate samples were taken from the cage implanted devices 48 hours after each activation. One direct implant device was removed after each activation for histological evaluation of the fibrous capsule, and the remaining devices were removed and analyzed 3 days after the final activation. Electrochemical data for samples with gold membranes were collected during each activation. Gold devices induced a consistent inflammatory response during the activation phase, with a decrease in the inflammatory response after activation. The platinum controls, however, showed a steady decrease in leukocyte concentration. The inflammatory response seen in the gold devices is probably in response to the gold chloride produced during the activation phase. Activation of the membranes also exposes the inside of the wells, creating new surface area for an inflammatory response. There was no significant difference in the fibrous capsule thickness of activated devices and controls at each time point. The ability to remove the gold membrane through electrochemical activation did not change with time, although some changes in the electrochemical data were observed after long implantation times. The data suggest that repeated activation of MEMS drug delivery devices produces an acceptable biological response that will resolve over a period of 14 days at the most [10].

9.2.5 Release of Model Compounds

In vitro Release Our first proof-of-concept release experiments were to independently release two model compounds, sodium fluorescein and $^{45}Ca^{2+}$ (as $CaCl_2$), from a single microchip device [4]. These model compounds were chosen because they are easily detected using a fluorimeter or liquid scintillation counter (LSC), respectively. Reservoirs were filled with aqueous solutions of the model compounds using a microinjector, which is capable of depositing nanolitre quantities of solutions. The aqueous solutions also contained 15–20% (by volume) liquid polymer (polyethylene glycol (PEG), $MW = 200$) to minimize the drying stress on the membranes. The water quickly evaporated from the reservoirs, and the back of the devices were covered with squares of a thin adhesive plastic and sealed with a water-resistant and solvent-resistant epoxy.

The sealed devices were placed in saline solution for 1 day before activation. Samples of the saline solution were analyzed periodically for fluorescence and radioactivity, to ensure the model compounds were not leaking from the reservoirs. After 1 day, specific reservoirs were opened by applying $+1.04\,V$ with respect to saturated calomel electrode (SCE) to the appropriate anode. Figure 9.4 shows the pulsatile release profile for the two model compounds ($^{45}Ca^{2+}$, open triangles, units of $5 \times nCi/min$; sodium fluorescein, filled circles, units of ng/min). Complete release from the activated reservoirs was achieved after several hours. This proof-of-principle release demonstrates that each reservoir in the active device can be individually controlled, allowing multiple compounds to be released from a single device in a variety of release patterns [4].

In vivo Release The first in vivo releases from our silicon device were demonstrated subcutaneously in female Fisher 344 rats, using fluorescein dye

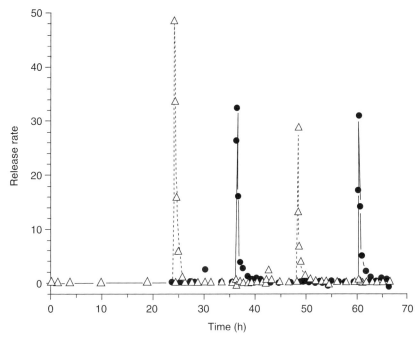

Figure 9.4. Pulsatile release of multiple substances from a single microchip device. The release of $^{45}Ca^{2+}$ ions (Δ; vertical scale in units of $5 \times nCi/min$) and sodium fluorescein (•; in units of ng/min) into 0.145 M NaCl solution over several hours is shown for each reservoir. Samples (1 mL) were taken every several minutes from the release medium, analyzed for radionuclide content in a scintillation counter, and replaced with an equal volume of fresh saline solution [4]. (Reproduced from *Nature* © 1999, with permission from Nature Publishing Group.)

and radiolabeled mannitol [2]. The fabrication and filling process for the active devices used in this in vivo study was described earlier. The spatial profile of fluorescein dye release from the drug delivery device was evaluated by fluorimetry and the temporal profile of ^{14}C-labeled mannitol release was evaluated by LSC.

Devices filled with dye were activated after 72 hours and the dye was allowed to diffuse into the surrounding tissue. The animals were sacrificed 1 hour after activation and tissue from the ipsilateral and contralateral flanks was sectioned and analyzed for fluorescein concentration. Figures 9.5a and 9.5b show a high concentration of fluorescein in the tissue surrounding the activated devices after 1 hour (filled circles). Contralateral tissue samples (open squares) were used as negative controls and showed only background fluorescence. An injected control (Figure 9.5c) and unactivated device control (Figure 9.5d) both served to contrast the results from the activated devices. The lower fluorescein concentration observed for the injected control is probably due to the rapid diffusion of fluorescein out of the tissue and into the systemic

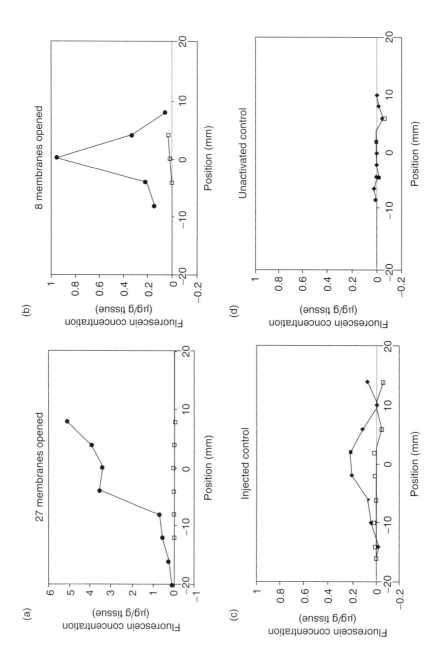

Figure 9.5. The spatial release profiles of fluorescent dye measured using spectroscopy in tissue sections from the ipsilateral (●) and contralateral flank (□) of rats. Animals had activated devices with (a) 27 and (b) 8 opened membranes, or (c) injected dye and (d) an unactivated device. The area under the curve per reservoir emptied was (a) 2.20 and (b) 1.27 μg/g tissue [2]. (Reproduced from *Journal of Controlled Release* © 2004, with permission from Elsevier.)

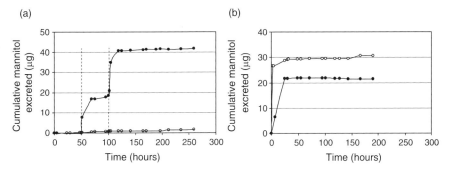

Figure 9.6. Cumulative ^{14}C-mannitol excreted from (a) packaged and (b) unpackaged devices measured by LSC of the urine samples. Packaged devices contained 100 μg mannitol; unpackaged devices contained 67 μg (●) and 74 μg (○), respectively. One device (●) in (a) was activated at 50 and 100 h after implantation (denoted by hatched lines), and the other device (○) acted as an unactivated control [2]. (Reproduced from *Journal of Controlled Release* © 2004, with permission from Elsevier.)

circulation. Within 5 minutes of injection, fluorescein was visibly detectable in the urine of these control animals. Animals with activated devices, however, did not have visible fluorescein in the urine until 1 hour after activation. This in vivo release study demonstrated that the active devices can achieve sustained high local concentrations [2].

Devices filled with ^{14}C-labeled mannitol were activated 50 and 100 hours after implantation. The rats were housed in individual metabolic cages, and urine samples were collected and analyzed for ^{14}C content. Figure 9.6a shows the cumulative mannitol excreted from an animal with an activated device (solid circles, activation times marked with dashed lines) and a negative control animal with an unactivated device (empty circles). Figure 9.6b shows the cumulative mannitol excreted from two animals with unpackaged control devices, where the mannitol was injected into the reservoirs (solid circles = 67 μg, empty circles = 74 μg), but the reservoirs were not sealed on the large square side, and openings were approximately 100 times those on the activated chips. Despite the much larger release area for the unpackaged devices, the release rates from the packaged and unpackaged devices were nearly identical. This indicates that the active device can achieve rapid release of highly soluble compounds [2].

9.2.6 Release of a Therapeutic Compound

In vitro Release Devices filled with ^{14}C-radiolabeled BCNU and PEG at different volume ratios were sealed, packaged, and placed in PBS for in vitro release [3]. Previous in vitro release studies with BCNU had shown slow release kinetics and incomplete release. Varying ratios of PEG were added to the BCNU formulation in an attempt to achieve rapid, complete release of the BCNU payload. The devices in this study were different from earlier devices in that they used a Pyrex package, shown in Figure 9.7. This package allowed an increase in the total capacity of the chip, at the expense of a reduced number of individual reservoirs. The increased total capacity was needed to accommodate the amount of BCNU necessary to be efficacious against a tumor, as determined in previous dose ranging studies. Half of the loaded reservoirs were activated almost immediately, and the rest were activated approximately 120 hours later. Samples of PBS were taken periodically and analyzed for radioactivity to quantify the amount of BCNU released [3].

Figure 9.8 shows the cumulative release of ^{14}C-BCNU from four devices in vitro. The device filled with 100% BCNU (filled diamonds) showed sluggish

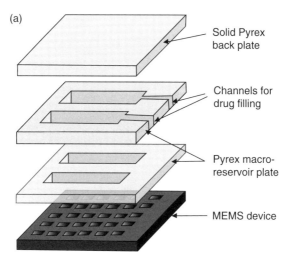

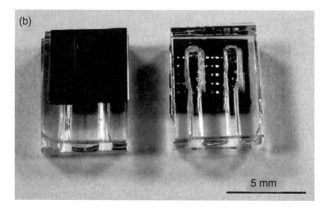

Figure 9.7. (a) Schematic showing the Pyrex package design. (b) Photograph showing the top and bottom of an assembled device [3]. (Reproduced from *Journal of Controlled Release* © 2005, with permission from Elsevier.) (*See color insert.*)

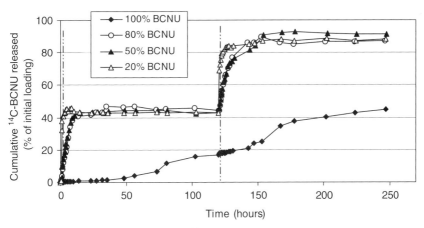

Figure 9.8. Cumulative percentages of ^{14}C-BCNU released from four Pyrex packaged devices. Each activation (denoted by the dashed line) corresponds to opening of 10 membranes with half of the initial loading. Each device was filled with a mixed solution of BCNU/PEG with different BCNU/PEG volume ratios. The BCNU loading was 1.2 mg in each of the three devices (100% BCNU, 80% BCNU, and 50% BCNU) and 0.96 mg in the device with 20% BCNU. Tests were performed at room temperature in PBS [3]. (Reproduced from *Journal of Controlled Release* © 2005, with permission from Elsevier.)

release kinetics and only 40% payload release after 250 hours. Addition of as little as 20% PEG (open circles) significantly enhanced the BCNU release kinetics, and all three devices filled with a BCNU/PEG coformulation showed nearly 100% recovery of the total radioactivity. The device filled with 20% BCNU (open triangles) had the fastest release kinetics, reaching equilibrium after approximately 6 hours. The 50% (filled triangles) and 80% (open circles) BCNU formulations took slightly longer to reach equilibrium ^{14}C levels (15–20). This experiment underlines the importance of formulation as a tool to control drug release kinetics. The start of release is controlled by activation of the device, and the release profile of this drug is easily controlled by adjusting the PEG volume ratio [3].

In vivo Release Radiolabeled BCNU was released from our silicon device after subcutaneous implantation in female Fisher 344 rats [2]. A total of five animals were used in this experiment, two of which were control animals. One control animal received a subcutaneous injection of ^{14}C-BCNU and the other received an unactivated device. Three devices were activated twice, at 24 and 27 hours postimplantation, with half the reservoirs being activated each time. Plasma samples were collected and analyzed for ^{14}C-BCNU by accelerator mass spectrometry (AMS). Figure 9.9 shows release profiles obtained from previous in vitro releases (Figure 9.9a) and the subcutaneous injected control (Figure 9.9b) [2]. Figure 9.10 shows the release profiles from the three activated

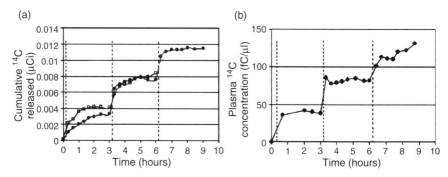

Figure 9.9. (a) Cumulative ^{14}C released from devices activated in vitro in saline. Each activation (denoted by a hatched line) corresponds to the opening of one row of reservoirs. (b) Plasma ^{14}C concentration measured by AMS from a subcutaneous injected control. Each injection (denoted by the hatched line) corresponds to 0.014-μCi loading. Each data point represents means of 3-7 replicate measurements with 25-μL plasma samples [2]. (Reproduced from *Journal of Controlled Release* © 2004, with permission from Elsevier.)

devices (filled circles, activation times marked with dashed lines) and the unactivated control device (open circles). Figure 9.10c shows that the second activation was not successful in opening the reservoirs, due to faulty wiring. The activated devices took slightly longer to reach steady-state BCNU plasma concentrations than the injected and in vitro controls. Note that the devices used in this experiment were not Pyrex packaged, as this experiment was performed before the dose ranging studies, which indicated a need for higher capacity [2].

MicroChips, Inc. recently demonstrated in vivo release of leuprolide, a polypeptide, from a silicon-based device very similar to the one discussed here [11]. Remote control was used to release leuprolide via electrothermal activation from a subcutaneous implant in beagle dogs up to 6 months after implantation. A minimal fibrous capsule formed as expected, but the maximum serum concentration (C_{max}), time to maximal concentration (T_{max}), and area under the pharmacokinetic curve (AUC) were independent of the time since implantation even though a fully formed fibrous capsule is only established weeks after implantation. In addition, T_{max} was comparable to the time for maximum release rate during in vitro testing where no fibrous capsule exists. This work supports the hypothesis that in vivo release of therapeutic agents will not be significantly hindered by the formation of a fibrous capsule [11].

Efficacy Against a Tumor Model The use of the Pyrex package and coformulation of BCNU with polyethylene glycol (PEG) led to complete and rapid BCNU release in vitro and in vivo, as well as increased device capacity. BCNU was thus delivered from our device against a tumor in a rodent model (female Fisher 344 rats), with doses varying between 0.67 and 2 mg [3]. The rats

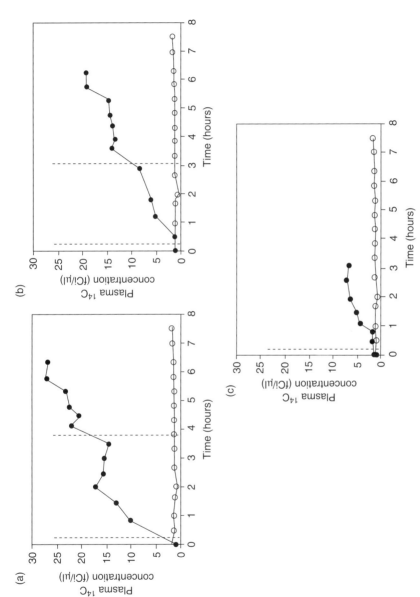

Figure 9.10. Plasma ^{14}C concentration measured by AMS from devices activated in vivo, with two sequential activations in (a) and (b), and one activation in (c). Plasma ^{14}C concentration from an unactivated device is plotted in each graph (○) as control. Each activation (denoted by a hatched line) corresponds to opening of one row of reservoirs with 0.01-μCi loading. Each data point represents the mean of 3–7 replicated measurements with 25-μL plasma samples [2]. (Reproduced from *Journal of Controlled Release* © 2004, with permission from Elsevier.)

were implanted with a 2-mm^3 piece of 9L gliosarcoma tumor from a carrier animal 10 days before device implantation. Eighteen rats received active devices, filled with a 50:50 volume ratio of BCNU and PEG, at the tumor site. The BCNU doses were 0.67, 1.2, or 2 mg (six animals for each dose). Half of the reservoirs were opened 11 days after tumor implantation, and the rest of the reservoirs were opened 5 days later. Thirty animals were used as controls. Eighteen received subcutaneous injections of the 50:50 BCNU/PEG mixture, six received active devices that were filled with 2 mg BCNU but not activated, and six received no treatment. The total dosage of the injected controls was intended to be 0.67, 1.2 or 2 mg (six animals for each dose), but the injections were done manually with a 10-μL syringe and it was difficult to control the total amount injected. The three doses for the injected controls ended up being 1.4, 1.5, and 2 mg. Tumor size was measured three times a week, using calipers to estimate the length, width and height of each tumor. These measurements were used to calculate tumor volume, assuming that the tumor was an ellipsoid [3].

Figure 9.11 shows tumor volume measurements up to 22 days after tumor implantation. The activated devices showed dose-dependent inhibiting effect on the tumor growth. No significant difference in tumor volume was observed between activated devices and injected controls, which suggests that the therapeutic effect of BCNU is not hindered by electrochemical activation of the gold membranes [3]. The ability to locally deliver an efficacious BCNU dose against a tumor, while a significant achievement, is but a stepping stone to the next level. Further optimization using this device to deliver BCNU in combination with other therapeutic agents, such as interleukin-2 (IL-2), against a tumor challenge, is the true goal of this device. This drug combination will

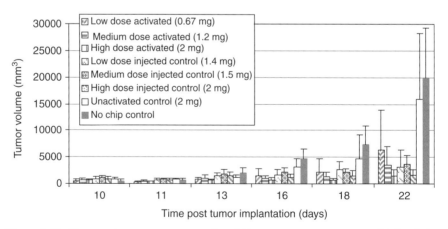

Figure 9.11. Tumor size measurements for different treatment groups. Half of the reservoirs were opened 11 days after tumor implantation and the rest were opened 5 days later. Values represent mean ± SD of measurements from six rats. Numbers in parentheses represent BCNU dosages [3]. (Reproduced from *Journal of Controlled Release* © 2005, with permission from Elsevier.) (*See color insert.*)

take full advantage of the potential of the active device, due to the temporal control that can be exerted on the release of each drug in order to obtain the most potent effect.

9.3 PASSIVE POLYMERIC MICROCHIP

9.3.1 Fabrication

Figure 9.1c is a schematic of the passive microchip device. The substrate of the device is poly(L-lactic acid) (PLLA) and the membranes are 50:50 copolymers of poly(D,L-lactic-*co*-glycolic acid) (PLGA). The substrate is 1.2 cm in diameter, approximately 500 µm thick, and contains 36 truncated conical reservoirs (arranged in a 6 × 6 array). Each reservoir is capped with a 150-µm thick degradable polymer membrane and can hold up to 100 nL of drug. Membrane degradation and drug release in the passive polymer device is based on device design and constituent materials of the membrane and is not externally controlled.

Figure 9.12 depicts the fabrication process for the passive microchip. The process begins with compression-molding of approximately 0.4 g of PLLA powder at room temperature into a preform that is 1.1 cm in diameter. This tablet is placed on an aluminum die with conical protrusions and compression molded at 180 °C. At this stage the reservoirs are conical in shape and protrude partially through the substrate (Figure 9.12b). Then the substrate is polished to remove PLA from the front of the device, turning the reservoirs into truncated cones that completely penetrate the substrate. The substrate is then placed with the large opening of the reservoirs facing up and a 12% solution (v/v) of PLGA in an organic solvent is microinjected into each reservoir to form the polymer membrane. The devices are dried in a vacuum oven at 80 °C for at least 48 hours to remove any residual solvent from the membranes. Finally, the desired drug is microinjected into each reservoir on top of the polymer membrane and the chip is sealed on the back with a pressure sensitive adhesive [1]. Figure 9.13 shows a photograph of a polished passive device (1.2 cm in diameter).

9.3.2 Membrane Degradation

Release of drug from the polymer microchip is controlled by degradation of polymeric timing membranes that cover the reservoir openings (see Figure 9.1d). The polymer degradation times are determined by the thickness and chemical composition of the timing membranes. These characteristics are fixed once the device is fabricated, so drug release cannot be externally controlled after device implantation. Release of the drug payload at the desired time therefore depends on accurate predictions of membrane degradation rates. In vitro and in vivo studies were performed to determine the degradation characteristics of PLGA thin films and these results were compared with in

(a) Compression molding at elevated temperature

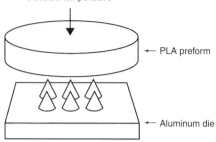

← PLA preform

← Aluminum die

(b) Device with conical reservoirs

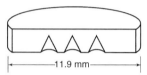

|←————11.9 mm————→|

(c) Cutting and polishing

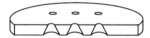

(d) Formation of membranes via microinjection

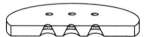

(e) Chemical loading via microinjection

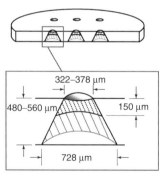

322–378 μm

480–560 μm

150 μm

728 μm

(f) Sealing

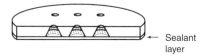

← Sealant layer

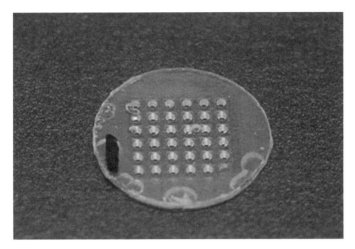

Figure 9.13. Photograph of a polished passive device (1.2 cm in diameter).

vitro membrane swelling and drug release data to better understand the mechanism of membrane degradation.

In vitro Thin Film Degradation Experiments Thin films of 50:50 PLGA copolymers with molecular weights of 4.4, 11, 28, and 64 kDa were solvent cast to a final thickness of 50 or 150 µm. The films were placed in PBS and stored at 25 or 37 °C. Some samples had the media changed periodically while other samples were kept in the same media for the duration of the experiment, to allow local accumulation of acidic degradation products. Samples were removed from the media at different times (up to 49 days), dried, and weighed. Gel-permeation chromatography (GPC) analysis determined the polymer molecular weight of each sample [12].

The thin film degradation experiments confirmed that the polymer degradation rate is determined by the initial molecular weight and thickness of the polymer film and the release media temperature and pH. Films with lower initial molecular weights displayed faster degradation rates. The degradation rate also increased as the film thickness increased, suggesting that acidic degradation products were trapped inside the thicker films but were able to diffuse out of the thinner films. Increased temperature and decreased pH of the

---

Figure 9.12. Fabrication process for the passive microchip device. (a) Compression molding of PLLA tablet on aluminum die, (b) PLLA substrate with conical reservoirs, (c) device substrate after the polishing step, (d) device after injection of polymer membranes, (e) device after injection of drug solution, with a close-up showing typical dimensions of a single reservoir, and (f) sealed device, ready for use in an in vitro or in vivo release study [1]. (Reproduced from *Nature Materials* © 2003, with permission from Nature Publishing Group.)

release media also resulted in an increase in the degradation rate. The decrease in pH was most notable in samples with no media change. In these samples, acidic degradation products, which were released into the media, further catalyzed degradation of the polymer films.

In vivo Thin Film Degradation Experiments Thin films (50–100 μm thick) of poly(glycolic acid) (PGA), PLA, a low molecular weight (LMW) 50:50 PLGA copolymer, and a high molecular weight (HMW) 50:50 PLGA copolymer were solvent cast on Mylar® films. Mylar is known to be biocompatible and was used to increase the mechanical strength of the thin films. Some films were placed in cylindrical stainless steel wire mesh cages, sterilized, and implanted subcutaneously in female Fisher 344 rats. These animals were sacrificed after 21 days and GPC was used to determine the molecular weight of the remaining thin film. Other films were sterilized and directly implanted subcutaneously. These films were explanted after 4, 7, 14, 21, 28, 35, 42, or 49 days. Half the film was removed from the Mylar backing layer and analyzed using GPC to determine the molecular weight. Thin film in vitro controls were submerged in PBS and kept at 37 °C in a humidified atmosphere. These films were dried at the same time that the directly implanted samples were explanted and GPC analysis was used to calculate the film molecular weight. Fibrous capsule thickness on the other half of the explanted sample and total leukocyte concentration (TLC) of the cage sample exudates were analyzed to determine the biocompatibility of the materials (see Section 4) [13].

The in vitro and in vivo degradation rates of the four polymers are ranked as LMW PLGA ≫ PGA > HMW PLGA > PLA. The degradation rate of each polymer seemed to increase slightly in vivo. Local accumulation of acidic degradation products and presence of hydrolytic enzymes are likely the cause of the increased in vivo degradation rates [13, 14].

Membrane Degradation Mechanism The mechanism of drug release from the microchip device was explored by comparing in vitro thin film degradation studies with in vitro release studies [12, 15]. Polymer microchip devices were prepared as described previously and sealed with PLGA membranes (molecular weights of 4.4, 11, 28, or 64 kDa). The predicted membrane thicknesses, based on injected volume, were between 150 and 250 μm. Each device was loaded with a radiolabeled chemical (glucose, glycerol, glycerol phosphate, glycerol trioleate, or dextran) and placed in PBS. These model compounds were chosen for their range of hydrophilic/hydrophobic properties and molecular weights. The release media were sampled periodically and a liquid scintillation counter was used to quantify the amount of radioactivity in the release media at each time point. The maximum height of the membranes of some devices was also measured periodically during the release experiment, and converted to a swollen membrane volume by assuming that the membrane swelled in a spherical section above the device surface. Devices were inspected using optical microscopy to confirm reservoir opening [12, 15]. Figure 9.14 shows pictures of

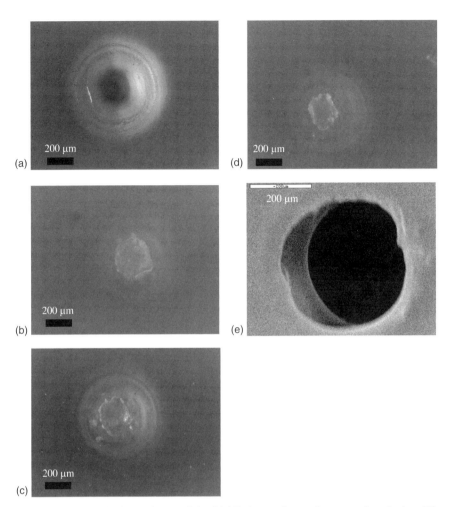

Figure 9.14. Degradation of a PLGA (11 kDa) membrane in a passive device. The membrane was approximately 150 μm thick and the reservoir was loaded with ^{14}C-dextran. The device was placed in PBS and images were taken with an optical microscope on (a) day 0, (b) day 12, (c) day 15, and (d) day 28. (e) SEM of the membrane after 30 days in PBS [16]. (Reproduced with permission from MIT © 2003.)

a PLGA membrane (11 kDa) as it undergoes degradation in PBS. Figures 9.14a to 9.14d are images from optical microscopy 0, 12, 15, and 28 days after being immersed in PBS. Figure 9.14e is an SEM of the reservoir after 30 days in PBS [16].

The thin film degradation and in vitro release experiments suggest that membrane rupture and subsequent release of the drug loaded in the reservoir are correlated with a critical membrane molecular weight of 5–15 kDa. The data did not show a correlation, however, between drug release and the amount of mass remaining in the membrane [12]. PLGA degradation is characterized by water uptake and polymer swelling, both of which increase as degradation progresses. It is likely that membrane rupture occurs when the tensile strength of the membrane can no longer withstand the force exerted on it by the membrane swelling. Chain hydrolysis causes a decrease in the molecular weight, and therefore a decrease in the tensile strength, until a critical molecular weight is reached and the membrane ruptures. The membrane swelling measurements showed a correlation between the observed maximum membrane swelling and model compound release. The maximum membrane swelling and drug release was relatively independent, however, of the compound chemistry and molecular weight [15].

9.3.3 Biocompatibility

One of the most important features of any implantable drug delivery device is its biocompatibility. Section 9.3.2 describes the materials and methods for an in vivo thin film degradation experiment. Samples from this study (PGA, PLA, LMW PLGA, and HMW PLGA films cast on Mylar) were also analyzed for fibrous capsule formation and total leukocyte concentration, which are measures of in vivo inflammatory response. Histological analysis was used to determine the thickness of the fibrous capsule formed around the directly implanted polymer thin films, compared to the fibrous capsule formed around control Mylar films. Several empty control cages were also sterilized and implanted as controls for the TLC exudates analysis [13].

All four of the polymer materials showed acceptable biocompatibility. Figure 9.15 shows a general TLC trend of amplified inflammatory response (compared to empty cage controls) for the faster degrading polymers at early time points and for the slower degrading polymers at later time points. The increased inflammatory response could be due to accumulation of acidic degradation products, which would be expected to peak earlier for the fast degrading polymers (LMW PLGA and PGA) and later for the slow degrading polymers (HMW PLGA and PLA). Figure 9.16 shows that the fibrous capsule thickness of the faster degrading polymers peaked around day 21 and then slowly decreased to the Mylar control value. The slower degrading polymers, however, show a steady, gradual increase in fibrous capsule thickness over the 49-day time period. These trends can also be explained by accumulation of acidic degradation products. The slower degrading polymers continue to release acidic degradation products over the 49 day period, which delays resolution of the fibrous capsule into a thinner, mature fibrous capsule consisting mostly of dense collagen [13].

9.3.4 Release of Model Compounds

Proof-of-principle in vitro release studies have shown release of radiolabeled dextran, heparin, human growth hormone (hGH), iodoantipyrine, glucose,

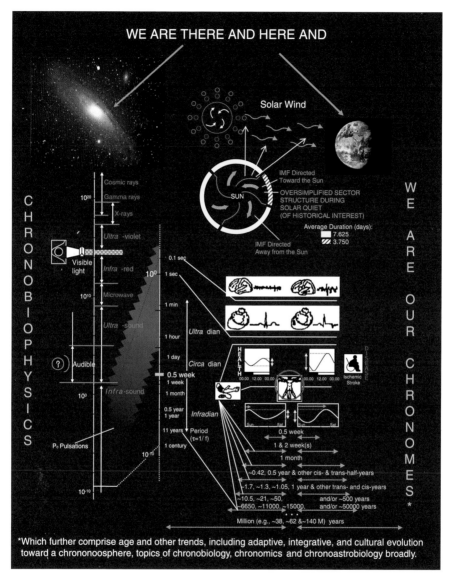

Figure 4 (Introduction). Chronoastrobiology strives to elucidate the past and present integration of organisms into their largely wavy environment. Reciprocal periods in the chronomes of variables in us and around us came about by the eventual genetic coding of the latter in the former. Internal–external interactions await further exploration in health care, notably for stroke prevention in individuals and for the prevention of war, crime, and other diseases of societies and nations.

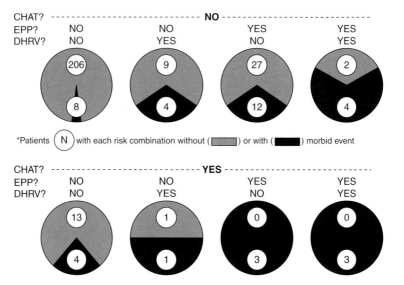

Decreased Heart Rate Variability (DHRV), Circadian Hyper Amplitude Tension (CHAT) and Elevated Pulse Pressure (EPP) are Separate Cardiovascular Disease Risks*

CHAT?	----------------------------	**NO**	----------------------------
EPP?	NO	NO	YES	YES
DHRV?	NO	YES	NO	YES

206 / 8   9 / 4   27 / 12   2 / 4

*Patients (N) with each risk combination without (▦) or with (▰) morbid event

CHAT?	----------------------------	**YES**	----------------------------
EPP?	NO	NO	YES	YES
DHRV?	NO	YES	NO	YES

13 / 4   1 / 1   0 / 3   0 / 3

*Results from 6-year prospective study on 297 (adding all N's) patients classified by 3 risks (8 circles), supported by findings on total of 2,807 subjects for total of over 160,769 sets of blood pressure and heart rate measurements.   Data from K Otsuka.

Figure 6 (Introduction). Abnormalities in the variability of blood pressure and heart rate, impossible to find in a conventional office visit (the latter aiming at the fiction of a "true" blood pressure), can raise cardiovascular disease risk in the next 6 years from <4% to 100%. As compared to an acceptable variability, the relative vascular disease risk associated with a circadian hyperamplitude tension (CHAT), a decreased circadian heart rate variability (DHRV), and/or an around-the-clock elevated pulse pressure (EPP) is greatly and statistically significantly increased. These silent risks are very great, even in the absence of hypertension. They can often be reversed, notably the risk of CHAT, by a nondrug (relaxation) or drug (specified in timing as well as in kind and dose) approach; and the need for intervention can be found when it occurs by the combination of a closed-loop diagnostic and therapeutic system for chrono-theranostics [28]. (See Chapter 11 in this volume.)

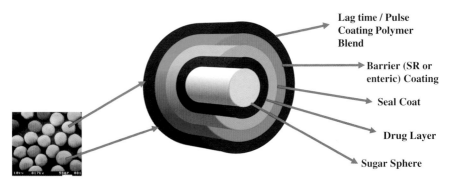

Lag time / Pulse Coating Polymer Blend

Barrier (SR or enteric) Coating

Seal Coat

Drug Layer

Sugar Sphere

Figure 5.1. Scanning electron micrographs and schematic of Diffucaps beads.

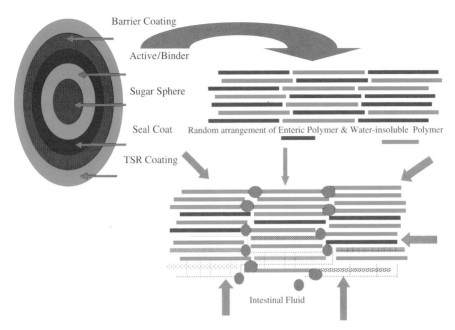

Figure 5.4. Mechanism of drug release from Diffucaps-based TPR beads.

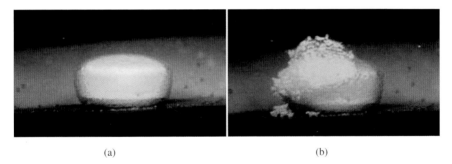

(a)   (b)

Figure 6.3. Morphological changes undergone by the release-controlling HPMC coating in aqueous medium: (a) formation of a gel layer and (b) disruption of said layer along with disintegration of the tablet core.

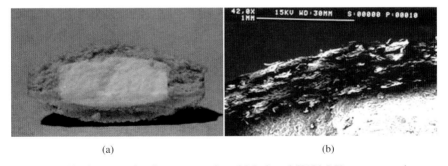

(a)   (b)

Figure 6.4. (a) Photograph of a cross-sectioned Methocel K100 LV press-coated system and (b) SEM photomicrograph (magnification 42.0X) of a coating detail.

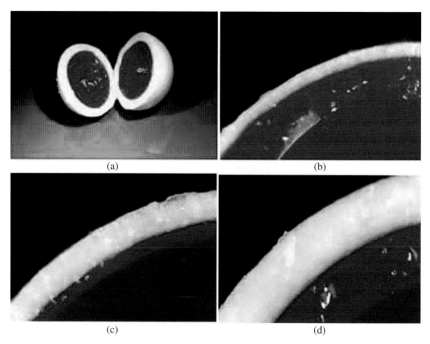

Figure 6.13. (a) Cross-sectioned Methocel E50-coated system based on soft-gelatin capsule (size 2 round C) core and (b–d) details of coatings with increasing thickness.

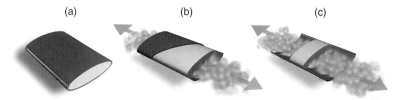

Figure 7.1. Egalet constant release (2K): (a) intact unit, (b) onset or erosion, and (c) further erosion showing the unit retaining the surface area for erosion.

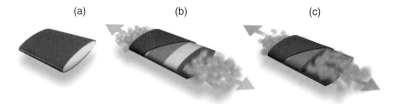

Figure 7.2. Delayed release (3K) form of Egalet: (a) intact unit (b) erosion of the time-delay inert plugs, and (c) drug release.

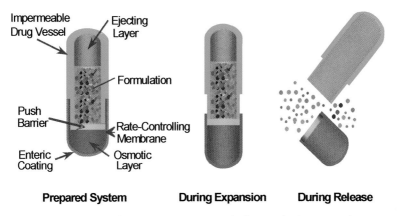

Impermeable Drug Vessel
Ejecting Layer
Formulation
Push Barrier
Rate-Controlling Membrane
Enteric Coating
Osmotic Layer

Prepared System   **During Expansion**   **During Release**

Figure 8.1. Cross section of CHRONSET system before and after operation.

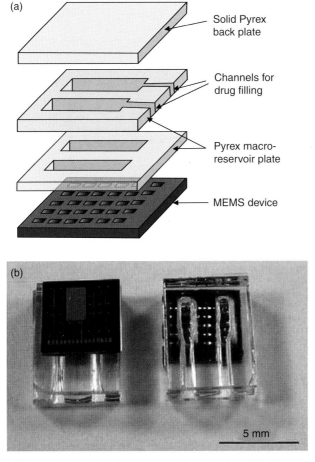

(a)

Solid Pyrex back plate

Channels for drug filling

Pyrex macro-reservoir plate

MEMS device

(b)

5 mm

Figure 9.7. (a) Schematic showing the Pyrex package design. (b) Photograph showing the top and bottom of an assembled device [3]. (Reproduced from *Journal of Controlled Release* © 2005, with permission from Elsevier.)

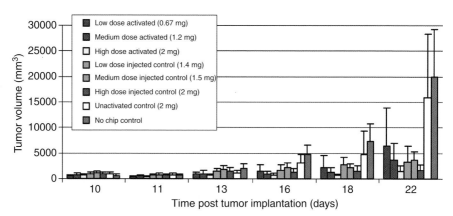

Figure 9.11. Tumor size measurements for different treatment groups. Half of the reservoirs were opened 11 days after tumor implantation and the rest were opened 5 days later. Values represent mean ± SD of measurements from six rats. Numbers in parentheses represent BCNU dosages [3]. (Reproduced from *Journal of Controlled Release* © 2005, with permission from Elsevier.)

Calorie-restricted meal offered evenings only slightly advances phase (no antiphase versus controls, as seen with morning meals), lowers MESOR and amplifies circadian eosinophil rhythm in C₃H mice with high breast cancer incidence that can be reduced by calorie restriction (CR)

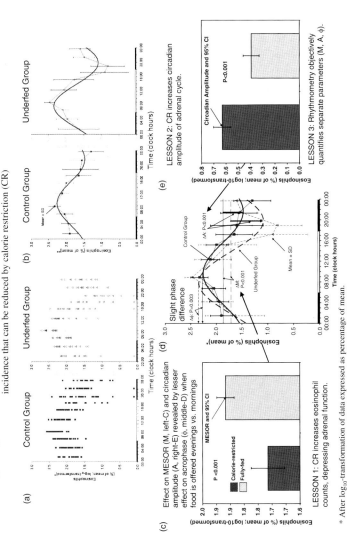

Figure 10.1. Effect of food restriction on circulating eosinophil counts in mice. Follow-up study on Figure 3 in the Introduction to this book, with a phase difference greatly reduced by offering the restricted diet in the evening. (a) Even after $\log_{10}$-transformation of the data expressed as percentage of mean, great interindividual variability is apparent in the raw data. (b) Plots of timepoint mean for mice in each group reveal different circadian patterns. (c–e) Parameter tests quantify differences, indicating that calorie restriction is associated with a lower MESOR (c,d), a larger circadian amplitude (d,e), and only a slight difference in acrophase (d). The difference in acrophase in this study, where calorie-restricted mice were fed in the evening, is much smaller than the almost antiphase observed in prior studies (Figure 3 in the Introduction to this book), where calorie-restricted mice were fed in the morning [1].

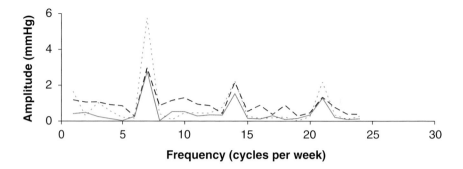

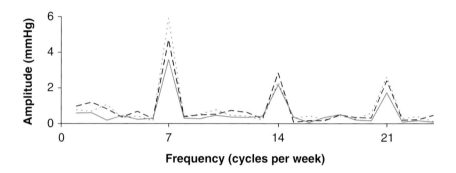

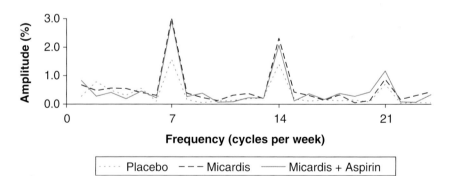

Placebo   ─ ─ ─ Micardis   ─── Micardis + Aspirin

Figure 10.10. Least squares spectra of blood pressure and ejection fraction reveal peaks at frequencies of 7, 14, and 21 cycles per week, corresponding to periods of 24, 12, and 8 hours. Results reflect drug-induced changes in the prominence of the circadian component. The presence of harmonic terms (with periods of 12 and 8 hours) indicates that the circadian waveform differs from sinusoidality. Note that the circadian rhythm of blood pressure has a reduced circadian amplitude on treatment with Micardis, alone or with low-dose aspirin, as compared with placebo. Micardis affected the circadian BP amplitude, being associated with a decrease of 2.1 ± 0.3 mm Hg ($t = 7.138$; $P < 0.001$) in the case of SBP and of 1.3 ± 0.3 mm Hg ($t = 4.224$; $P < 0.001$) in the case of DBP. Micardis was also associated with an increase in the circadian amplitude of EF by $0.57 \pm 0.16\%$ ($t = 3.593$; $P < 0.001$). (From Ref. 77.)

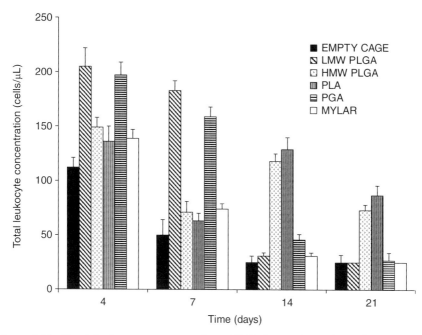

Figure 9.15. Total leukocyte concentration (TLC) in exudates from four polymer samples implanted subcutaneously in wire cages in rats and two controls (Mylar film and empty cage) [13]. (Reproduced from *Journal of Biomaterials Science – Polymer Edition* © 2004, with permission from VSP Publishers.)

glycerol, glycerol 3-phosphate, and glycerol trioleate from the polymer microchip [1, 12, 15, 16]. The purpose of these initial in vitro studies was to first demonstrate release of multiple pulses of a single compound, and then multiple pulses of multiple compounds from a single device. Preliminary in vivo studies released radiolabeled mannitol from polymer microchips implanted subcutaneously in rat flanks [16].

In vitro Release of Multiple Compounds   In vitro release studies have shown release of two compounds (dextran and heparin) from a single polymer microchip device [1]. The devices were fabricated as described in Section 9.3.1. Each device contained four reservoirs that were sealed with different molecular weight PLGA membranes (4.4, 11, 28, or 64-kDa) and loaded with drug. ^{14}C-dextran (70 kDa) was loaded in reservoirs with 11- or 64-kDa PLGA membranes and ^{3}H-heparin was loaded in reservoirs with 4.4- or 28-kDa PLGA membranes. The devices were sealed on the backside with a pressure sensitive adhesive, placed in PBS, and stored at 28–33 °C. Aliquots of PBS were removed periodically and the amount of each radioisotope was quantified using a liquid scintillation counter [1].

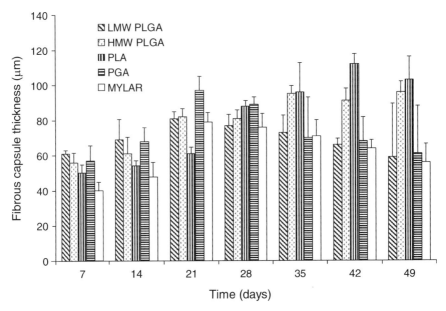

Figure 9.16. Fibrous capsule thickness of four polymer thin films directly implanted subcutaneously in rats and one control Mylar film [13]. (Reproduced from *Journal of Biomaterials Science – Polymer Edition* © 2004, with permission from VSP Publishers.)

Figure 9.17 shows the release profile for a representative device in this proof-of-principle study. This figure shows four distinct pulses of drug corresponding to the degradation of the four different molecular weight PLGA membranes. Burst release of dextran occurred on days 1 and 32, from the 4.4- and 28-kDa PLGA membranes, respectively. Burst release of heparin occurred on days 15 and 37, from the 11- and 64-kDa PLGA membranes, respectively. These results demonstrate that the passive microchip can achieve controlled pulsatile release of multiple chemicals simply by controlling the membrane characteristics (molecular weight, composition, and thickness) [1].

In vivo Release   Proof-of-principle in vivo release studies with radiolabeled mannitol were performed in a rodent model [1]. Each device contained two reservoirs filled with 0.1 μCi of ^{14}C-mannitol and capped with a membrane that was approximately 325 μm thick. One reservoir had an 11-kDa PLGA membrane and the other reservoir had a 64-kDa PLGA membrane. Female Fischer 344 rats were used as the animal model for this initial in vivo release study. After fabrication, drug loading, and sealing, the devices were gamma irradiated and surgically implanted subcutaneously in the rat flank. Control animals received a subcutaneous injection of 0.1 μCi ^{14}C-mannitol. The rats were kept in individual metabolic cages for the duration of the release study and urine and feces collections were analyzed periodically for radioactivity [1].

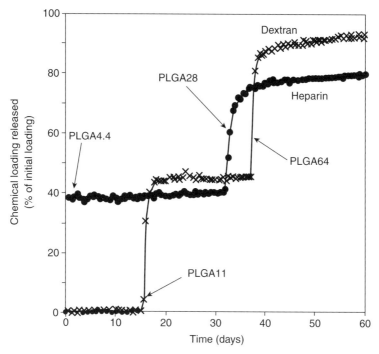

Figure 9.17. In vitro pulsatile release of multiple compounds (dextran and heparin) from a single passive microchip device [1]. (Reproduced from *Nature Materials* © 2003, with permission from Nature Publishing Group.)

Figure 9.18 shows cumulative ^{14}C-mannitol recovered in the rat excretions, compared to the initial loading [1]. This in vivo release profile shows release from the reservoir with the 11-kDa PLGA membrane between days 2 and 4 (compared to release on day 15 in vitro), and release from the reservoir with the 64-kDa membrane around day 5 (compared to release on day 37 in vitro). This significant increase in PLGA degradation rates in vivo is most likely due to higher temperatures (37 °C in vivo compared to 28–33 °C in vitro), local accumulation of acidic degradation products, and presence of hydrolytic enzymes [1, 13, 14]. The cumulative amount of radioactivity recovered from a control animal (subcutaneous bolus injection) is also included in Figure 9.18. The cumulative amount of radioactive recovered from the control (75%) is significantly higher than from the device (32%). This difference can be explained by differences in drug form and diffusion area. The liquid injection (0.3 mL) forms a subcutaneous bolus with a large surface area for diffusion of the mannitol. The devices are loaded with solid mannitol, which must dissolve and then diffuse out of the reservoir opening (approximately 250-μm diameter) [16].

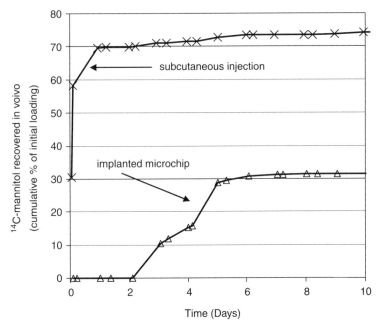

Figure 9.18. In vivo release of ^{14}C-mannitol from the passive microchip (containing 11- and 64-kDa PLGA membranes) compared to an injected control [1]. (Reproduced from *Nature Materials* © 2003, with permission from Nature Publishing Group.)

9.3.5 Release of a Therapeutic Compound

In vitro release of BCNU, a small, hydrophobic chemotherapy drug, has been demonstrated with the passive microchip [16]. Devices were prepared as described earlier and the reservoirs capped with 4.4-, 11-, 28-, or 64-kDa PLGA membranes. The devices were loaded with ^{14}C-BCNU, sealed with a pressure sensitive adhesive, and placed in PBS at 37 °C. Samples of PBS were removed periodically and analyzed on a liquid scintillation counter for radio-activity. Figure 9.19 shows the release profile for four different passive microchip devices. The BCNU release profile is characterized by an immediate, steady release of BCNU from all the devices, not the burst release observed during previous in vitro release studies with model compounds. Accelerated membrane swelling is also observed in reservoirs loaded with BCNU, compared to reservoirs loaded with 70-kDa dextran. This suggests that the release of BCNU is governed by diffusion of the molecule into the membrane, which could also lead to increased water uptake and accelerated membrane swelling [16].

Separation of the polymer membrane and the BCNU drug depot with a barrier layer may be able to achieve a burst release of BCNU from the passive device. The ideal barrier layer material will be biodegradable, nontoxic, and biocompatible. The barrier layer must also be able to make a conformal coating

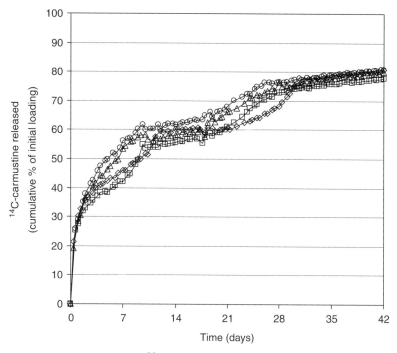

Figure 9.19. In vitro release of ^{14}C-BCNU from the passive microchip device [16]. (Reproduced with permission from MIT © 2003).

on the inside surface of the polymer membrane, be able to withstand the microinjection and drying of a drug solution on top of it, and have low diffusion/partition coefficients for BCNU. In vitro release studies with various organic barrier layer materials are currently in progress. In vivo BCNU dose ranging studies and efficacy studies against a 9L glioma animal tumor model are also currently in progress with the passive microchip.

9.4 CONCLUSION

In vitro and in vivo release studies have demonstrated repeated pulsatile release of multiple compounds from active or passive microchip devices. The active device has also demonstrated efficacy against a 9L glioma rat tumor model. The materials of construction and the operation of the devices have been shown to be biocompatible. Advancement of these microchip devices to clinical use in chronotherapy (e.g., delivery of gonadotropin, growth hormone, or thyrotropin) will require several further major preclinical developments and studies.

One issue that will require further investigation is the effect of fibrous capsule formation on drug release kinetics in a chronotherapy application.

Formation of a minimal fibrous capsule around the drug delivery device had no measurable effect on leuprolide release kinetics or bioavailability up to 6 months after implantation in beagle dogs [11]. Further testing will need to be done to see if the fibrous capsule becomes an issue when the desired dosing regimen is repeated release on a daily basis. Characterization of the transport properties of the fibrous capsule and knowledge of methods for modulating the inflammatory response will aid in proper dosing strategies. Knowledge of the rate at which substances are transported through the fibrous capsule to their therapeutic target, as well as any degradation that occurs during transport, will also aid in interpreting the pharmacokinetics of the substances.

An issue specific to the passive device is precise control over membrane degradation rates to allow release at nearly any time after implantation. The four PLGA copolymers (4.4, 11, 28, and 64 kDa) used in previous in vitro release studies result in burst release on approximately days 1, 15, 32, and 37, respectively. Biodegradable membranes capable of releasing drugs on the days between these four PLGA copolymer burst days will need to be developed and characterized. Current understanding of the PLGA copolymer membrane degradation allows prediction of release times within 1–2 days. This predictive time frame will need to be narrowed significantly to allow the passive microchip to reliably deliver compounds on a daily basis.

REFERENCES

1. Grayson ACR, Choi IS, Tyler BM, Wang PP, Brem H, Cima MJ, Langer R. Multi-pulse drug delivery from a resorbable polymeric microchip device. *Nat Mater*. 2003; 2: 767–772.

2. Li Y, Shawgo RS, Tyler B, Henderson PT, Vogel JS, Rosenberg A, Storm PB, Langer R, Brem H, Cima MJ. In vivo release from a drug delivery MEMS device. *J Control Release*. 2004; 100: 211–219.

3. Li Y, Ho Duc HL, Tyler B, Williams T, Tupper M, Langer R, Brem H, Cima MJ. In vivo delivery of BCNU from a MEMS device to a tumor model. *J Control Release*. 2005; 106: 138–145.

4. Santini JT Jr, Cima MJ, Langer R. A controlled-release microchip. *Nature*. 1999; 397: 335–338.

5. Li Y Cima MJ. Bulge test on free-standing gold thin films. In: Corcoran SG, Joo Y, Moody NR, Suo, Z, (ed.), *Thin Films—Stresses and Mechanical Properties*. X. *Proceedings of the Fall 2003 Materials Research Society Symposium; Materials Research Society*; 2003; 795:U10.3.1–U10.3-6.

6. Johnson AM, Sadoway DR, Cima MJ, Langer R. Design and testing of an impedance-based sensor for monitoring drug delivery. *J Electrochem Soc*. 2005; 152: H6–H11.

7. Johnson AM. Noninvasive quantification of drug delivery from an implantable mems device [dissertation]. Cambridge, MA: Massachusetts Institute of Technology; 2004. Available at: http://hdl.handle.net/1721.1/28765.

8. Voskerician G, Shive MS, Shawgo RS, von Recum J, Anderson JM, Cima MJ, Langer R. Biocompatibility and biofouling of MEMS drug delivery devices. *Biomaterials.* 2003; 24: 1959–1967.

9. Voskerician G, Shawgo RS, Hiltner PA, Anderson JM, Cima MJ, Langer R. In vivo inflammatory and wound healing effects of gold electrode voltammetry for MEMS micro-reservoir drug delivery device. *IEEE Trans Biomed Eng.* 2004; 51: 627–635.

10. Shawgo RS, Voskerician G, Ho Duc HL, Li Y, Lynn A, MacEwan M, Langer R, Anderson JM, Cima MJ. Repeated in vivo electrochemical activation and the biological effects of microelectromechanical systems drug delivery device. *J Biomed Mater Res Part A.* 2004; 71A: 559–568.

11. Prescott JH, Lipka S, Baldwin S, Sheppard NF Jr, Maloney JM, Coppeta J, Yomtov B, Staples MA, Santini JT Jr. Chronic, programmed polypeptide delivery from an implanted, multireservoir microchip device. *Nature Biotech.* 2006; 24: 437–438.

12. Grayson ACR, Cima MJ, Langer R. Size and temperature effects on poly(lactic-*co*-glycolic acid) degradation and microreservoir device performance. *Biomaterials.* 2005; 26: 2137–2145.

13. Grayson ACR, Voskerician G, Lynn A, Anderson JM, Cima MJ, Langer R. Differential degradation rate in vivo and in vitro of biocompatible poly(lactic acid) and poly(glycolic acid) homo- and co-polymers for a polymeric drug-delivery microchip. *J Biomater Sci Polym Ed.* 2004; 15: 1281–1304.

14. Lu L, Peter SJ, Lyman MD, Lai H, Leite SM, Tamada JA, Uyama S, Vacanti JP, Langer R, Mikos AG. *In vitro* and *in vivo* degradation of porous poly(DL-lactic-*co*-glycolic acid) foams. *Biomaterials.* 2000; 21: 1837–1845.

15. Grayson ACR, Cima MJ, Langer R. Molecular release from a polymeric micro-reservoir device: influence of chemistry, polymer swelling, and loading on device performance. *J Biomed Mater Res Part A.* 2004; 69A: 502–512.

16. Grayson ACR. A resorbable polymeric microreservoir device for controlled drug delivery [dissertation]. Cambridge, MA: Massachusetts Institute of Technology; 2003. Available at: http://hdl.handle.net/1721.1/17036.

CHAPTER 10

IMPLICATIONS AND APPLICATIONS OF CIRCADIAN SUSCEPTIBILITY RHYTHMS: CHRONOMICS AND ANESTHESIA*

FRANZ HALBERG, GERMAINE CORNÉLISSEN, and OTHILD SCHWARTZKOPFF

"The only reason for time is so that everything doesn't happen at once... Make everything as simple as possible, but no simpler."

— *Albert Einstein (1879–1955)*

CONTENTS

*Dedicated to the memory of James H. Matthews and Egon Marte, late associate and assistant professors of anesthesiology at the University of Minnesota, who in the early 1960s visualized a then-budding chronoanesthesiology. We trust they would have welcomed not only the now-feasible ambulatory preoperative monitoring of the blood pressure and heart rate variabilities but in particular their chronomic interpretation before administering anesthesia, rather than relying on a single spotcheck measurement that obviously cannot gauge the time structures involved. Chronomics detects vascular disease risks greater than that of hypertension, even in the presence of an average blood pressure that is neither too high nor too low.

Chronopharmaceutics: Science and Technology for Biological Rhythm-Guided Therapy and Prevention of Diseases, edited by Bi-Botti C. Youan
Copyright © 2009 John Wiley & Sons, Inc.

10.1 INTRODUCTION

In any anesthesiologic or other biomedical investigation, familiarity with chronomes (i.e., time structures in and around us) constitutes an often indispensable aspect of control information. This is best documented for about 24-hour or circadian and about-calendar-yearly or circannual rhythms, that is, photic genetic adaptations to the well-seen changes from day to night and with the seasons. Information also accumulates in living matter, in our circulation, in hormones, and at the cellular level about unseen nonphotic signatures of the Earth, the solar wind, and/or more distant influences. Beyond accounting for rhythms, if blunders are to be avoided, the use of information on circadian rhythms has proved its merit in timing certain treatments in research and in practice. Still more important for anesthesiology could be the preoperative detection and treatment of an elevated cardiovascular disease risk by a chronomic (time-structural) interpretation of monitoring pre- and postoperative care.

10.2 AVOIDING BLUNDERS

By ignoring any rules of variation within the so-called normal range, concepts such as the constancy of the natural environment or homeostasis draw a curtain of ignorance over everyday physiology. Two circadian or any other rhythms with the same frequency may happen to be out of phase, or two rhythms may differ in frequency. When these facts are not recognized, blunders of interpretation are unavoidable (Figure 10.1) (see also Figure 3 in the Introduction to this book) [1]. By estimating parameters of the underlying rhythms (Figures 10.2–10.5 (see also Figure 2 in the Introduction to this book), blunders can be prevented and reliable information can be obtained. The solution of puzzles in Minnesota illustrated in Figures 10.1 and 10.2 (and Figure 3 in the Introduction to this book) led us to chronobiology, as a sine qua non to avoid three different, including opposite conclusions drawn from a comparison of the same two concomitantly sampled groups, only because they were compared, in replications, inadvertently at different, then-convenient clock hours. Unrecognized differences in frequency (Figures 10.2 and 10.3) can also play havoc, yielding faulty interpretations until resolved. By contrast, when the rhythms are recognized, a set of new rules (nomos) of behavior in time (chronos) emerges as chronomics (see Figure 2 in the Introduction to this book) [1].

10.3 OVERVIEW

The caveat in Figures 10.1–10.5 also applies to largely ignored or unknown nonphotics such as cycles with periods, τ, among others, of a near-transyear $(1.00 \, yr < [\tau - CI, \text{ where } CI = 95\% \text{ confidence interval}] < [\tau + CI] < 1.2 \, yr)$, longer than a year by weeks and/or of a far-transyear $(1.200 \, yr \leq [\tau - CI] < [\tau + CI] < 1.9 \, yr)$. Biological transyears [2–5] are signatures of ionized particles streaming past satellites, dubbed the solar wind [6].

Transyears in blood pressure as yet are basic science, but an influence of hypotensive drugs upon them is already documented [7]; their importance is suggested by far-transyear τ values in the incidence pattern of sudden cardiac death, at least in certain geographic locations [2, 8, 9], found after cardiac arrest associated with myocardial infarctions was separated from sudden cardiac death that constitute electrical accidents of the heart—by ICD10 (International Classification of Diseases, 10th revision), code I46.1. It is also demonstrated that environmental spectral components with a τ of 6 months, corresponding to geomagnetism [10, 11], and with a τ shorter than a half-year, a cis-half-year of about 0.42 year, first described in hard solar flares detected by γ-radiometry via satellite [12], have signatures in biology, including sudden cardiac death [8], while they also modulate the circadian rhythms of human systolic blood pressure [13].

The recognition that the circadians in particular, the past main focus from the viewpoint of therapy, can differ in phase or frequency among individuals requires a chronotherapy dependent on marker rhythms. The literature focusing on timing only by clock hour is beyond our scope whenever marker rhythmometry is applicable. This review of transdisciplinary findings on susceptibility rhythms and the disciplines to which they led, chronobiology, the study of mechanisms underlying biological rhythms, and chronomics, the mapping of aligned chronomes (time structures) in and around us, is limited mainly to Minnesota studies; these preceded and were beyond the scope of a recent review of timing in anesthesiology [14] and of time of day effects, reported in the incidence of anesthetic adverse events [15].

After a historical introduction to susceptibility rhythms, including data on halothane (fluothane), we turn to methods for testing in the laboratory and assessing and displaying parameters of rhythms and of uncertainties such as CIs by the cosinor method [16, 17]. The dramatically changing susceptibility of the central nervous system as a function of circadian time to agents such as ethanol, under conditions of continuous darkness [18], among others [1], led to the recognition that circadians in susceptibility are partly built-in. They can be synchronized in humans by their social routine and in the laboratory by manipulating lighting and feeding, while magnetic storms can override other effects in the species examined thus far, that is, rabbits [19], rats [20, 21], and humans [22–24]. We conclude with clinical trials and putative chronomic clinical applications for monitoring high cardiovascular risk states in the hands of anesthesiologists.

Without duplicating, we complement Chassard and co-workers' [14] introduction of timing to anesthesiologists, by noting earlier (missed) investigations [25], including systematic six-timepoint surveys [26]. We emphasize partly endogenous aspects of circadian and other rhythms, recording the importance of chronopharmacodynamics as compared to chronopharmacokinetics, and the merit of assessing in future studies possible nonphotic as well as photic influences on a much broader chronome than circadian. We also advocate aligning biological monitoring with ongoing physical government-supported environmental surveillance to detect alterations of chronomes, not only around but also in us, and external–internal interactions, to arrive at preventive measures, by treating any reversible pathogenic abnormality in the range of everyday physiology.

10.4 SUSCEPTIBILITY RHYTHMS

For a few variables, there is already a very broadly mapped spectrum of rhythms with a range of τ values from 1 cycle in a second, a minute, a day, a year, and a decade or 1 cycle with still longer τ values in populations. Not all serial data can be sampled over many cycles with different frequencies in the same variable; usually the data cannot be collected densely enough to document all aspects of the stage dependence of effects of stimuli upon the cycles

Figure 10.1. Effect of food restriction on circulating eosinophil counts in mice. Follow-up study on Figure 3 in the Introduction to this book, with a phase difference greatly reduced by offering the restricted diet in the evening. (a) Even after $\log_{10}$-transformation of the data expressed as percentage of mean, great interindividual variability is apparent in the raw data. (b) Plots of timepoint mean for mice in each group reveal different circadian patterns. (c–e) Parameter tests quantify differences, indicating that calorie restriction is associated with a lower MESOR (c,d), a larger circadian amplitude (d,e), and only a slight difference in acrophase (d). The difference in acrophase in this study, where calorie-restricted mice were fed in the evening, is much smaller than the almost antiphase observed in prior studies (Figure 3 in the Introduction to this book), where calorie-restricted mice were fed in the morning [1]. (*See color insert.*)

Calorie-restricted meal offered evenings only slightly advances phase (no antiphase versus controls, as seen with morning meals), lowers MESOR and amplifies circadian eosinophil rhythm in C₃H mice with high breast cancer incidence that can be reduced by calorie restriction (CR)

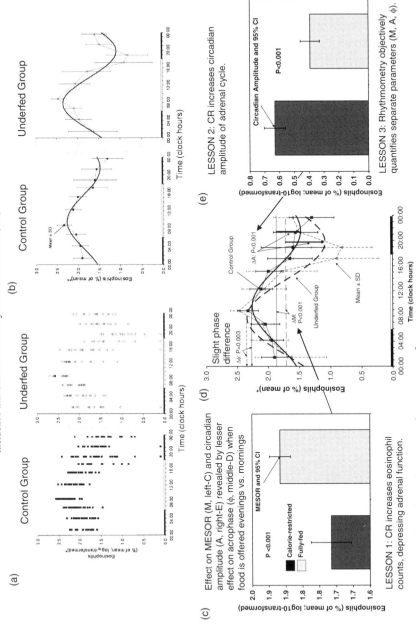

* After log₁₀-transformation of data expressed as percentage of mean.
From Halberg F & Visscher MB. Endocrinology 1952; 51: 329–335.

221

involved. Single surveys are usually done along a system time of 24 hours or of a year or along other time scales, sampled over one or at most a few cycles, such as one or a few days, weeks, or decades, whereby a cycle stage-dependent set of responses is invariably found. Such sampling suffices to document that timing accounts for a within-cycle difference between a large and a small, versus no or even versus an opposite response to the identical stimulus. The importance of these findings for new drug development seems obvious. Many promising molecules may be discarded because they were tested at the wrong time. Testing for timing should precede the regular three phases of drug testing and has hence been called a phase-zero design.

10.5 LIFE OR DEATH FROM THE SAME STIMULUS AT DIFFERENT CIRCADIAN TIMES

Periodicity in the nervous system was known for centuries as epilepsy occurring only during waking versus only during sleep or mostly on awakening, if not diffusely during 24 hours [1]. Hence it was hardly surprising for us to be able to demonstrate circadian rhythms in the human electroencephalogram in disease by 1952 and in health in 1966 [1]. That noise of a fixed intensity to which mice of susceptible strains were exposed can induce convulsions and death at one circadian stage but not at another was reported in the 1950s [27, 28].

Some inbred strains of mice are susceptible to noise-induced convulsions that can be fatal. To assess any role of timing in the central nervous system, separate groups of such comparable rodents can be exposed to the identical stimuli at different clock hours. Lighting regimens and other laboratory conditions can be standardized to synchronize what has been dubbed "circadian time" with an environmental cycle, the synchronizer. The lighting cycle is only a clock-time or calendar-time giver, since physiologic (body) time prevails in the synchronizers absence, so that a zeitgeber is a clock- or calendar-time giver, but not a body-time giver [1, 17]. Once this standardization in the animal room was introduced

————————————————————————————▶

Figure 10.2. Importance of assessing the rhythm's period. Whereas circadian rhythms are usually synchronized by environmental schedules, they may desynchronize, for example, in the absence of the eyes, thereby assuming a period that deviates slightly but statistically significantly from precisely 24 hours. When such free-running occurs, results from two-timepoint studies may yield confusing results. (a) This is illustrated for circulating eosinophil counts of mice sampled twice a day, during daytime and nighttime, after a sham-operation or bilateral optic enucleation. Results from four different (nonconsecutive) days postoperation are shown. Whereas sham-operated mice display a consistent pattern of higher daytime and lower nighttime counts, blinded mice exhibit erratic patterns, the nighttime counts being sometimes higher than, sometimes lower than, and sometimes almost equal to daytime counts. (b) Abstract illustration of two components with slightly different periods accounts for the changing relation between the two curves depending on whether they are in or out of phase with one another [1].

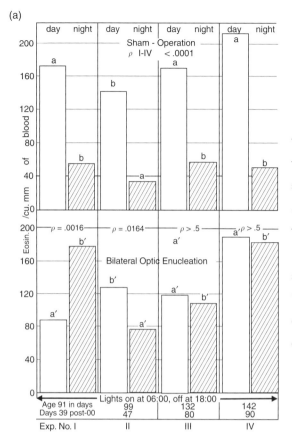

(a)

Mean eosinophil counts at two times of day in tail blood from blinded and from sham-operated male CBC mice, during the 3 months following the operation. (Serially independent sampling.) Note that the blinded mice (below) do not exhibit the regular behavior of sham-operated mice (above).

(b)

Changes in time relations of two circadian rhythms with different periods (Halberg F, Loewenson R, Winter R, Bearman J, Adkins GH. Physiologic circadian systems (differences in period of circadian rhythms or in their component frequencies; some methodologic implications to biology and medicine). Proc Minn Acad Sci 1960; 28, 53–75).

in the 1950s [1], it was also found that the same audiogenic stimulus—noise from bells in a tub where the mice of a sensitive strain were placed [27] or more specialized apparatus [28]—can induce a sequence of dashing, often followed by clonic and then tonic convulsions, some ending in the death of these inbred animals (brother–sister mated for dozens of generations) at one exposure time while the same stimulus at another predictable time was compatible with the superficially unimpaired survival of most of the tested separate groups of comparable mice [1, 27, 28]. Moreover, a shift in the timing of the synchronizing lighting regimen results in a shift of the timing of high versus low susceptibility, a result demonstrating that we are not dealing with an effect of clock hour (as illustrated in Figure 1A in the Introduction to this book).

Many other agents were thereafter tested [1]. In our laboratory alone, another physical stimulus was whole-body X-ray irradiation. The LD_{50} was first shown to be circadian stage dependent, as noted in the discussion of Ref. [29 cf. 30]. This finding in turn led to a doubling of 2-year survival rate by the timed radiotherapy of patients with very advanced perioral cancers

---

Figure 10.3. Blinding studies (I) led to the concept of free-running, as shown in chronograms of rectal temperature of sham-operated and blinded mice (Ia), seen to peak earlier and earlier each day in the blinded mice. Accordingly, the circadian acrophases of the blinded mice gradually drift as a function of time whereas those of the control mice remain about the same, an original hint of partial endogenicity that led to the coining of a "circadian" system (Ib) [1]. Histograms of best-fitting periods estimated from records of groups of mice show that, on average, the circadian period of blinded mice is slightly shorter than 24 hours (Ic). Internal phase relations among several variables are also shown (Id). The components of the chronome are internally coordinated through feedsideward, in a network of spontaneous, reactive, and modulatory rhythms (II). Apart from the spontaneous rhythms characterizing variables such as serum corticosterone (IIa) or melatonin (IIb) , reactive rhythms are found in response to a given stimulus applied under standardized controlled conditions of the laboratory: the adrenal response to ACTH is a case in point (broken line in IIa). Such response rhythms have been named β-rhythms, the spontaneous rhythms being called α-rhythms, whether they are 24 hour or otherwise synchronized. Much controversy can be resolved by studying the effect of the interaction by more than two variables at different rhythm stages. A third entity may modulate, in a predictable insofar as rhythmic way, the effect of one entity on the other. Predictable sequences of attenuation, no-effect, and amplification can then be found. A case in point is corticosterone production by bisected adrenals stimulated by ACTH 1-17 in the presence versus absence of pineal homogenate (IIc). Such chronomodulation is also observed for the effect of ACTH 1-17 on the metaphyseal bone DNA labeling in the rat (IId). Some of these multiple entity interactions involve more than one frequency; this is the case for the effect of the immunostimulator cefodizime (HR221) on corticosterone production by the adrenals stimulated by ACTH 1-17 (IIe). Chronomodulations involving one or several frequencies are known as γ- or δ-rhythms, respectively. They are part of feedsidewards, rhythmic sequences of attenuation, amplification, and no-effect by a modulator on the interaction of an actor and a reactor (III).

Endogenous time structure (Chronome) of internally coordinated free-running rhythms (TOP) through (feedsidewards) in network of spontaneous (α), Reactive (β) and Modulatory (γ, δ) Rhythms (Bottom)

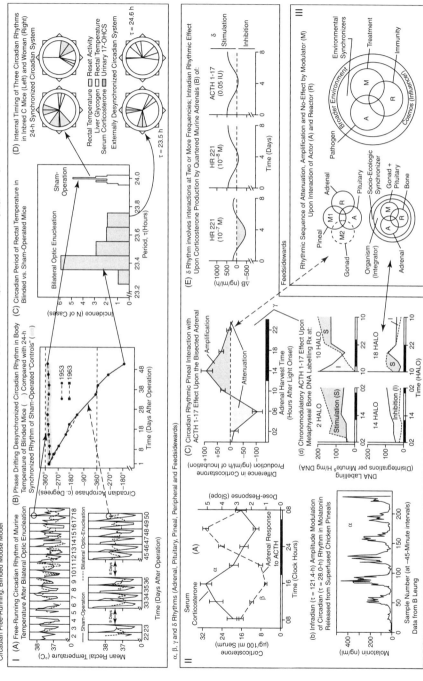

225

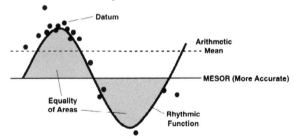

(a) **Higher Accuracy (Smaller Bias) in the Presence of Unequidistant Data**

The arithmetic mean does not represent true average for rhythm (defined, e.g., by cosine curve) when sampling is unequispaced and/or does not cover integral number of cycles.

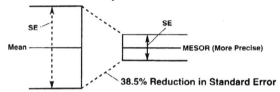

(b) **Higher Precision (Smaller Error) in the Presence of Equidistant Data**

The SE of the mean depends on the total variability; a large portion of this variability can be ascribed to the rhythmic time structure; fitting an approximating cosine curve can reduce the residual variance, which determines how small the SEs of the MESOR and other parameters are. The better the cosine model fits the data, the greater the reduction in SE.

Figure 10.4. The MESOR usually provides a more accurate estimate of location than the arithmetic mean (a). When sampling is denser near the maximum (or minimum) of a periodic function than at other times, the arithmetic mean is biased toward that extremum, whereas the MESOR tends to be closer to the true average value of the given function (obtained when sampling is equidistant over an integer number of cycles). The MESOR usually also provides a more precise estimate of location than the arithmetic mean, notably when the data are characterized by a large-amplitude rhythm (b). This stems from the fact that the error around the MESOR is estimated after the variability accounted for by the rhythmic behavior of the data has been portioned out.

(Figure 10.6) [31, 32]. By 1960, bacteriological substances like the endotoxins of *Brucella melatensis* [33] or *Escherichia coli* [34], chemicals like ethanol [35; cf. 18, 36] and a drug, ouabain (Figure 10.7 bottom) [37], were all shown to have circadian stage-dependent effects [cf. 1]. Soon, the importance of susceptibility rhythms to another drug, Librium (chlordiazepoxide; 7-chloro-2-methylamino-5-phenyl-3H-1,4-benzodiazepine-4-oxide HCl) was also demonstrated [38].

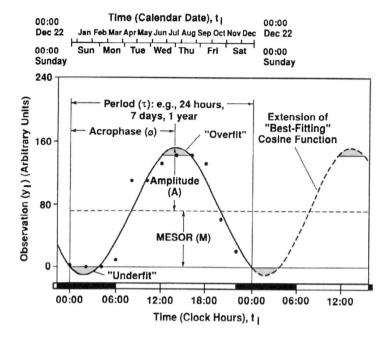

* $y_i = M + A\cos(\omega t_i + \emptyset) + e_i$; where $\omega = \frac{2\pi}{\tau}$, t_i = time; y_i = observation at t_i and e_i = error at t_i; assumed as a first approximation to have the same independent normal distribution with mean zero and unknown variance σ^2, regardless of time; F statistic from zero-amplitude test compares sum of squares (SS) accounted for by fitted model either with the residual SS (original or pooled cosinor) or with the SS due to pure error, uncontaminated by lack of fit (unpooled cosinor).

Figure 10.5. Illustration of the single-cosinor method. One or several cosine curves with known (or approximately known) periods* are fitted by least squares to the data, yielding estimates for the following parameters: the MESOR, a rhythm-adjusted (or rather chronome-adjusted) mean value; the amplitude, a measure of half the extent of predictable change within a cycle; and the acrophase, a measure of the timing of overall high values recurring in each cycle. When a multiple-component model is fitted, estimates of the amplitude and acrophase are obtained for each component. When the different components are harmonically related, the amplitudes and acrophases of the harmonic terms qualify the waveform of the fundamental component, which can in turn be characterized by a magnitude (rather than amplitude) and orthophase (rather than acrophase), measures of the predictable extent and timing of change of the complex waveform. If the period is not known a priori, nonlinear least squares are needed to estimate M and (A, φ) of each component together with its respective period, the period being defined as the duration of one cycle. The acrophase is usually expressed in (negative) degrees, with 360° equated to the period length and 0° being set to the reference time (such as midnight preceding the start of data collection or the time of light onset in the case of circadian rhythms assessed in laboratory experiments, notably when staggered lighting regimens are used to facilitate the work during office hours without the need for around-the-clock sampling).

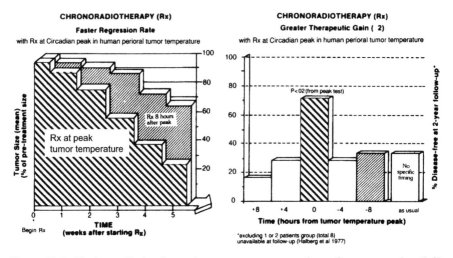

Figure 10.6. Timing radiation by peak tumor temperature shows faster regression (left) and doubling of disease-free 2-year survival rate.

Mortality and/or survival time from an intraperitoneal (IP) injection of Librium was tested on inbred D_8 and B_1 mice. In each of several experiments, separate groups, each of 21–65 mice, were given a fixed dose of Librium at 4-h intervals, the first group injected at 0800 h of one day, the last at 0400h or 0800h of the next. The number of survivors was recorded at 4-hour intervals for the first 48 hours postinjection and then at 12-hour intervals up to 1 week. Mortality was higher in mice injected during the daily dark span (1800h to 0600h) than during the light span, with a peak usually at 0000h, but occasionally at 2000h or 0400h on an $L_{06-18}D_{18-06}$ schedule (Figure 1 in Introduction to this book). The statistical significance of susceptibility rhythms below a 1% level was ascertained by a procedure for locating the peak of a time series [39; cf. 17]. Circadian changes in susceptibility interact with age effects, susceptibility changing statistically significantly with age, in this case increasing or, in the case of the susceptibility of D_8 mice to audiogenic convulsions, decreasing with age. The circadian peak in susceptibility to this psychotherapeutic drug has a timing similar to some but not all other susceptibility rhythms involving the central nervous system (e.g., to ethanol, acetylcholine [40], and to audiogenic abnormality); it falls into a span of increased electrocerebral and gross motor activity. The stage for studies on halothane was thus set by the foregoing findings as well as by the pioneering investigations of Yngve Edlund and Hjalmar Holmgren in Stockholm [25].

10.6 SUSCEPTIBILITY TO ANESTHESIA

In studies published in 1939, Edlund and Holmgren [25] gave Avertin and Evipan to groups of mice at 0600h or 1100h. They reported differences in the time elapsed between an intraperitoneal injection and the assumption of a position lying on one side, spontaneously or passively, and recorded when the pain reflex was lost and when it was recovered, any convulsions, and recovery time, that is, the time between injection and the resumption of the normal motility of the animals.

Edlund and Holmgren [25] ascertained a within-day difference (between the two test times) in the time to falling asleep for Avertin, and they concluded that at 0600h the animals were more resistant to Avertin than at 1100h. Similar results were found for Evipan. The authors consider the possibility that the detoxifying role of the liver may be involved. Edlund and Holmgren [25] cautiously propose a parallel between the "work of the liver" and the speed of onset of anesthesia, its depth, and its length.

Against this background, a quarter century later, in 1964, the dependence of halothane toxicity on the circadian system phase was seen in three surveys on male C_{57} black mice of three age groups [41]: 137 mice in a first study, 147 in a second, and 125 in a third. The lighting regimen on which mice were kept for a week prior to study and up to a minute prior to testing is also indicated in Figure 1 in the Introduction to this book. During anesthesia and thereafter, the mice were kept in light at all times. In each survey, the 10-minute exposure of separate groups of comparable animals to 3.5% halothane was associated with differences in mortality as a function of exposure time. P-values derived according to a procedure developed for analyzing the statistical significance of crests in physiological time series [39] were eventually complemented or replaced by cosinor.

Mortality at a given test time was expressed as a percentage of the average mortality at the end of a given study, with the latter mean equated to 100%. These relative values for each test time were then averaged to obtain the mean relative change, plotted in Figure 10.7 (top). The bottom of Figure 10.7 time-macroscopically aligns the susceptibility rhythm to halothane (fluothane) with other susceptibility-resistance cycles mapped earlier. This figure conveys the degree of generality of changes in response to toxic doses of several drugs as a function of circadian system phase. Evidence in Figure 10.7, in the Introduction's Figure 1, and elsewhere [1] may be used further to suggest that crests and troughs in susceptibility to different agents do not all occur at the same time: circadian synchronization occurs with differences in phase, some of which are positive or negative as well as zero, and there is no alternative to mapping the rhythms' characteristics with their uncertainties, that can be readily computed, for example, by drawing tangents to each consecutive 95% elliptical confidence region.

The Introduction's Figure 1 shows results in C_{57} mice for a single study on halothane [41]. Mortality within the 10 minutes of anesthesia (as curve A) is presented separately from mortality after 10 minutes of exposure (curve B). The times of highest susceptibility are seen to differ for mortality during and after anesthesia. Mortality from halothane, analyzed by the single cosinor method, yielded an acrophase at $-172°$ from midlight for all deaths or those occurring

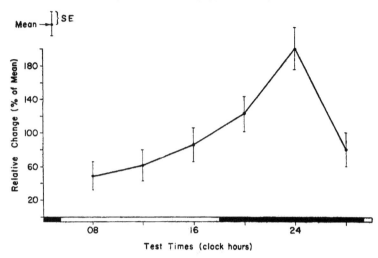

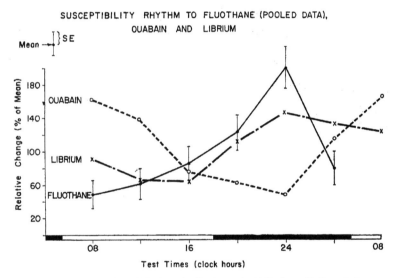

Top: Conversion of pooled data into "relative changes", with estimates of variability also provided for results from each test time.

Bottom: Concept of hours of changing resistance can be further documented by data on Fluothane (•——•). Data aligned with some obtained on other susceptibility-resistance cycles earlier. This figure conveys the degree of generality of changes in response to toxic doses of several drugs as a function of circadian system phase. The same figure may be used further to suggest that crests and troughs in susceptibility to different agents do not all occur at the same time; circadian synchronization occurs with differences in phase, some of which are positive or negative, as well as zero (Cold Spr Harb Symp quant Biol 1960; 25: 524).

From Matthews JH, Marte E, Halberg F. A circadian susceptibility-resistance cycle to fluothane in male B1 mice. Canad Anesthesiol Soc J 1964; 11: 280-290.

Figure 10.7. Halothane studies on 409 mice in 1964 were subsequently extended by two studies on methohexital IP on 407 mice (not here shown), also revealing circadian periodicity with a different timing and showing further that "in no case was the time of highest mortality associated with the time of highest blood concentrations," an argument for chronopharmacodynamic precedence over pharmacokinetics [41]. For timemicroscopy, see Figure 1 in the Introduction to this book [41].

only during exposure to halothane; a rhythm in deaths after exposure to anesthesia ($P < 0.01$) was in antiphase with that during exposure. The former may be more important than the latter; the depression of the central nervous system beyond respiratory arrest is reversible by artificial ventilation.

The clinically more important periodicity appears to be that encountered during relatively light anesthesia. For this, curve B may constitute a model. It should be emphasized that the number of animals exposed at each timepoint was 20 or 21; at no point were all animals dead. At two timepoints there were no deaths after exposure to the anesthetic, even though plenty of animals were alive, a circumstance which applies to the timepoints of 2, 6, and 10 hours after the start of the daily light span. By contrast, at four times mortality during exposure to halothane was zero, but at four times there were some deaths after discontinuance of exposure. These results suggest the operation of different mechanisms in the mortality at different times in relation to anesthesia, as supported further by results expressed as percentage change in the series mean. The out-of-phase character of the two curves is readily seen. A third curve shows the average recovery time in minutes and appears to be close in phase to the curve for death after anesthesia.

The foregoing impression is quantified in the three cosinors in the Introduction's Figure 1. The elliptical areas are 95% confidence regions and do not cover the center of the cosinor display, the pole, a finding that indicates a nonzero amplitude and thus the statistical significance of the rhythm in each case. The cosinor also shows the circadian rhythm of deaths during anesthesia as being about 180° out of phase with the rhythms of (1) deaths after anesthesia and (2) recovery times of survivors. On this more rigorous basis, it seems reasonable to suggest that we are dealing with different mechanisms underlying the differently timed susceptibility rhythms [41].

In another set of two surveys, methohexital was injected intraperitoneally in a dose of 1.5 mg/20 g of body weight to 201 C_{57} black mice or in a dose of 1.6 mg/20 g of body weight to 206 C mice, 4–6 months of age. The mice were continuously observed in the chamber and thereafter until death or recovery from anesthesia (judged by return of righting reflex) [41]. Thus a circadian rhythm was demonstrated for methohexital. A macroscopic peak in mortality (not shown) occurred at 1600 h for mice of both strains. It was statistically significant in each strain, when tested by χ^2, the χ^2 values being 12.7 and 12.1 for C_{57} and C mice, respectively. Drug concentrations in plasma were determined in separate studies for each survey. Whether or not the blanks were subtracted from the results at each timepoint or whether the blood concentrations as such were examined, in no case was the time of highest mortality associated with the time of highest blood concentrations, an early demonstration of the greater importance of chronopharmacodynamics versus chronopharmacokinetics.

The circadian stage dependence of pentobarbital is shown in the Introduction's Figure 1 in terms of disappearance rates and by reference to the desired effect of the drug, an extension of chronotoxicology to chronopharmacology

[42]. Within-day differences in the disappearance rate of ouabain at the previously reported times of high and low lethal response were demonstrated earlier [43] but are not shown here. With the recognition not only of many more rhythms than circadians in us [1] and the observations that these circadian and other physiological rhythms are subject to a matching set of environmental cycles, the interaction of chronomes in and around us prompted their mapping in the discipline of chronomics, documented by publications in a series of conferences [44–46].

Chronopharmacology [47], with its phase-zero exploration [48], was a dividend of these developments. At a certain circadian time, but not at other times, the same molecule, an ACTH analogue, ACTH 1-17 enhanced DNA labeling for 24 hours, while at another time it enhanced first and then inhibited, at a third time it inhibited DNA labeling for 24 hours, and at still another time it first inhibited and then enhanced DNA labeling, all during the same 24 hours after injection into separate groups of comparable inbred mice 6 hours apart (Figure 10.3, part II) [49]. Epinephrine can also have circadian stage-dependent effects on cell division in rodents [50] and in urodeles [51]; cf. [52]. An immunomodulator, lentinan, as a function of circadian, circaseptan, and circannual schedules, can enhance the growth of a subsequently implanted cancer or inhibit it [53]. Beyond drugs, even a nutriceutical, ubiquinone, can act preferentially at one time, when it is tested to treat a circadian blood pressure overswing (CHAT, circadian hyper *amplitude-t*ension), that carries a risk of stroke greater than an elevation of the MESOR, *M*, of blood pressure, *M*-hypertension [54]. Melatonin effects are circadian and circannual stage dependent [55–58]. Opposite effects as a function of timing of melatonin upon tumor growth are confirmed [59].

10.7 WHY AN INITIAL SIX-TIMEPOINT APPROACH

Why, in preference to two timepoints, was a six-timepoint approach chosen in most of the studies reported here? From a conventional viewpoint, "six groups are just too many" [60]. For exploiting rhythms in optimizing treatment timing, by estimating their parameters with uncertainties, "two groups are too few" [61]. The difference in approach between classical and chronobiologic study designs results in part from differences in aim that require different methods of analysis. The classical approach as a rule places emphasis on a comparison among different treatments, irrespective of time, and relies on the analysis of variance (ANOVA) or other techniques based on similar assumptions. Only large changes are detected, since rhythms loom large, albeit hidden, in the noise term. By contrast, the chronobiologic approach aims to resolve a major component of what is otherwise buried in the noise term, namely, the very rhythms to be used for an optimization of treatment by timing. External information concerning the occurrence and importance of rhythms can now be advantageously used. The analysis of data relies on techniques such as the cosinor [16; cf. 17], which involve the least-squares fit of models consisting of components with anticipated (preferably already mapped) periods.

10.8 COVERING ALL RHYTHM STAGES VERSUS TWO SELECTED TIMEPOINTS

The chronobiologic approach recommends, at the outset, sampling at different timepoints to test different rhythm stages, since the extent and even the sign of the response to a given treatment may depend on the rhythm stage at which the treatment was administered. If prior information is available as to the times at which the outcome is minimal and maximal and the uncertainties of the phase estimates are also known and small, a two-timepoint approach (at the times of the peak and the trough) can be preferred, since the difference between treatment is then the largest and each timepoint's mean can be more precisely defined.

In many critical pilot studies, however, only seldom is there prior information concerning the precise temporal (phase) location of the underlying rhythm and about the CIs of its characteristics. In the case of the chronotherapy of advanced ovarian cancer according to the circadian salivary CA125 or CA130 rhythms, for instance, we do not know of any lags between the time of highest cancer cell proliferation and the shedding of antigen and the latter's arrival in saliva, nor do we know the contributions and timing of any nontumoral sources of CA125 or CA130 [62]. A two-timepoint approach may inadvertently be carried out at the midline crossings of a rhythm. Even if that rhythm is of very large amplitude, differences will then be negligible and erroneous conclusions are inescapable. From the viewpoint of curve fitting, the acrophase (from a single-component fit) or orthophase (from a multiple-component fit) will be more accurately estimated the more sampling times are covered by the experimental design.

10.9 POWER CONSIDERATIONS

One of the reasons for advocating as small a number of groups as possible in a conventional experimental design stems from the inverse relationship between power [63] and the number of groups. The reduction in power with an increased number of groups comes about at least in part from the fact that in the numerator of the F-test (e.g., in an ANOVA), the sum of squares is divided by the number of groups minus 1. The mean squares for a time effect will thus be lower the larger the number of groups. This is not the case for chronobiologic approaches relying on curve-fitting procedures. When the single cosinor method is used, the number of degrees of freedom associated with the sum of squares accounted for by the model (entering the numerator of the F-test) is always 2, irrespective of the number of groups (timepoints); it is determined by the number of parameters to be estimated in the fitted model. This parsimony of the cosinor method is at the origin of the enhanced power of a chronomic approach.

More specifically, let us compare the cosinor and analysis of variance for testing a time effect, that is, for a comparison of test groups differing only by the timing of a given treatment. Let us consider the case where data (y_{ij}) are collected at k timepoints ($i = 1, \ldots, k$), with n_i replications at each timepoint ($j = 1, \ldots, n_i$). Both the ANOVA and single cosinor partition the total residual sum of squares around the overall mean

$$\bar{\bar{y}} = \sum_i \sum_j y_{ij} / \sum_i n_i \qquad (10.1)$$

into an "explained" and "unexplained" sum of squares (SS).

For the ANOVA, the total residual sum of squares (TSS) is partitioned as follows:

$$\sum_i \sum_j (y_{ij} - \bar{\bar{y}})^2 = \sum_i n_i (\bar{y}_i - \bar{\bar{y}})^2 + \sum_i \sum_j (y_{ij} - \bar{y}_i)^2 \qquad (10.2)$$

where

$$\bar{y}_i = \sum_j y_{ij} / n_i \qquad (10.3)$$

is the mean at the ith timepoint. This can also be written

$$TSS = GSS + WSS \qquad (10.4)$$

where GSS stands for the among-groups SS and WSS for the within-groups SS. The test statistic is

$$F_A = \frac{GSS/(k-1)}{WSS/(N-k)} \sim F(k-1; \ N-k) \qquad (10.5)$$

with

$$N = \sum_i n_i \qquad (10.6)$$

For the single cosinor, the total sum of squares (TSS) is partitioned with respect to values predicted according to the fitted model at each timepoint ($\hat{y}_i$)

rather than to group means:

$$\sum_i \sum_j (y_{ij} - \bar{\bar{y}}_i)^2 = \sum_i n_i(\hat{y}_i - \bar{\bar{y}})^2 + \sum_i \sum_j (y_{ij} - \hat{y}_i)^2 \qquad (10.7)$$

where

$$\hat{y}_i = \hat{M} + \hat{A}\cos(\omega t_i + \hat{\phi}) \qquad (10.8)$$

if the model is a cosine curve with angular frequency $\omega = 2\pi/\tau$, where τ is the assumed period; M is called the MESOR, A the amplitude, and ϕ the acrophase. Again, this can be written

$$TSS = CSS + ESS \qquad (10.9)$$

where CSS stands for the SS accounted for by the cosine curve and ESS stands for the SS around the predicted values or error sum of squares. The test statistic is

$$F_C = \frac{CSS/2}{ESS/(N-3)} \sim F(2; \ N-3) \qquad (10.10)$$

The numbers of degrees of freedom are determined as a function of the number of estimated parameters. In the case of the single-component cosine model, this number of degrees of freedom is 2 (3 parameters-1). In the case of the ANOVA, however, it is $(k-1)$; that is, it is a function of the number of timepoints considered.

Moreover, since both methods partition the same TSS,

$$GSS + WSS = CSS + ESS \qquad (10.11)$$

In the single cosinor, the error sum of squares (ESS) is computed by reference to the predicted value at each sampling time, $\hat{y}_i$ ($i = 1, \ldots, k$). By definition of the sample mean, this error sum of squares will necessarily be larger than that intervening in the ANOVA (WSS), where it is computed by reference to the mean at each sampling time, $\bar{y}_i$ ($i = 1, \ldots, k$). Let the difference be denoted as Δ^2:

$$\Delta^2 = ESS - WSS = \sum_i n_i(\bar{y}_i - \hat{y}_i)^2 \qquad (10.12)$$

From Eqs. (10.11) and (10.12), it can be seen that

$$\Delta^2 = GSS - CSS \qquad (10.13)$$

It follows that the F-ratio used in the single cosinor can be related to the F-ratio used in the ANOVA by

$$\frac{CSS/2}{ESS/(N-3)} = \frac{GSS/(k-1)}{WSS/(N-k)} \left[\frac{\frac{k-1}{2}}{\frac{N-k}{N-3}} \frac{(GSS - \Delta^2)/GSS}{(WSS + \Delta^2)/WSS} \right] \qquad (10.14)$$

For $N \gg k$, which is often the case,

$$F_C = \frac{k-1}{2} F_A \delta \tag{10.15}$$

with

$$\delta = \frac{(GSS - \Delta^2)/GSS}{(WSS + \Delta^2)/WSS} \tag{10.16}$$

It follows that the cosinor method is more sensitive for

$$\delta > \frac{2}{k-1} \frac{F_{1-\alpha}(2, N-3)}{F_{1-\alpha}(k-1, N-k)} \tag{10.17}$$

If the data are well approximated by the cosine model, Δ^2 is small and δ is close to 1. In this case, for $k > 3$, the single cosinor is more powerful (more sensitive) than the ANOVA since the critical level for F decreases less rapidly as a function of k than does $2/(k-1)$ [63]. This is often the case since most biologic variables exhibit large rhythmic variations with periods that can be anticipated from their environmental counterparts, serving as synchronizers.

10.10   MERITS OF THE CHRONOBIOLOGIC APPROACH FROM THE VIEWPOINT OF PARAMETER ESTIMATION

Even though the two approaches are equally powerful in the case of $k = 3$ (the test statistics from both methods are identical since the cosine curve is determined by three points: the fitted curve will thus pass exactly through the means of each of the three test times ($\hat{y}_i \equiv \bar{y}_i$; $i = 1, 2, 3$)), preference should be given to the cosinor since the latter method will also provide point and interval estimates of rhythm parameters, useful in their own right. Moreover, if an individual is being tested only once at each of three different times, the ANOVA is not applicable, whereas point estimates of rhythm characteristics are obtained by cosinor [63]. These may later be useful as imputations in a population-mean cosinor approach [16], even if the different individuals sampled in the population are each tested at different times.

The single cosinor was specially designed for rhythm detection and assessment of effects from sparse and short data series. Its power comes in part from the fact that the method relies on external information, namely, that biological functions are usually rhythmic with (approximately) known periods. The ubiquity of circadian rhythms in biology and medicine is a case in point. By including at least five or six timepoints in a study design, not only can the hypothesis of a time effect be tested, but also rhythm characteristics useful in their own right can be estimated. The MESOR, a rhythm-adjusted mean, is more accurate as compared to the arithmetic mean as a location index (i.e., determining the overall effectiveness of a drug) when the timepoints are unequally spaced (Figure 10.4). For equidistant test times, the MESOR is identical to the arithmetic mean in a balanced design consisting of the same number of measurements at each timepoint. It is again superior, being characterized by a smaller standard error since a large portion of the variability of the data ascribed to their rhythmic time structure is accounted for by fitting an approximating cosine curve (Figure 10.4). In addition to the MESOR, the acrophase and amplitude describing the rhythmic variation provide a measure of when to treat to optimize treatment efficacy as well as a measure of the potential gain in therapeutic effect that can be obtained by treating at the right time (Figure 10.5).

10.11 ILLUSTRATIVE CHRONOBIOLOGIC CLINICAL TRIALS

10.11.1 N-of-5 Study of the Urinary Free-Cortisol Response to ACTH by Patients with Rheumatoid Arthritis

Figure 10.8 shows, with five timepoints, that a response rhythm not only can be suspected, but also is detected with statistical significance [64]. This is achieved in a study of only one subject at each of five timepoints, 4.8 hours apart, that is, with five subjects who, for the fit of a cosine curve, could be viewed as "replications." If the five subjects were all tested at the same timepoint, 0600h, as may be picked by an eager early-morning investigator, this effect could not have been detected. The effect of an ACTH analogue, ACTH 1-17, can be quite different at five different circadian stages. We are dealing with results of chronobiologic pilots that, of course, await extension to larger samples. It should be emphasized that the Figure 10.8 test situation is particularly favorable. The circadian cortisol rhythm is one of large amplitude; its response can be studied as a change in amplitude, in timing, in waveform, and in the mean, with the same subject serving as longitudinal control. What also appears to be critical is that the adrenal cortex is well known to respond to ACTH, even if it does so in a circadian stage-dependent fashion [64, 65]. There are distinct advantages to the point that, in a chronobiologic pilot, even only one subject per timepoint can be meaningfully studied. With this minimal number of five subjects, not only is the given dose found to be active, an answer to the major question raised, but the same survey also reveals when the dose is most active and by how much it is more active at the best time as compared to the worst time [64; cf. 65].

10.11.2 N-of-6 Study of Low Doses of Aspirin on Prostaglandin and Adrenergic Pathways

Figure 10.9 shows the circadian stage dependence of effects of daily low doses of aspirin (ASA) on lipoperoxides in platelet-rich plasma [66]. Six clinically

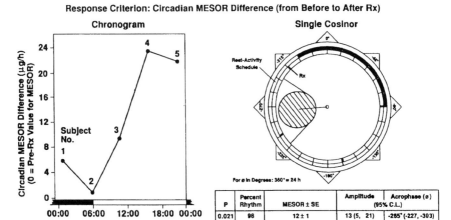

N-OF-5 STUDY: CIRCADIAN RHYTHMIC URINARY FREE CORTISOL RESPONSE TO ACTH 1-17 BY HETEROGENEOUS SMALL GROUP OF PATIENTS WITH RHEUMATOID ARTHRITIS*

Response Criterion: Circadian MESOR Difference (from Before to After Rx)

P	Percent Rhythm	MESOR ± SE	Amplitude (95% C.L.)	Acrophase (ø)
0.021	98	12 ± 1	13 (5, 21)	-265° (-227, -303)

CL = Confidence Limits

* 5 men, 45-75 years of age, with rheumatoid arthritis, each provided 6 urine samples in unequal daily fractions (19:30-06:00, 06:00-08:30, 08:30-11:30, 11:30-13:15, 13:15-17:30 and 17:30-19:30) for 24h before and after Rx. MESOR determined from fit of 24-h cosine curve to each man's data before and after Rx. PR = Percent Rhythm; P = P-value from zero amplitude test. Günther et al., 1980.

CC 7/92

Figure 10.8. The effect of placebo and ACTH 1-17 (Synchrodyn®, Hoechst) upon urinary free cortisol was examined at five different circadian stages on 10 men with Steinbrocker Stage II–III rheumatoid arthritis. A mean cosinor analysis of urinary cortisol data from the subjects prior to treatment with either ACTH or placebo revealed a statistically highly significant rhythm. The response of the MESOR (midline-estimating statistic of rhythm, or rhythm-adjusted circadian average) of urinary free cortisol to ACTH 1-17 by patients with rheumatoid arthritis is circadian rhythmic. This reactivity rhythm is out of phase with the spontaneous rhythm in urinary cortisol acrophases.

healthy women, 20–30 years of age, volunteered to participate in a randomized pilot study consisting of a reference stage (lasting 2 days, starting after a 5-day adjustment to hospital conditions) followed by a 7-day span during which aspirin (100 mg/day) was administered at one of six different circadian stages: upon awakening, at 3, 6, 9, or 12 hours after awakening, or at bedtime. During the reference stage and during the last 2 days of the low-dose aspirin test span, venous blood samples were collected every 4 hours for the determination of, among others, lipoperoxide (LP) concentration in platelet-rich plasma.

Whereas lipoperoxides are invariably depressed by aspirin, the extent of this effect varies as a function of the circadian stage of its administration. Aspirin use upon awakening (top row left) is associated with a clear (desired) inhibition. Inhibition is also seen when aspirin is taken 3 hours after awakening. By comparison, the effect is very greatly reduced if aspirin is taken 12 hours after awakening. The extent of lipoperoxide depression associated with aspirin use at a given circadian stage is depicted as vertical bars. The differences in mean

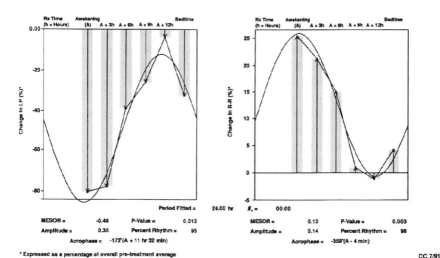

Figure 10.9. Aspirin effect on lipoperoxides (LPs) in platelet-rich plasma (left panel) and lymphocyte β-adrenergic receptors (B-Rs) (right panel) may be predictably present or absent as a function of timing (circadian rhythm stage). Easily implemented and cost-effective timing of aspirin critically determines two of the drug's major effects. Last timepoint, labeled bedtime, corresponds to approximately 15 hours after awakening. Change in LPs and B-Rs are expressed as a percentage of the overall pretreatment average. MESOR indicates *m*idline-*e*stimating *s*tatistic *o*f *r*hythm. (From Ref. 66.)

value between the low-dose aspirin test span and the reference stage computed for each subject were assigned to the circadian stage of treatment administration and fitted by least squares with a 24-hour cosine curve to assess the response (rhythm) to aspirin. The circadian stage dependence of the effect is statistically significant by cosinor analysis ($P = 0.012$).

10.11.3 Aspirin and Blood Pressure

In addition to lipoperoxides in platelet-rich plasma, the six women participating in the study also had their blood pressure and heart rate measured by staff at hourly intervals throughout the study [67]. Each data series was analyzed by cosinor. Self-starting CUSUMs and parameter tests served to compare the MESOR and circadian amplitude and acrophase between the spans of ASA or placebo administration. Aspirin was found to depress the systolic and diastolic blood pressure MESOR at 6 or 9 hours after awakening but not at other test times [67]. As a follow-up in clinically healthy subjects, the possibility was examined that effects of ASA upon blood pressure could indeed be time dependent. Hermida et al. [68] studied the systolic, mean arterial, and diastolic blood pressures and heart rates of 55 healthy subjects (35 men and 20 women), 19–24 years of age, automatically monitored every 30 min for 48 h with an

ABPM-630 Colin (Komaki, Japan) device before and after a 1-week course of ASA (500 mg/day). Subjects were randomly assigned to one of three groups, according to the circadian timing of administration of the daily dose of ASA: within 2 hours of awakening (Rx1), 7–9 hours after awakening (Rx2), or within 2 hours before bedtime (Rx3). The second blood pressure profile was obtained during the sixth and seventh days of treatment.

A statistically significant blood pressure reduction was obtained only when aspirin was given 7–9 hours after awakening (Rx2; $P = 0.012$, 0.003, and 0.006 for systolic, mean arterial, and diastolic blood pressure, respectively). These results were corroborated by a nonparametric (sign) test, also indicating the significant reduction in systolic and diastolic BP for Rx2 ($P = 0.003$ and 0.010, respectively) [68]. The study was followed by an extensive documentation of within-day differences in aspirin effect, started at bedtime (presumably for the sake of compliance), rather than at 7–9 hours after awakening [69–72]; cf. [73].

10.12 CHRONOBIOLOGIC BLOOD PRESSURE TRIALS

A first chronobiological trial to optimize the circadian timing of an antihypertensive drug was conducted with prazosin at the U.S. National Institutes of Health and revealed large differences from the same dose of the drug [74]. A trial by Rina Zaslavskaya [75], the pioneer in chronocardiology, compared a three-times-a-day administration schedule with the timing of a single dose given about 2 hours before the daily time-macroscopic peak in systolic and/or diastolic blood pressure for propranolol, clonidine, and α-methyldopa: the single-dosing schedule was associated with an enhanced hypotensive effect, obtained with a lesser dose, and was accompanied by fewer side effects. In a double-blind, placebo-controlled N-of-1 study, six test times, equally distributed along the 24-hour scale during the waking span, were successfully used to determine the best administration time of the diuretic hydrochlorothiazide, the tests showing further, however, that the patient did not need the medication [76].

Effects of Micardis (telmisartan), an oral angiotensin II receptor (type AT_1) antagonist, alone or with low-dose aspirin, on blood pressure and other cardiovascular endpoints were examined on 20 patients with MESOR-hypertension in a crossover, double-blind, randomized study consisting of three stages, each lasting 7 days: (I) placebo, (II) Micardis, and (III) Micardis with low-dose aspirin. Treatment was administered each day at a different circadian stage, upon awakening and 3, 6, 9, 12, 15, and 18 hours after awakening. Each data series was analyzed by single cosinor and were further summarized by population-mean least-squares spectra [77]. At matched treatment times, the MESOR and circadian amplitude of each variable were compared among the three treatments by paired t-tests. A prominent circadian rhythm characterizes all variables. Micardis was associated not only with a lowering of blood pressure, but also with a reduction of the circadian blood pressure amplitude, as seen in the spectra of Figure 10.10. The decrease in circadian amplitude of BP may be of importance for patients diagnosed with a circadian blood pressure overswing, CHAT [78]. Such a drug effect on an endpoint of variability is usually not considered and if large enough may underlie the benefits conferred by angiotensin II receptor antagonists in reducing cardiovascular morbidity and mortality, beyond their ability to decrease blood pressure. The daily alternation of the treatment time in this study [77] was too fast to assess the merits of timing. For the purpose of examining the effect of the given treatment time in a patient, an interval of 17 days was used initially for systematically changing the timing of medication, as seen in Figures 10.11 and 10.12, with a check of the results as sequential testing [78], a procedure recommended for the initiation of treatment.

10.13 LIMITS TO INTERPRETATION

In 1987, Moore and Goo [79] reported that the severity of gastric mucosal injury produced by aspirin was endoscopically viewed greater in the morning as compared to the evening. Their study was based on the administration of 1300 mg of ASA, involving 14 subjects. In 1995, Nold et al. [80] reported that, based on a randomized double-blind double-dummy crossover trial, the "degree of gastric mucosal injury seen with both doses [1000 and 75 mg ASA] did not differ after morning and evening application." In the same year, another abstract by Nold et al. [81], however, presents numerical scores in two ways, as actual scores and video scores, and made the important observations that the use of a video may be more suitable to assess the severity of drug-induced gastrointestinal injury. Numerically, however, in 3 out of 4 comparisons of any difference in timing, numerically the values are higher at 2000h as compared to 0800h. No statistical significance was found for the day–night difference, and the authors' interpretation is that none exists, a view in agreement with a personal communication by John Moore, who regards the approach by Nold et al. [81] to be the more rigorous. The possibility remains, however, that chance, if not the larger dose used by Moore Goo [79], 1300 versus 1000 tested by Nold et al. [80], may have contributed to the detection or not of a within-day difference in the former versus the latter study by two-timepoint approaches. It also seems critical to note that the findings at two or three-timepoint studies, while they suffice to rule in a within-day difference, cannot be used to rule one out. The probability remains that two timepoints happen to be chosen incidentally at midline crossings of a rhythm with a large amplitude.

Likewise, even a six-timepoint approach, notably when it is based on single individuals at each timepoint, has its limitations and must be checked further, notably when its results are of borderline significance. Phase-zero studies are an efficient start, but not a definitive end to drug development.

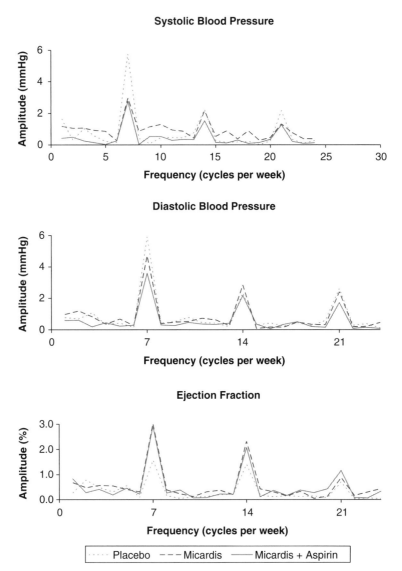

Figure 10.10. Least squares spectra of blood pressure and ejection fraction reveal peaks at frequencies of 7, 14, and 21 cycles per week, corresponding to periods of 24, 12, and 8 hours. Results reflect drug-induced changes in the prominence of the circadian component. The presence of harmonic terms (with periods of 12 and 8 hours) indicates that the circadian waveform differs from sinusoidality. Note that the circadian rhythm of blood pressure has a reduced circadian amplitude on treatment with Micardis, alone or with low-dose aspirin, as compared with placebo. Micardis affected the circadian BP amplitude, being associated with a decrease of 2.1 ± 0.3 mm Hg ($t = 7.138$; $P < 0.001$) in the case of SBP and of 1.3 ± 0.3 mm Hg ($t = 4.224$; $P < 0.001$) in the case of DBP. Micardis was also associated with an increase in the circadian amplitude of EF by $0.57 \pm 0.16\%$ ($t = 3.593$; $P < 0.001$). (From Ref. 77.) (*See color insert.*)

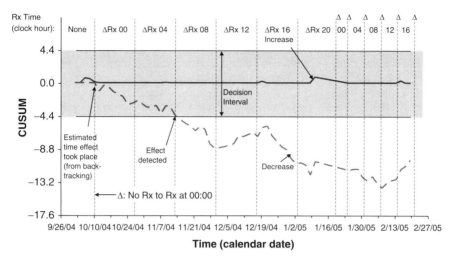

Figure 10.11. Changing timing of medication (ΔRx) during consecutive spans shows efficacy of treatment. An empirical approach to chronotherapy: immediately after diagnosis, one should ascertain that the treatment is effective. Optimization of treatment effects by timing can be achieved for the individual patient by systematically changing (e.g., advancing the time of treatment). Successful treatment of MESOR-hypertension assessed by a self-starting cumulative sum control chart [78]. To optimize his hypotensive treatment (Rx), a just-diagnosed 24-year-old individual (TT) switched his Rx first every 17 days by 4 hours and then mostly at shorter intervals. Note statistically significant decrease in MESOR, evidenced by the breakout outside the decision interval of the negative CUSUM line. With continued Rx, the blood pressure MESOR leaves the decision interval, indicating a statistically significant decrease in overall blood pressure [9]. The extent and even direction of effect is circadian stage-dependent.

10.14   DETECTION OF BLOOD PRESSURE AND HEART RATE VARIABILITY DISORDERS: CHALLENGE ALSO IN PROSPECTIVE PROCEDURES IN ANESTHESIOLOGY?

A time-structural (chronomic) interpretation of half-hourly blood pressure and heart rate records, monitored around the clock for a week, detects disease risk conditions such as the following:

1. MESOR-hypertension.
2. MESOR-hypotension, each defined more reliably in the 7-day summary than by a 24-hour record's analysis (Figures 10.13 and 10.14, upper half).
3. A circadian overswing or CHAT, short for **c**ircadian **h**yper**a**mplitude-**t**ension, that is for a double circadian amplitude, 2A, exceeding a gender- and age-matched peer group's reference limit [8, 9]. This predictor of cardiovascular complications is associated with a numerically higher risk

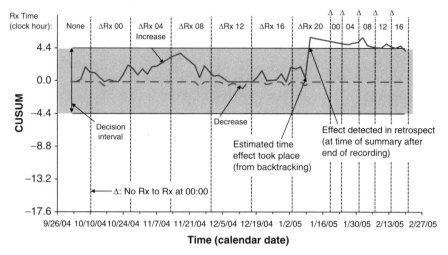

Figure 10.12. Changing timing of medication (ΔRx) during consecutive spans shows risk of iatrogenic CHAT. An empirical approach to chronotherapy: immediately after diagnosis, one should ascertain that one does not induce circadian hyperamplitu-detension (CHAT) by inappropriate timing of antihypertensive medication. In this 24-year old man (TT) who advanced the time of treatment by 4 hours every 17 days initially and at shorter intervals thereafter, treatment in the evening was associated with an increase in circadian amplitude, which could bring about CHAT iatrogenically when the circadian amplitude is high at the outset. This possibility raises the question of whether the risk of MESOR-hypertension may not have been traded for the even higher risk of stroke that CHAT represents [1, 8, 9]. Iatrogenic CHAT, putatively induced by treatment at 2000 h daily, was silent to office visits. With treatment at 2000 h, TT may have traded benefit (lowering of the MESOR of blood pressure, Figure 10.11) for something worse (circadian overswinging of blood pressure). This danger applies to some hypertensives (who tend to have a large circadian amplitude of blood pressure) to whom treatment time is not specified by the care provider, as was the case for TT (or is specified for a time that is not validated by monitoring). A few among many others who took a given hypotensive medication at bedtime have been found to have CHAT. The figure also shows the assessability of otherwise undetected harm by as-one-goes sequential analysis [9, 78].

than that of a high blood pressure [82, 83] and again is better assessed in a week-long, as compared to ~24-hour data analysis, as seen in the lower halves of Figures 10.13 and 10.14.

4. An above-adult threshold (of 60 mm Hg) circadianly assessed pulse pressure, yet to be gender- and age-specified.

5. An odd timing of the circadian rhythm in blood pressure but not in heart rate (circadian blood pressure ecphasia).

6. A below-adult threshold reduced circadian heart rate variability.

All these risk conditions, if diagnosed in several consecutive weekly overall summaries, should not be missed (see Figure 6 in Introduction to this book). Patients are in need of treatment, since evidence is available to show that a reduction, at least of the excessive M and the $2A$ of blood pressure, can result in a halving of hard events [84]. Some drugs that act selectively on one or more risk conditions, such as pulse pressure or circadian heart rate variability, are already reported [85]. Even when daily measures of a week's monitoring show abnormality, in view of the current limitation in the availability of instrumentation for monitoring, if the overall summary of the week's data as a whole is acceptable, no intervention is recommended and the subject can be advised to return in a year. If abnormality is found in the week's summary as a whole, another 7 days' or longer monitoring is recommended. When this second 7-day monitoring and summary shows no abnormality, this is satisfactory. In general practice, longer monitoring is warranted when the 2-week summary shows abnormality, with reference values for seasonal and other longer-than-yearly (transyearly) variability still to be collected in the future along with improved

CONSECUTIVE AVERAGES (above) and CIRCADIAN SWINGS (below) of SYSTOLIC BLOOD PRESSURE (SBP) DURING ~8 YEARS ALTERNATE BETWEEN MOSTLY ACCEPTABLE and PARTLY UNACCEPTABLE*

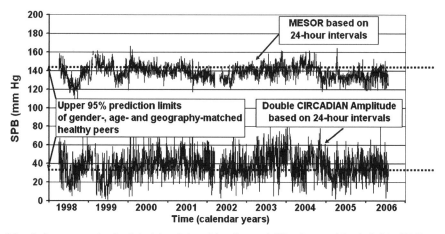

* Results from non-overlapping 1-day intervals in serial sections on half-hourly around the clock data; GK (M, 72-80 y) on varying treatments. ** MH = MESOR-Hypertension, CHAT = Circadian Hyper-Amplitude Tension.

Figure 10.13. Record of a physician under treatment with hypotensive drugs for several decades, who automatically recorded his blood pressure half-hourly with few gaps for about 8.5 years. In office spotchecks, his blood pressure seems acceptable. In one-day summaries in the upper half of the graph for the chronome-adjusted mean or MESOR, a dotted line showing the upper limit of acceptability is often exceeded, as is, in the bottom half of the graph, the dotted line showing the upper limit of acceptability of the double amplitude. Under treatment, in daily summaries, the patient has MESOR-hypertension 33.7%, and CHAT 60% of the time.

reference values for circadian and infradian variation. Definitive reference values will eventually have to be provided by peers screened for a disease-free lifetime record and will be specified for ethnicity as well as gender and age.

For some individuals, whether MESOR-normotensive or MESOR-hypertensive, monitored half-hourly around the clock for years or even decades, it is now documented in a yearly or much longer perspective, that opposite diagnoses in daily and even weekly summaries can occur so that weeks with a high M alternate with weeks with an acceptable M. The same finding applies to acceptable versus overswinging circadian double amplitudes, $2A$, of blood pressure: a week of CHAT can alternate with many weeks of acceptable $2A$ values (Figures 10.13 and 10.14).

Chronomically interpreted automatic ambulatory blood pressure monitoring, C-ABPM, reveals the extent of any efficacy of antihypertensive medication throughout the 24 hours and as a function of drug administration time, as assessed by sequential (e.g., CUSUM) testing [78]. Chronotherapy in the

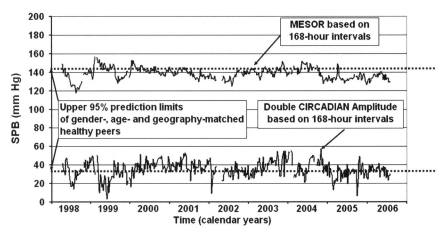

CONSECUTIVE AVERAGES (above) and CIRCADIAN SWINGS (below) of SYSTOLIC BLOOD PRESSURE (SBP) DURING ~8 YEARS ALTERNATE BETWEEN MOSTLY ACCEPTABLE and PARTLY UNACCEPTABLE*

* Results from non-overlapping 7-day intervals in serial sections on half-hourly around the clock data; GK (M, 72-80 y) on varying treatments. ** MH = MESOR-Hypertension, CHAT = Circadian Hyper-Amplitude Tension.

Figure 10.14. When the same record as that in Figure 10.13 is summarized on a weekly basis, transient MESOR-hypertension lasting only one or a few days, or transient CHAT, is somewhat washed out by the 24-hour cosine curve best-fitting all data; and hence based on the weekly summaries, MESOR-hypertension is largely successfully treated, but not the patient's CHAT. The merit of the 7-day summary has also been documented in a study on several hundred 7-day/24-hour profiles by Kuniaki Otsuka in Urausu, where the 7-day record in a 5-year perspective allowed the prediction of outcomes when omission of the last 6 days' data and sole reliance on the first 24-hour monitoring failed to predict outcomes (unpublished data).

treatment of MESOR-hypertension can play a major role, and just by changing the timing of treatment, blood pressure variability can be better controlled. CHAT, a great risk of stroke, can sometimes be eliminated, simply by a change of the timing of treatment instituted in the light of the results of monitoring [82–84]. The importance of C-ABPM and of the indices derived from its chronomic interpretation are just beginning to be documented and need greater appreciation and exploration, as a minimum to ascertain that we do not trade for an acceptable M an unacceptable $2A$ (Figures 10.13 and 10.14), a topic for assessment of outcomes in already available data from completed clinical trials.

Chronomics predict vascular disease risks and can treat some of them to prevent consequences such as stroke [84], heart attack, kidney disease, retinopathy, and depression, by prompting primary preventive action (pre-habilitation), specifically tailored to the abnormal patterns found (preventive chronotheranostics), that may be missed in current practice, since they often occur within the usual range of physiologic variation. These conditions constitute a great burden in terms of suffering and in health care cost. The use of preoperative ambulatory monitoring of blood pressure and heart rate and of postoperative temperature monitoring to detect alterations of parameters before fever (Figure 10.15) [86] remains to be tested.

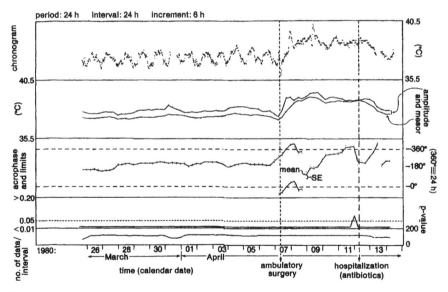

Figure 10.15. Retrospectively computed chronobiologic serial section of automatically recorded rectal temperature before, during, and after hospitalization for nosocomial infection following ambulatory surgery (D + C, 60-year-old woman). Note a change in acrophase (in row 3) preceding the onset of fever. If this were seen prospectively in other cases, it could serve as a putative early indicator for preventive treatment (e.g., to avoid sepsis) [86].

10.15 OPPORTUNITY

The foregoing evidence constitutes the working hypothesis of a group of volunteering engineers, the Phoenix Group (www.phoenix.tc-ieee.org), endeavoring eventually to offer cuffless, cheap blood pressure and heart rate hardware and software for self-help in health care. In the interim, the current generation of hardware for automatic monitoring is available via the BIOCOS project with an 80% reduction in cost (for a protocol and a copy of the data, with identity coded whenever the monitored individual wishes to guard anonymity). For both current hardware, at reduced cost, and analyses, interested parties may contact corne001@umn.edu.

10.16 CONCLUSION

Medical care delivery factors such as case load, fatigue, and care transitions are cited as influencing the rate of anesthetic adverse events for cases that start anesthesia in the late afternoon by Melanie C. Wright et al. [15]: "Post hoc inspection of data revealed that the predicted probability [of adverse events] increased from a low of 1.0% at 9 AM to a high of 4.2% at 4 PM. The two most common event types (pain management and postoperative nausea and vomiting) may be primary determinants of these effects … clinical outcomes may be different for patients anesthetized at the end of the work day compared with the beginning of the day."

Indeed, as early as 1929, different outcomes of surgery were reported as a function of time of day [87; cf. 29]. Laboratory experiments suggest that patient-related factors such as partly built-in circadian (and probably other) rhythms in response to anesthetics can play a critical role, tipping the scale between death and survival, with follow-up evidence subsequently reviewed along similar lines [14].

Much more broadly, we advocate the following:

1. Switching emphasis from the impact of the time of day in studies devoted to periodicity and timing of anesthesia, or any other drug treatment, to that of body time, detected by now-feasible physiological monitoring.
2. Giving preference, over pharmacokinetics, required by the Food and Drug Administration, to the critical issue of chronopharmacodynamics; a drug may reach the highest blood concentration when it is inactive.
3. Considering rhythms with more than a single frequency, that is, extra-circadians as part of a very broad spectrum of rhythms and an even broader time structure [1].
4. Realizing that chronomes also contain, in long time series, trends with age and disease risk elevation, and in dense time series, probabilistic and other chaos, in addition to the rhythm spectrum, which constitutes just one element of time structures for use in diagnostics and otherwise.

5. Recognizing that chronomes in us, as open systems, continuously interact with the chronomes of our cosmos, in a spectrum of nearly matching rhythms, in and around us, which contains some new, non-photic components (such as now-confirmed rhythms longer than a year) (1–3, extended in scope by 4 and 5); and that points 1–5 could be the basis of a budding pharmacochronomics, in the service, among others, of anesthesiology, as "patient-related factors," critical to changing health care from a spotcheck-based medicine flying blind most of the time to one based on time series collected outside the operating room as well as inside. Assessing disease risk by chronomically interpreted ambulatory blood pressure and heart rate monitoring (e.g., by screening before anesthesia) is an immediate challenge.

In a rodent, core temperature, motor activity, blood pressure, heart rate, the ECG, and the EEG can all be monitored for long spans, with changes of sensors for a lifetime. Sooner or later, the single blood pressure measurement, which has helped an immense number of people and has led to saving many lives for many of those who are now treated for hypertension, will be replaced by monitoring and saving a probably equally large, if not much larger section of people who can benefit from a transition from a spotcheck medicine to one that does for humans what can be done routinely today for a mouse because there is a demand for it in the pharmaceutical industry.

The as-yet putative merits of blood pressure, heart rate, and temperature monitoring for a week before anesthesia sound futuristic, but they will be applicable in anesthesiology once they are also applied in internal medicine [88, 89]. In the context of a search for a reduced heart rate variability and an excessive heart rate variability, Chassard and Bruguerolle [90] also note that "the application of such a technique to detect patients at risk for vascular complications during the perioperative period is promising but remains to be proven." In many other perspectives, the interested reader can be referred to this review [90]. A test of any merits of preoperative ambulatory screening by anesthesiologists may well be the best follow-up on the studies in the 1960s by the late James Matthews and Egon Marte [26].

REFERENCES

1. Halberg F, Cornélissen G, Katinas G, et al. Transdisciplinary unifying implications of circadian findings in the 1950s. *J Circadian Rhythms.* 2003; 1(2): 1–61. Available at www.JCircadianRhythms.com/content/pdf/1740-3391-2-3.pdf.

2. Halberg F, Cornélissen G, Schwartzkopff O, Bakken EE. Cycles in the biosphere in the service of solar–terrestrial physics? In: Schroeder W, ed. *Case Studies in Physics and Geophysics.* Bremen: Wilfried Schroeder/Science Edition; 2006: 39–87. [*Beiträge zur Geophysik und Kosmischen Physik/Journal for the History of Geophysics and Cosmical Physics,* Special issue, 2006/2. ISSN 1615-2824.]

3. Cornélissen G, Masalov A, Halberg F, et al. Multiple resonances among time structures, chronomes, around and in us. Is an about 1.3-year periodicity in solar wind built into the human cardiovascular chronome? *Human Physiol*. 2004; 30(2): 86–92.

4. Mikulecky M, Florida PL. Daily birth numbers in Davao, Philippines, 1993–2003: Halberg's transyear stronger than year. Abstract, 26th Seminar, Man in His Terrestrial and Cosmic Environment, Upice, Czech Republic, May 17–19, 2005.

5. Kovac M, Mikulecky M. Secular rhythms and Halberg's paraseasonality in the time occurrence of cerebral stroke. *Bratisl Lek Listy*. 2005; 106(2): 423–427.

6. Richardson JD, Paularena KI, Belcher JW, Lazarus AJ. Solar wind oscillations with a 1.3-year period. *Geophys Res Lett*. 1994; 21: 1559–1560.

7. Watanabe Y, Cornélissen G, Katinas G, Schwartzkopff O, Halberg F. Case report: a drug for damping circannual and transannual amplitudes of blood pressure and heart rate. In: *2nd International Symposium, Problems of Rhythms in Natural Sciences*, Moscow, March 1–3, 2004. Moscow: Russian People's Friendship University; 2004: 18–20.

8. Halberg F, Cornélissen G, Katinas G, et al. Chronobiology's progress: season's appreciations 2004–2005. Time-, frequency-, phase-, variable-, individual-, age- and site-specific chronomics. *J Appl Biomed*. 2006; 4: 1–38. Available at http://www.zsf.jcu.cz/vyzkum/jab/4_1/halberg.pdf

9. Halberg F, Cornélissen G, Katinas G, et al. Chronobiology's progress: Part II, chronomics for an immediately applicable biomedicine. *J Appl Biomed*. 2006; 4: 73–86. Available at http://www.zsf.jcu.cz/vyzkum/jab/4_2/halberg2.pdf.

10. Grafe A. Einige charakterische Besonderheiten des geomagnetischen Sonneneruptionseffektes. *Geofis Pura Appl*. 1958; 40: 172–179.

11. Russell CT, McPherron RL. Semiannual variation of geomagnetic activity. *J Geophys Res*. 1973; 78: 92–108.

12. Rieger A, Share GH, Forrest DJ, Kanbach G, Reppin C, Chupp EL. A 154-day periodicity in the occurrence of hard solar flares? *Nature*. 1984; 312: 623–625.

13. Sothern SB, Sothern RB, Katinas GS, Cornélissen G, Halberg F. Sampling at the same clock-hour in long-term investigation is no panacea. In: *Proceedings of the International Conference on the Frontiers of Biomedical Science: Chronobiology*, Chengdu, China, September 24–26, 2006, pp. 208–211.

14. Chassard D, Allaouchiche B, Boselli E. Timing is everything: the pendulum swings on. *Anesthesiology*. 2005; 103: 454–456.

15. Wright MC, Phillips-Bute B, Mark JB, et al. Time of day effects on the incidence of anesthetic adverse events. *Quality Safety Health Care*. 2006; 15: 258–263.

16. Halberg F. Chronobiology. *Annu Rev Physiol*. 1969; 31: 675–725.

17. Refinetti R, Cornélissen G, Halberg F. Procedures for numerical analysis of circadian rhythms. *Biol Rhythm Res*. 2007; 38(4): 275–325.

18. Halberg F. Symposium on "Some current research methods and results with special reference to the central nervous system." Physiopathologic approach. *Am J Ment Defic*. 1960; 65: 156–171.

19. Chibisov SM, Cornélissen G, Halberg F. Magnetic storm effect on the circulation of rabbits. *Biomed Pharmacother*. 2004; 58 (suppl 1): S15–S19.

20. Jozsa R, Halberg F, Cornélissen G, et al. Chronomics, neuroendocrine feedside-wards and the recording and consulting of nowcasts — forecasts of geomagnetics. *Biomed Pharmacother*. 2005; 59 (suppl 1): S24–S30.

21. Halberg F, Cornélissen G, Schwartzkopff O, et al. Chronometaanalysis: magnetic storm associated with a reduction in circadian amplitude of rhythm in corneal cell division. In: Proceedings of the International Conference on the Frontiers of Biomedical Science: Chronobiology, Chengdu, China, September 24–26, 2006, pp. 40–42.

22. Cornélissen G, Halberg F, Schwartzkopff O, et al. Chronomes, time structures, for chronobioengineering for "a full life." *Biomed Instrum Technol*. 1999; 33: 152–187.

23. Otsuka K, Oinuma S, Cornélissen G, et al. Alternating-light–darkness-influenced human electrocardiographic magnetoreception in association with geomagnetic pulsations. *Biomed Pharmacother*. 2001; 55 (suppl 1): 63s–75s.

24. Oinuma S, Kubo Y, Otsuka K, et al. Graded response of heart rate variability, associated with an alteration of geomagnetic activity in a subarctic area. *Biomed Pharmacother*. 2002; 56 (suppl 2): 284s–288s.

25. Edlund Y, Holmgren HJ. Experimentelle Studien des Verhaltens der Narkose zu verschiedenen Zeiten der 24Stundenperiode. *Z Gesamte Exp Med*. 1939; 107: 26–52.

26. Matthews JH, Marte E, Halberg F. A circadian susceptibility-resistance cycle to fluothane in male B_1 mice. *Can Anaesthetists' Soc J*. 1964; 11: 280–290.

27. Halberg F, Bittner JJ, Gully RJ, Albrecht PG, Brackney EL 24-Hour periodicity and audiogenic convulsions in I mice of various ages. *Proc Soc Exp Biol (NY)*. 1955; 88: 169–173.

28. Halberg F, Jacobson E, Wadsworth G, Bittner JJ. Audiogenic abnormality spectra, 24-hour periodicity and lighting. *Science*. 1958; 128: 657–658.

29. Halberg F. Temporal coordination of physiologic function. *Cold Spring Harb Symp Quant Biol*. 1960; 25: 289–310. Discussion on LD_{50}, p 310.

30. Haus E, Halberg F, Loken MK, Kim US. *Circadian rhythmometry of mammalian radiosensitivity*. In: Tobias A, Todd P, eds. *Space Radiation Biology*. New York: Academic Press; 1973: 435–474.

31. Halberg F. Biological as well as physical parameters relate to radiology. Guest Lecture, Proceedings of the 30th Annual Congres on Radiology, January 1977, Post-Graduate Institute of Medical Education and Research, Chandigarh, India.

32. Halberg F, Cornélissen G, Wang ZR, et al. Chronomics: circadian and circaseptan timing of radiotherapy, drugs, calories, perhaps nutriceuticals and beyond. *J Exp Ther Oncol*. 2003; 3: 223–260.

33. Halberg F, Spink WW, Albrecht PG, Gully RJ. Resistance of mice to *Brucella* somatic antigen, 24-hour periodicity and the adrenals. *J Clin Endocrinol*. 1955; 15: 887.

34. Halberg F, Johnson EA, Brown BW, Bittner JJ. Susceptibility rhythm to *E. coli* endotoxin and bioassay. *Proc Soc Exp Biol (NY)*. 1960; 103: 142–144.

35. Haus E, Halberg F. 24-Hour rhythm in susceptibility of C mice to a toxic dose of ethanol. *J Appl Physiol*. 1959; 14: 878–880.

36. Nagayama H, Cornélissen G, Pandi-Perumal SR, Halberg F. Time-dependent psychotropic drug effects: hints of pharmacochronomics, broader than circadian time structures. In: Lader M, Cardinali DP, Pandi-Perumal SP, eds. *Sleep and Sleep Disorders: A Neuropsychopharmacological Approach.* Georgetown, TX: Landes Bioscience; 2005: 34–71.

37. Halberg F, Stephens AN. Susceptibility to ouabain and physiologic circadian periodicity. *Proc Minn Acad Sci.* 1959; 27: 139–143.

38. Marte E, Halberg F. Circadian susceptibility rhythm of mice to librium. *Fed Proc.* 1961; 20: 305.

39. Savage IR, Rao MM, Halberg F. Test of peak values in physiopathologic time series. *Exp Med Surg.* 1962; 20: 309–317.

40. Jones F, Haus E, Halberg F. Murine circadian susceptibility-resistance cycle to acetylcholine. *Proc Minn Acad Sci.* 1963; 31: 61–62.

41. Marte E, Nelson DO, Halberg F, Matthews JH. Circadian rhythms in murine susceptibility to the anesthetics halothane and methohexital. In: Walker CA, Winget CM, Soliman KFA, eds. *Chronopharmacology and Chronotherapeutics.* Tallahassee, FL: Florida A&M University Foundation; 1981: 89–94.

42. Nelson W, Halberg F, mathematical appendix by Hwang DS. An evaluation of time-dependent changes in susceptibility of mice to pentobarbital injection. *Neuropharmacology.* 1973; 12: 509–524.

43. Nelson W, Kupferberg H, Halberg F Dose–response evaluations of a circadian rhythmic change in susceptibility of mice to ouabain. *Toxicol Appl Pharmacol.* 1971; 18: 335–339.

44. Halberg F, Cornélissen G, Regal P, et al. Chronoastrobiology: proposal, nine conferences, heliogeomagnetics, transyears, near-weeks, near-decades, phylogenetic and ontogenetic memories. *Biomed Pharmacother.* 2004; 58(suppl 1): S150–S187.

45. Halberg F, Bakken EE, Katinas GS, et al. Chronoastrobiology: Vernadsky's future science ? Benefits from spectra of circadians and promise of a new transdisciplinary spectrum of near-matching cycles in and around us. Opening keynote. In: Proceedings, III International Conference, Civilization Diseases in the Spirit of V. I. Vernadsky, October 10–12, 2005. Moscow: People's Friendship University of Russia; 2005: 4–25.

46. Halberg F, Cornélissen G, Watanabe Y, et al. Transient circadian blood pressure overswing (CHAT), an intermediate stage between MESOR-normo- and –hypertension. In: Proceedings of the International Conference on the Frontiers of Biomedical Science: Chronobiology, Chengdu, China, September 24–26, 2006, pp. 6–10.

47. Halberg F. From aniatrotoxicosis and aniatrosepsis toward chronotherapy: Introductory remarks to the 1974 Capri Symposium on timing and toxicity: the necessity for relating treatment to bodily rhythms. In: Aschoff J, Ceresa F, Halberg F, eds. *Chronobiological Aspects of Endocrinology.* Stuttgart: FK Schattauer Verlag; 1974: 1–34.

48. Cornélissen G, Halberg E, Haus E, et al. Chronobiology pertinent to gynecologic oncology. University of Minnesota/Medtronic Chronobiology Seminar Series, #5, July 1992, 25 pp. text, 7 tables, 30 figures.

49. Walker WV, Russell JE, Simmons DJ, Scheving LE, Cornélissen G, Halberg F Effect of an adrenocorticotropin analogue, ACTH 1-17, on DNA synthesis in murine metaphyseal bone. *Biochem Pharmacol.* 1985; 34: 1191–1196.

50. Chaudhry AP, Halberg F, Bittner JJ Epinephrine and mitotic activity in pinnal epidermis of the mouse. *J Appl Physiol.* 1956; 9: 265–267.

51. Chiakulas JJ, Scheving LE, Winston S The effects of exogenous epinephrine and environmental stress stimuli on the mitotic rates of larval urodele tissues. *Exp Cell Res.* 1966; 41: 197–205.

52. Halberg F, Cornélissen G, Salti R, et al. Chronoauxology. Chronomics: trends and cycles in growth and cosmos rather than secularity. In: Proceedings, 10th Auxology Congress: Human Growth in Sickness and in Health, Florence, July 4–7 2004.

53. Halberg E, Halberg F Chronobiologic study design in everyday life, clinic and laboratory. *Chronobiologia.* 1980; 7: 95–120.

54. Cornélissen G, Halberg F, Schwartzkopff O, et al. Coenzyme-Q10 effect on blood pressure variability assessed with a chronobiological study design. In: *Noninvasive Methods in Cardiology,* Brno, Czech Republic, September 14, 2005, p 10.

55. Bartsch C, Bartsch H, Jain AK, Laumas KR, Wetterberg L Urinary melatonin levels in human breast cancer patients. *J Neur Trans.* 1981; 52: 281–294.

56. Langevin T, Hrushesky W, Sanchez S, Halberg F Melatonin (M) modulates survival of CD_2F_1 mice with L1210 leukemia. *Chronobiologia.* 1983; 10: 173–174.

57. Halberg F, Cornélissen G, Conti A, et al. The pineal gland and chronobiologic history: mind and spirit as feedsidewards in time structures for prehabilitation. In: Bartsch C, Bartsch H, Blask DE, Cardinali DP, Hrushesky WJM, Mecke W, eds. *The Pineal Gland and Cancer: Neuroimmunoendocrine Mechanisms in Malignancy.* Heidelberg: Springer; 2001: 66–116.

58. Cornélissen G, Halberg F, Perfetto F, Tarquini R, Maggioni C, Wetterberg L. Melatonin involvement in cancer: methodological considerations. In: Bartsch C, Bartsch H, Blask DE, Cardinali DP, Hrushesky WJM, Mecke W, eds. *The Pineal Gland and Cancer: Neuroimmunoendocrine Mechanisms in Malignancy.* Heidelberg: Springer; 2001: 117–149.

59. Sanchez de la Pena S The feedsideward of cephalo-adrenal immune interactions. *Chronobiologia.* 1993; 20: 1–52.

60. Peto R, Pike MC, Armitage P, et al. Design and analysis of randomized clinical trials requiring prolonged observation of each patient. I. Introduction and design. *Br J Cancer.* 1976; 34: 585II. Analysis and examples. *Br J Cancer.* 1977;35:1.

61. Cornélissen G, Halberg F. The chronobiologic pilot study with special reference to cancer research: Is chronobiology or, rather, its neglect wasteful? In: Goldson AL, ed. *Cancer Growth and Progression,* vol. 9, Chap 9, Kaiser H, series ed. Dordrecht: Kluwer Academic Publishers; 1989: 103–133.

62. Ames T, Portela A, Cornélissen G, et al. Species difference in the salivary vs. serum concentration of the proliferation marker CA130 in human vs. ruminant. Combined Meeting of American Association of Bovine Practitioners and World Buiatrics Congress, St Paul, MN, August 29–September 4, 1992. In: Cornélissen G, Halberg E, Bakken E, Delmore P, Halberg F, eds. Toward Phase Zero Preclinical and Clinical Trials: Chronobiologic Designs and Illustrative Aapplications. University

of Minnesota Medtronic Chronobiology Seminar Series, #6, September 1992. p. 357–361.

63. Cornélissen G, Halberg E, Haus E, O'Brien T, Berg H, Sackett-Lundeen L, Fujii S, Twiggs L, Halberg F, *International Womb-to-Tomb Chronome Initiative Group.* Chronobiology pertinent to gynecologic oncology. University of Minnesota/Medtronic Chronobiology Seminar Series, #5, July 1992, 25 pp. text, 7 tables, 30 figures.

64. Günther R, Herold M, Halberg E, Halberg F Circadian placebo and ACTH effects on urinary cortisol in arthritics. *Peptides.* 1980; 1: 387–390.

65. Halberg F, Cornélissen G, Katinas GS, et al. Feedsidewards: intermodulation (strictly) among time structures, chronomes, in and around us, and cosmo-vasculo-neuroimmunity. About ten-yearly changes: what Galileo missed and Schwabe found. *Ann NY Acad Sci.* 2000; 917: 348–376.

66. Cornélissen G, Halberg F, Prikryl P, et al. Prophylactic aspirin treatment: the merits of timing. *JAMA.* 1991; 266: 3128–3129.

67. Siegelova J, Cornélissen G, Dusek J, et al. Aspirin and the blood pressure and heart rate of healthy women. *Policlinico (Chrono).* 1995; 1(2): 43–49.

68. Hermida RC, Fernandez JR, Ayala DE, Iglesias M, Halberg F Time-dependent effects of ASA administration on blood pressure in healthy subjects. *Chronobiologia.* 1994; 21: 201–213.

69. Hermida RC, Ayala DE, Calvo C, et al. Administration time-dependent effects of aspirin on blood pressure in untreated hypertensive patients. *Hypertension.* 2003; 41: 1259–1267.

70. Hermida RC, Ayala DE, Iglesias M. Administration time-dependent influence of aspirin on blood pressure in pregnant women. *Hypertension.* 2003; 41(3 Pt 2): 651–656.

71. Hermida RC, Ayala DE, Calvo C, et al. Differing administration time-dependent effects of aspirin on blood pressure in dipper and non-dipper hypertensives. *Hypertension.* 2005; 46: 1060–1068.

72. Hermida RC, Ayala DE, Calvo C, Lopez JE. Aspirin administered at bedtime, but not on awakening, has an effect on ambulatory blood pressure in hypertensive patients. *J Am Coll Cardiol.* 2005; 46: 975–983.

73. Messerli FH. Aspirin: a novel antihypertensive drug? Or two birds with one stone? *J Am Coll Cardiol.* 2005; 46: 984–985.

74. Güllner HG, Bartter FC, Halberg F. Timing antihypertensive medication. *Lancet.* 1979; Sep 8: 527.

75. Zaslavskaya. RM Chronodiagnosis and Chronotherapy of Cardiovascular Diseases, 2nd edition. Translation into English from Russian. Moscow: Medicina; 1993.

76. Little J, Sanchez de la Peña S, Cornélissen G, Abramowitz P, Tuna N, Halberg F. Longitudinal chronobiologic blood pressure monitoring for assessing the need and timing of antihypertensive treatment. *Prog Clin Biol Res.* 1990; 341B: 601–611.

77. Prikryl P, Cornélissen G, Neubauer J, Prikryl P Jr, Karpisek Z, Watanabe Y, et al. Chronobiologically explored effects of telmisartan. *Clin Exp Hypertension.* 2005; 2 & 3: 119–128.

78. Cornélissen G, Halberg F, Hawkins D, Otsuka K, Henke W. Individual assessment of antihypertensive response by self-starting cumulative sums. *J Med Eng Technol.* 1997; 21: 111–120.

79. Moore JG, Goo RH. Day and night aspirin-induced gastric mucosal damage and protection by ranitidine in man. *Chronobiol Int.* 1987; 4: 111–116.

80. Nold G, Drossard W, Lehmann K, Lemmer B. Daily variation of acute gastric mucosal injury after high- and low-dose acetylsalicylic acid. *Biol Rhythm Res.* 1995; 26: 428.

81. Nold G, Drossard W, Lehmann K, Lemmer B. Gastric mucosal lesions after morning versus evening application of 75 mg or 1000 mg acetylsalicylic acid (ASA). *Naunyn-Schmiedeberg's Arch Pharmacol.* 1995; 351: R17.

82. Otsuka K, Cornélissen G, Halberg F. Predictive value of blood pressure dipping and swinging with regard to vascular disease risk. *Clin Drug Invest.* 1996; 11: 20–31.

83. Halberg F, Cornélissen G, International Womb-to-Tomb Chronome Initiative Group. Resolution from a meeting of the International Society for Research on Civilization Diseases and the Environment (New SIRMCE Confederation), Brussels, Belgium, March 17–18, 1995: *Fairy Tale or Reality?* Medtronic Chronobiology Seminar #8, April 1995, 12 pp. text, 18 figures. Available at http://www.msi.umn.edu/~halberg/.

84. Shinagawa M, Kubo Y, Otsuka K, Ohkawa S, Cornélissen G, Halberg F. Impact of circadian amplitude and chronotherapy: relevance to prevention and treatment of stroke. *Biomed Pharmacother.* 2001; 55(suppl 1): 125–132.

85. Fok BSP, Cornélissen G, Halberg F, Chu TTW, Thomas GN, Tomlinson B. Different effects of lercanidipine and felodipine on circadian blood pressure and heart rate among hypertensive patients. Abstract 15, HK College of Cardiology, 12th Annual Science Congress. *J Hong Kong Coll Cardiol.* 2004; 12: 33.

86. Halberg E, Fanning R, Halberg F, et al. Toward a chronopsy: Part III. Automatic monitoring of rectal, axillary and breast surface temperature and of wrist activity; effects of age and of ambulatory surgery followed by nosocomial infection. *Chronobiologia.* 1981; 8: 253–271.

87. Frey S Der Tod des. Menschen in seinen Beziehungen zu den Tages und Jahreszeiten. *Dtsch Z Chir.* 1929; 218: 366–369.

88. Cornélissen G, Halberg F, Otsuka K, Singh RB, Chen CH. Chronobiology predicts actual and proxy outcomes when dipping fails. *Hypertension.* 2007; 49: 237–239.

89. Halberg F, Cornélissen G, Halberg J, Schwartzkopff O. Pe-hypertensive and other variabilities also await treatment. *Am J Medicine.* 2007; 120: e19–e20.

90. Chassard D, Bruguerolle B. Chronobiology and anesthesia. *Anesthesiology.* 2004; 100: 413–427.

CHAPTER 11

TREATMENT WITH OPEN EYES: MARKERS-GUIDED CHRONOTHERANOSTICS*

GERMAINE CORNÉLISSEN, and FRANZ HALBERG

"I must govern the clock (treating by marker rhythms), not be governed by it."
— *Golda Meir (1969–1974), paraphrased*

CONTENTS

*Dedicated to Earl E. Bakken, who started chronotheranostics over half a century ago by restoring a failing heart rhythm and who led the way to closing the loop between diagnosis and treatment by his development of implantable devices.

Chronopharmaceutics: Science and Technology for Biological Rhythm-Guided Therapy and Prevention of Diseases, edited by Bi-Botti C. Youan
Copyright © 2009 John Wiley & Sons, Inc.

11.1   INTRODUCTION

Chronobiological trials have demonstrated the merits of assessing the time structure of marker variables to recognize a heightened risk of disease, to specify the kind and timing of treatment, and to evaluate and optimize the patient's response [1, 2]. By so doing, abnormalities in the pattern of the circadian (or other) rhythm are part of the diagnosis (and prognosis) (chronodiagnosis) [2]. Because such abnormalities are usually observed within the physiological range, before there is overt disease, preventive measures can be initiated in a timely fashion. Correcting an ongoing treatment plan can also be carried out earlier, in order to avoid excessive toxicity and most importantly to improve efficacy [3]. Chrono-biological trials have also demonstrated the merit of timing the administration of treatment (chronotherapy), even for 24-hour formulations [4]. Very often, how-ever, the desire to generalize and to seek "the optimal time (or schedule)" to administer a given treatment overlooks the even greater necessity of individualiz-ing the therapeutic plan. Therein lies a major merit of marker-rhythmometry. Adjusting the scheduling of treatment according to the kind of abnormal pattern diagnosed, a procedure referred to as chronotheranostics, addresses this need of individualized temporal and all other therapeutic optimization.

Markers-guided chronotheranostics is best implemented when the following requirements are met:

1. One or several marker variables are available and can easily and cost-effectively be measured repeatedly. Longitudinal around-the-clock mea-surements of variables directly pertinent to the medical problem on hand are ideal but may not always be feasible or cost-effectively practicable.

2. Protocols can be designed to effectively determine optimal treatment schedules. It is often thought that chronotherapeutic trials are much more costly than usual trials because the cost needs to be multiplicd by the number of treatment schedules tested. This misconception will be dispelled. More difficult to achieve but not impossible is the

implementation of *N*-of-1 designs that make the individualization of timed treatment feasible.

3. Outcome measures are available that can shed light on the efficacy of treatment and identify the presence of any undesired effects.

4. Statistical methods can be applied not only for groups of patients but also for individual subjects, to recognize abnormality, to assess whether treatment was efficient, and to determine whether one treatment schedule is superior to another.

While chronotherapy has been used successfully in different medical specialties, applications in relation to blood pressure disorders will be emphasized herein, for the simple reason that, in this case, blood pressure is a most pertinent variable easily monitored around the clock for long spans. It also has the merit that it can be used as a multiple-purpose marker, to assess the efficacy of a given intervention, to guide the optimization of its timing, and to survey its continued efficacy. Before turning to medical applications, a brief, generally relevant methodological overview introduces chronobiological concepts for study designs and for data analysis.

11.2 METHODOLOGICAL OVERVIEW

Currently, no general provisions are made for defining what the optimal circadian (or other) rhythm stages are at which to administer a given pharmacological or nonpharmacological treatment, despite much evidence suggesting that timing is important [5, 6]. For drugs found to be effective preclinically, Phase I clinical trials are designed to determine tolerated doses associated with acceptable side effects, at times usually dictated by convenience rather than pertinence [7]. Timing, the critical ingredient of chronobiological designs, is not just another factor like genetics and nutrition that can be ignored, when under the standardized conditions of the experimental laboratory, it has been repeatedly shown that timing can tip the scale between health and disease and even between death and survival after exposure to a fixed dose of a potentially noxious agent (Figure 11.1) [8]. While timing remains an essential factor in Phase II and Phase III trials focusing on treatment efficacy and a comparison with the current best treatment, respectively, the case has been made to incorporate "Phase 0" chronobiological pilot designs at the outset [9–11]. These would aim at detecting, sooner and with smaller sample sizes [12], desired or undesired effects that may otherwise be missed.

The misconception that chronobiological designs are too expensive, assuming that the needed sample size should be multiplied by the number of rhythm stages to be tested, is easily dispelled by the following considerations:

1. Most biological variables are characterized by a ubiquitous time structure composed of multifrequency rhythms, chaos, and trends. Rather than

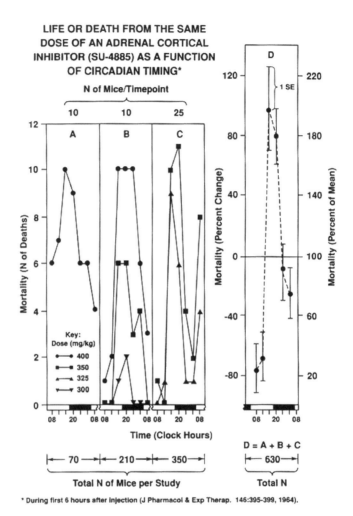

Figure 11.1. Dose affects circadian amplitude of neuron susceptibility resistance cycle to SU-4885, assessed by single component model.

unnecessarily inflating the error term by ignoring rhythms, their assessment is incorporated into study designs, samples being spread uniformly to cover several stages of the rhythm under consideration rather than collecting samples without time specification. Circadian rhythms are usually prominent. Ignoring such large-amplitude predictable variation by sampling at any time during usual office hours yields estimates of mean values associated with an inflated dispersion index, as illustrated in Figure 11.2.

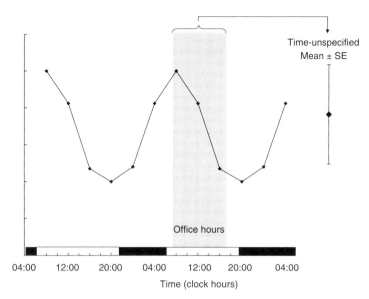

Figure 11.2. Large dispersion when measurements are not time-specified. Physiological variables such as cortisol are characterized by large-amplitude circadian rhythms. Ignoring the rhythmic structure of this variable may unduly inflate the dispersion index, notably when measurements are taken during only a portion of the cycle such as regular office hours (e.g., from 0700h to 1700h), a span that covers most of the predictable range of variation assumed by this variable.

2. When the merits of two treatments need to be compared, the lack of time specification is associated with the need for large sample sizes to detect a difference in view of the inflated standard deviation (Figure 11.3, top).
3. With large sample sizes, however, some spurious differences may result from a phase difference when sampling is limited to part of the cycle (e.g., during office hours; Figure 11.3, bottom). This situation may arise when two anticancer drugs that act on a different stage of the cell cycle are compared: their mechanism of action being different, the circadian stage of highest efficacy and/or tolerance is likely to differ accordingly. While the two drugs are administered during the same subspan of the 24-hour day, differences in effect may hence not reflect a true difference in treatment efficacy. Figure 11.4 summarizes results from 35 studies on 5266 rodents investigating the tolerance of seven different anticancer drugs, with corresponding therapeutic gains shown in Figure 11.5 [13].
4. Failure to account for the rhythmic behavior of the variable investigated may further lead to controversial results, large differences in opposite directions being reported by investigators working at two different times (e.g., in the morning or in the late afternoon or evening). As illustrated in

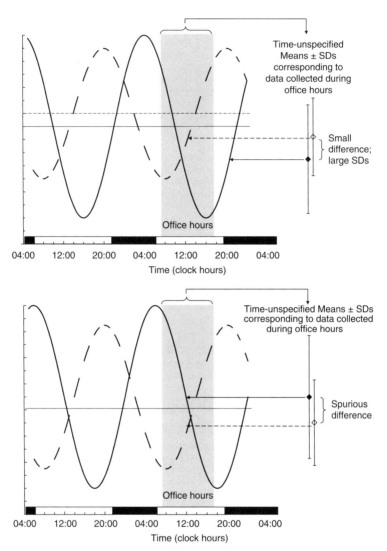

Figure 11.3. A heavy price for ignoring the chronome's rhythms in current Phase III trials. Top: The need for large sample sizes may arise from the following situation: When rhythmic variables are sampled during "regular" hours (e.g., from 0700h to 1700h) and are characterized by large-amplitude circadian rhythms with different phases, the dispersion indices around the mean value of each variable will be very large, much larger than the difference in mean value between the two rhythmic variables. A large sample size is hence needed to detect such a difference, which may be small compared to the dispersion index. Bottom: There is also the danger that in the absence of a real difference, large sample sizes may detect spurious differences. This situation may arise from a phase difference between two rhythmic variables sampled during the same span (e.g., from 0700h to 1700h), corresponding to only a subspan of the full cycle of variation of these variables.

CIRCADIAN TIMING OF TOLERANCE OF ANTI-CANCER DRUGS

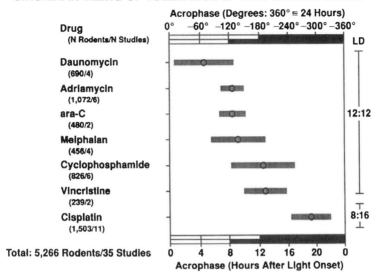

Figure 11.4. Different times of optimal resistance to the toxicity of a few anticancer drugs. Acrophase chart of cosinor results.

Figure 11.6, controversial differences may stem from a difference in amplitude, phase, or period.

5. When treatments are being compared, concern about statistical power usually prompts investigators to limit the comparison to two or as few groups as possible [14–17]. Whereas statistical power is indeed greater with fewer groups when relying on conventional tests such as the one-way analysis of variance, it is not the case when results are assessed in the light of a model such as the cosinor, used in chronobiology to find optimal times of treatment administration [9]. As illustrated in Figure 11.7, limiting the design to two test times may be optimal when the times of highest and smallest responses are known a priori (top left), but if this is not the case, there is the risk of inadvertently selecting two test times corresponding to the midline crossings, thereby failing to detect differences of potential great benefit to the patients (top right). Whereas three timepoints are sufficient to determine a rhythmic pattern if it does not deviate too much from sinusoidality (bottom left), six timepoints are usually sufficient to define a rhythm (bottom right). In this case, estimates of uncertainties for all parameters involved can also be obtained.

6. Critical for the individualized optimization of treatment timing is the availability of statistical procedures applicable to the individual patient providing a longitudinal record of one or several marker variables. As illustrated later for the case of blood pressure, parameter tests [18] can detect not only a change in the mean value but also differences in

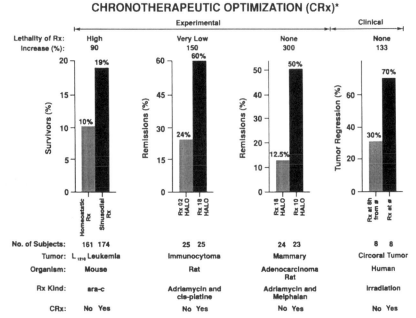

Figure 11.5. Chronotherapeutic optimization of cancer treatment in experimental animals (first 6 columns), and in clinical radiotherapy research (last 2 columns). In each pair, the column on the right shows the gain from timing, with the column on the left in each pair serving as reference standard.

other rhythm characteristics such as the amplitude and acrophase (timing of overall high values recurring in each cycle). Cumulative sum (CUSUM) control charts [19, 20]; see also Ref. [21] can also determine whether a desired therapeutic goal has been achieved, insofar as a given endpoint departs from a decision interval, the latter corresponding to "no statistically significant change." When used to assess a patient's response to treatment, a directional change can be anticipated. Since the time of intervention is known, the CUSUM can further relate the effectiveness of the treatment to the time of its administration, thereby providing an inferential statistical approximation of causality.

11.3   APPLICATIONS IN ONCOLOGY

11.3.1   Chronoradiotherapy of Perioral Tumors

It had been shown in the laboratory that subgroups of mice responded differently to the exposure to 400, 450, or 500 roentgens of total body X-irradiation at one of six different circadian stages, 4 hours apart [22].

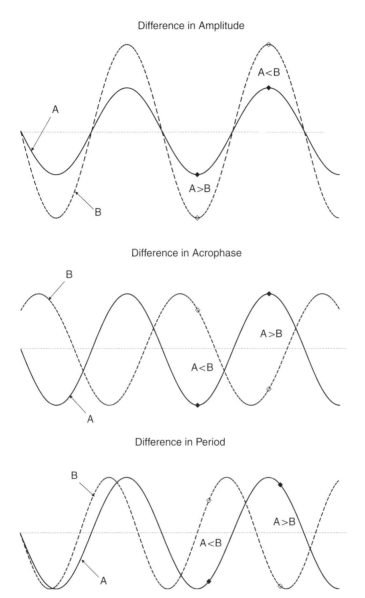

Figure 11.6. Opposite results may be obtained at two different test times when the underlying rhythmic patterns of two groups being compared are characterized by a difference in amplitude, acrophase, or period.

From mortality at each dose and at each test time, a dose was computed that killed 50% of the animals within 30 days. The highest tolerance was found to occur during the second half of the light (rest) span [22]. Against this background, a study in India sought the optimal circadian stage to administer

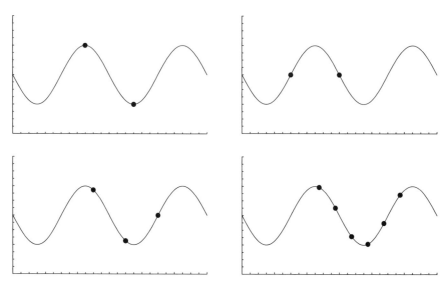

Figure 11.7. A two-test-time approach on a cycle is often carried out and thought to be optimal (top left). This is true only when the times of spontaneous minima and maxima or of the minimal and maximal response are known. The spread of the observations is then maximal. Correspondingly, the power may also be maximal. If, however, the exact timing of the rhythmic function is not known, or is likely to be altered in certain circumstances or may differ among individuals, then one takes the risk of sampling at the midline crossings (top right). A prominent rhythm may hence remain undetected and unexploited. Major gain is obtained by adding single subjects and test times, for example, from three to six equidistant experimental units (bottom) such as patients per cycle investigated. Three test times per cycle allow the estimation of rhythm characteristics (#1) but do not suffice for hypothesis testing (#2) or for the derivation of confidence intervals for the parameters (#3). A design involving six test times per cycle is parsimonious and powerful for achieving all three purposes.

radiotherapy in patients with large cancers of the oral cavity amenable to temperature measurement around the clock for a few days prior to treatment [13, 23]. The response to radiotherapy could also be readily assessed at least semiquantitatively by measuring tumor size. Groups of 8 patients each were scheduled for 5 weeks of radiotherapy, 5 days per week. Patients were randomly assigned to be treated at the time of peak tumor temperature, or 4 or 8 hours before or after that time. Another control group was treated "as usual," with no regard for timing. As seen in Figure 11.8 (left), the average tumor regression rate was much higher for patients treated at the optimal time of peak tumor temperature than for patients treated at the worst time (8 hours after the time of peak tumor temperature). Moreover, the tumor regression rate follows a predictable circadian pattern depending on the circadian stage of treatment administration in relation to the patient's circadian temperature variation used as marker rhythm ($P = 0.042$); see Figure 11.8 (right) [13, 23]. These short-term results based on tumor regression rate are in keeping with longer-term outcomes, as shown elsewhere (see Chapter 10 in this volume). Patients treated at the time of peak tumor temperature had the highest 2-year disease-free survival rate, which was about twice as high as for patients treated at other times or for patients treated as usual, without regard for timing [13, 23].

11.3.2 Unspecific Markers Preferred to Clock Hour: Successful *N*-of-1 Chronochemotherapy

An earlier attempt focusing on reducing toxicity while relying on results from the experimental laboratory for efficacy was successful, the patient being alive 30 years later [24]. In this patient (CN) diagnosed with a rare and highly malignant ovarian endodermal sinus tumor with spillage into the peritoneal cavity, who is alive and well more than 30 years after subsequent individualized chronochemotherapy, the timing of drug administration was varied from month to month for the first 4 months and autorhythmometry (mood, vigor, nausea, temperature) and complete blood counts were followed to determine the patient's time of highest tolerance. Prior to each course of medication, blood samples were drawn every 4 hours for 24 hours at specific timepoints to determine the circadian rhythm of circulating platelets, white blood cells (WBCs), and differential, hemoglobin, hematocrit, and red blood cell (RBC) indices. Core temperature, blood pressure, pulse, mood, and vigor were also assessed around-the-clock every 4 hours for months. Then, at scheduled times subsequent to medication, WBCs were obtained to assess bone marrow suppression. Oral temperature was measured five or more times a day, on most days, mostly during wakefulness. Regularly, around the clock, mood and vigor were self-rated by admittedly subjective criteria. In March, the medications were given between 0800h and 1100h, in April between 2000h and 2200h, in May at 0400h, and in June again at 2200h. After the fourth course, 0400h was chosen as the preferred time of administration based on criteria for the patient's drug tolerance, as well as by extrapolation of optimal cyclophosphamide timing from mice (correcting for differences in diurnality vs. nocturnality of activity) [25]. CN received 20 courses of treatment covering 19 months.

11.3.3 Chronosensitivity Complements Chemosensitivity Tests: The Erna Test

More recently, several protocols were designed to seek optimal cancer treatment administration schedules to benefit a patient (EH) with advanced ovarian cancer focusing primarily on treatment efficacy [26]. Difficulties related to *N*-of-1 designs relate primarily to confounding effects due to the patient's response to prior treatment, any development of drug resistance, and to any progression of the disease [10, 27, 28]. Optimization of efficacy also requires repeated measurements of pertinent variables such as tumor markers that are usually invasive, when the validity of a treatment effect is to be ascertained. For treatment timing, however, serial blood samplings for several days can be substituted by determining tumor marker rhythms in urine (such as UGP) or saliva (such as CA125 or CA130) [29, 30]. The fact that some markers (such as CA125 or CA130) can be determined in saliva, where they are characterized by a large-amplitude circadian rhythm and also by a circaseptan variation of lesser prominence, but where their pertinence may be limited to guiding the timing of treatment (since a determination in saliva is less specific than in blood), made it possible to obtain around-the-clock measurements before, during, and after a given course of chemotherapy in an unusually cooperative patient (EH) [11, 31–33]. Whereas around-the-clock determinations of tumor markers during treatment, such as taxol [31] or cisplatin [10, 32], administered at a constant rate for 24 hours, or time-specified differences in tumor markers during versus before treatment such as doxorubicin [33] administered differently from one day to the next over several days via a programmable pump may provide information regarding the individual patient's response to treatment, this approach is more problematic for treatment administered as a bolus. In the latter case, an answer may not be obtained until at least three courses have been administered, which may be too late to benefit that particular patient, unless it is done early, as in the case of CN [24]. In this case, treatment timing was guided with unspecific markers insofar as efficacy and resistance other than that to myelotoxicity are concerned.

Circulating CA125 was assayed in about 3-hourly samples during a 24-hour infusion of taxol ($135 \, \text{mg/m}^2/24 \, \text{h}$) [31]. A statistically significant decrease in the circulating marker concentration could be ascertained ($P = 0.007$). The largest decrease in CA125 in EH occurred at a time similar to that of largest tumor proliferation, which had been independently assessed by flow cytometry from intraperitoneal washings obtained on 30 patients with ovarian cancer [34]. A similar trend was observed for another ovarian marker, M-CSF, during this treatment [35], and for serum CA125 during another 24-hour infusion of taxol administered to the same patient [31]. CA125 was determined in around-the-clock unstimulated saliva samples collected during 7 days before treatment and during the 24-hour constant infusion of cisplatin ($25 \, \text{mg/m}^2/24 \, \text{h}$). A decrease in the MESOR of salivary CA125 ($P = 0.046$) suggests that, overall, the

Figure 11.8. Illustration of a five-timepoint chronobiologic design, with results analyzed by single cosinor. The original data (left) are tumor regression rates, expressed as a percentage per week, plotted as a function of the timing of radiotherapy in relation to peak tumor temperature. The five timepoints are the time of peak tumor temperature, 4 or 8 hours before the peak, or 4 or 8 hours after the peak, described by 0, $+4$, $+8$, -4, and -8, respectively. The 24-hour cosine curve best fitting these results is plotted together with the data (left). The cosinor results are also shown in a polar display (right). The fact that the 95% confidence ellipse for the joint estimation of the circadian amplitude and acrophase does not cover the pole (center of the plot) attests to the statistical significance of the fitted model (rejection of the zero-amplitude or no-rhythm assumption).

Validation of effectiveness of human chronoradiotherapy

Faster peri-oral tumor regression rate with radiotherapy at circadian peak in tumor temperature *

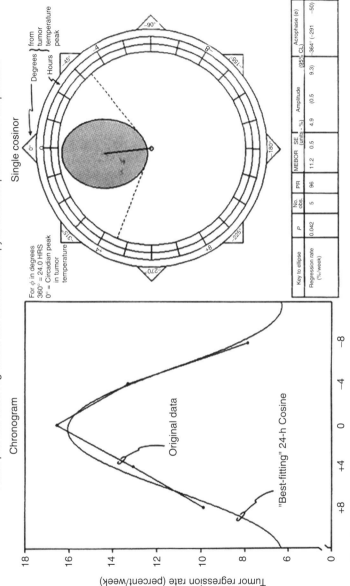

Chronogram

Tumor regression rate (percent/week)

Time (hours from macroscopic peak of tumor temperature)

Original data

"Best-fitting" 24-h Cosine

Single cosinor

Degrees } from tumor temperature peak
Hours }

For ϕ in degrees
$360° = 24.0$ HRS
$0° =$ Circadian peak in tumor temperature

Key to ellipse	P	No. obs.	PR	MEBOR	SE (units ·%)	Amplitude	(95% CL)	Acrophase (ø)	(95% CL)
Regression rate (%/week)	0.042	5	96	11.2	0.5	4.9	(0.5)	9.3)	-364° (-291 -50)

* Determined in a patients/group (total = 40 patients) receiving radiotherapy 5 days/week for 5 weeks at 1 of 5 treatment times in relation to macroscopic peak of tumor temperature (based on 2-hourly measurements taken around–the–clock for 1–5 days prior to treatment onset) (Helberg, et al., 1977).

269

treatment was effective. The depression in cancer marker occurred primarily between 0600h and 0900h with a further response of lesser extent lasting until 1600h [32].

A treatment course of doxorubicin administered continuously for 7 days by means of a programmable pump offered the opportunity to vary the infusion rate in a circadian stage-dependent manner and to vary the timing of the high rate infusion span from one day to the next [33]. After an about 2-day infusion of doxorubicin at a constant rate (0.6 mL/h of a 25 mg/100 mL solution), a high 6.6 ml dose was programmed to be administered over 4.8 hours followed by a low dose rate of 0.4 mL/h for the remainder of the 24-hour cycle. The 4.8-hour span of high infusion rate was shifted by 4.8 hours each day. The ovarian cancer marker UGP was assessed in fractionated urine samples collected around the clock before treatment and during the entire treatment span. Optimal timing of treatment could be assessed for efficacy by time-specified differences in UGP during constant infusion of doxorubicin as compared to values before treatment. Results in this case could also be compared with an assessment of treatment efficacy, gauged by UGP on days with highest infusion rate at five different circadian stages, analyzed by cosinor, the UGP response being assigned to the midpoint of the interval during which the high dose was administered. An overall decrease in both UGP and CA125 during treatment was noted, as an indication that it was effective. Conceivably, to the extent to which the marker reflects tumor metabolism, the time of largest marker response serves as an indication of the time of highest drug efficacy [33].

Chemosensitivity assays in vitro on tumor cells removed at surgery can help determine the most appropriate choice of treatment [36], its effectiveness being further checked in vivo by changes in noninvasively sampled marker rhythms in response to treatment [37]. The chemoresponse assay helps determine whether drug resistance has developed and accordingly secure the putatively most useful drug. A chemoresponse assay for nine antineoplastic agents found the patient to be sensitive to 5-FU. A 1-hour infusion of 5-FU (12 mg/kg) was administered at 2200h (given at the end of a 700-mg/m^2/day leucovorin infusion for 24 hours). During the first 2 days after treatment, UGP dropped markedly, this response being replicated after another similar treatment also administered at 2200h, but not when it was administered at 0600h or at 1400h [33]. The optimal timing determined in this N-of-1 study (in the Erna test) corresponds closely to the recommended infusion schedule for 5-FU (with maximal dosing at night) based on a subsequent large clinical trial [38].

11.3.4 Triangulation

Many anticancer drugs and radiation disrupt cell reproduction and have their greatest effect on tissues that are growing most rapidly. Drugs or radiation can destroy some cancer cells whenever they are administered. But, depending on the timing of treatment, a variable amount of healthy tissue is also destroyed. The healthy cells most sensitive to such treatment are the fast-growing cells in hair follicles, the lining of the intestine, and bone marrow. Hence the usual side effects of anticancer treatment are loss of hair, nausea, and a reduction in the red and white blood cells formed in bone marrow. By charting rhythms of cell division in healthy and cancerous tissue, it should be possible to find the time when chemotherapy or irradiation is least harmful to healthy cells. Such an approach has already been extensively used in the experimental laboratory [39, 40]. Extension of the findings to the clinic can thus shield healthy tissues of cancer patients by timing treatment [24], albeit without losing sight of the primary objective of optimizing treatment efficacy for the given patient. A rhythm in the concentration of a drug in blood (in bioavailability, the false gold standard), brought about by interactions within the body among effects of metabolic and excretatory mechanisms, may well be timed quite differently as compared to that desired for an optimal treatment effect. In the case of a carcinostatic drug, one strives to give a potentially toxic drug at a time that represents the most desirable compromise between the times when the drug is best tolerated by the host, insofar as this is compatible with a time when it is most effective against the tumor [28].

In a clinical trial of advanced ovarian and bladder cancer at the University of Minnesota [41, 42], combination chemotherapy consisted of about nine courses of doxorubicin followed 12 hours later by cisplatin. Patients were randomly assigned to one of two treatment times, doxorubicin being administered either about 1 hour before awakening or about 11 hours after awakening. Heart rate was monitored around the clock before each treatment course. The difference in heart rate MESOR between the last and first profiles served to assess the cardiotoxicity of doxorubicin for each patient. These differences in heart rate MESOR were then assigned to a time code representing the time of doxorubicin treatment in hours and minutes from the pretreatment heart rate acrophase. A cosinor analysis of these data (consisting of differences in heart rate MESOR assigned to the time of doxorubicin administration relative to the pretreatment heart rate acrophase, pooled over all patients and all treatment courses) indicated a statistically significant circadian rhythm in the cardiotoxicity of doxorubicin ($P = 0.043$), being highest about 10 hours after the heart rate acrophase. Accepting the possible increase in heart rate MESOR as unfavorable leads to the inference that treatment at the cardiosensitivity chronorisk (corresponding to the time of anticipated largest increase in heart rate MESOR) should be avoided [43].

Triangulation is defined as the location of a point in circadian (or other) time which is associated with the best compromise between desired and undesired effects [43]. First, optimal circadian stages may be evaluated by reference to several marker rhythms, each used for the double purpose of gauging the patient's response to treatment and the timing of treatment administration relative to that marker's acrophase. Each marker rhythm assesses the different toxicities of the drug(s) (such as cardiotoxicity, myelotoxicity, and nephrotoxicity) as well as any benefit derived therefrom (e.g., by tumor markers or tumor size and survival time). As such, they provide information concerning the merits and/or demerits of the treatment. Second, the marker rhythms can provide information concerning the timing of treatment by means of their acrophase. To investigate optimization by timing, treatment time is not specified only in terms of clock hours but also relative to the acrophases of the various marker rhythms. Thus the patient's responses to treatment (evaluated as an increase in heart rate MESOR for cardiotoxicity, as the area under the curve of weekly WBCs, neutrophils, and platelets for myelotoxicity, and by creatinine clearance for nephrotoxicity) can be referred as outcomes to the given patient's prospectively determined internal time structure. This approach allows the individualization of timed treatment. Triangulation is then based on a collateral hierarchy of estimates relating to the anticipated benefits from and risks of the treatment [43]. It has been suggested by the founder of the specialty of oncology in the United States, B. J. Kennedy, that this approach added a few years to the life of a patient with a very advanced ovarian cancer at the time of its diagnosis [44].

When relying on more than one marker rhythm, several indications of desired treatment time are obtained. These may or may not converge; that is, they may point toward a similar rhythm stage overall or toward conflicting rhythm stages. When there is convergence of desired times, an average optimal time can be derived from all estimates by "triangulation." In the case of divergence, however, optimization may be carried out by assigning different weights to the different marker variables in view of the given patient's strengths and weaknesses, more weight being given to the estimate thought to describe the risk to which the patient is thought to be most susceptible [43].

Studies by Blank et al. [45] of mitotic activity of bone marrow and tumor of sarcoma-bearing rats and of bone marrow of healthy controls indicate the possibility to achieve concomitantly near-maximal efficacy and near-minimal myelotoxicity, with similar results already observed in humans with different kinds of malignancies (Blank et al., unpublished). Indeed, whereas the circadian rhythm in mitotic activity of bone marrow was similar for intact and tumor-bearing rats, with a peak occurring shortly after the onset of the dark (activity) span, the circadian rhythm in mitotic activity of tumor had a much smaller amplitude and a different acrophase occurring late in the dark span (Figures 11.9 and 11.10). Also to be considered is a set of usually cyclic environmental conditions that may affect healthy cell division. For instance, corneal mitotic activity was found to be affected by magnetic storms [46]. Geomagnetic activity was also reported to influence hematotoxicity in cancer patients [47, 48].

11.4 APPLICATIONS IN INFECTIOUS DISEASE: IMPORTANCE OF CHRONOPHARMACOKINETICS

As an illustrative example of the chronoavailability of drugs (e.g., see Ref. [49]), three erythromycin test preparations were tested [50]. Twenty-four adult men were given 250 mg of erythromycin as one of three different preparations in a

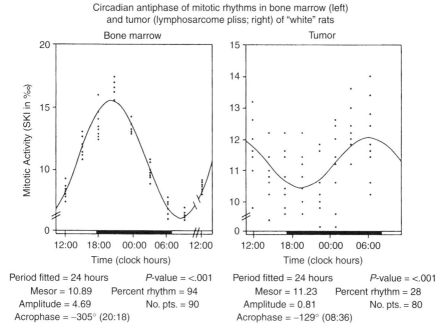

Figure 11.9. Comparison of circadian mitotic rhythm in bone marrow and tumor of rats bearing a lymphosarcoma. Note large difference in acrophase between the two circadian mitotic rhythms, suggesting the possibility of optimizing treatment efficacy without excessive toxicity. Data from M Blank.

crossover study with 1-week intertreatment intervals. All subjects were diurnally active and nocturnally resting, and fasted for 2 hours before each dose and for at least 2 hours after each medication. Dosing started at 0800h of one day and continued every 6 hours for 3 days. Blood concentrations of erythromycin were determined at 0, 1.5, 3, 4.5, and 6 hours in relation to each dose for 24 hours, and again with the same sampling schedule beginning 48 hours after the first dose. On a group basis, a circadian rhythm was invariably demonstrated with statistical significance for all endpoints considered, namely, the time to peak, the peak concentration, the area under the curve, and the nadir. The largest area, and hence the greatest coverage in terms of antimicrobial activity, was found with drug administration around noon [50].

11.5 APPLICATIONS IN TRANSPLANTATION

11.5.1 Chronopharmacodynamics Override Chronopharmacokinetics

Cyclosporine is a powerful immunosuppressive drug able to prevent or greatly delay the onset of acute allograft rejection both in experimental [51] and in

274

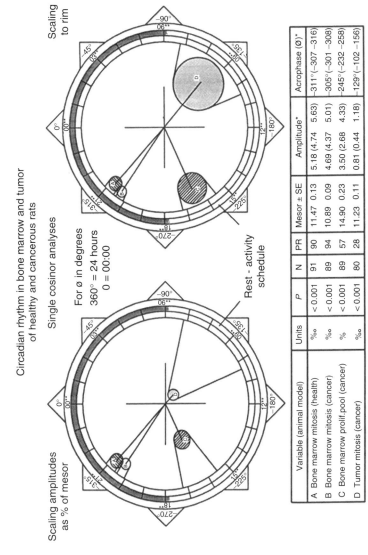

Circadian rhythm in bone marrow and tumor
of healthy and cancerous rats

Single cosinor analyses

For ø in degrees
360° = 24 hours
0 = 00:00

Scaling amplitudes
as % of mesor

Scaling
to rim

Rest - activity
schedule

Variable (animal model)	Units	P	N	PR	Mesor ± SE	Amplitude*	Acrophase (Ø)*
A Bone marrow mitosis (health)	‰	< 0.001	91	90	11.47 0.13	5.18 (4.74 5.63)	-311°(-307 -316)
B Bone marrow mitosis (cancer)	‰	< 0.001	89	94	10.89 0.09	4.69 (4.37 5.01)	-305°(-301 -308)
C Bone marrow prolif.pool (cancer)	%	< 0.001	89	57	14.90 0.23	3.50 (2.68 4.33)	-245°(-232 -258)
D Tumor mitosis (cancer)	‰	< 0.001	80	28	11.23 0.11	0.81 (0.44 1.18)	-129°(-102 -156)

P = Probability of hypothesis: amplitude = 0; N = number of observations

PR = Percent rhythm (percentage of variability accounted for by cosine curve)

* Conservative 95% confidence limits (parentheses) derived from cosinor ellipse

Figure 11.10. Polar representation of circadian mitotic rhythms in bone marrow and tumor of rats bearing a lymphosarcoma as compared to circadian mitotic rhythm in bone marrow of healthy control rats. Whereas mitotic activity of bone marrow peaks shortly after the onset of the dark (activity) span in both healthy and cancerous rats, the circadian rhythm in mitotic activity of tumor has a smaller amplitude and a different acrophase occurring late in the dark span. This difference has important implications for scheduling the administration of oncotherapy. Data from M. Blank.

clinical [52] transplantation. Cyclosporine's nephrotoxicity being dose-related, the optimization of this drug's immunosuppressive properties could lower the dosage needed to prevent acute graft rejection and thus reduce nephrotoxicity [53]. Studies on rats had shown that the toxicology of cyclosporine was circadian stage dependent [54]. Moreover, rejection of a heart allografted across a major histocompatibility barrier was delayed with low single IP daily doses of cyclosporine given during the daily dark (active) span. A circannual variation in the immunosuppressive effect of cyclosporine was also noted, manifested by a prolongation of graft function [55]. Studies with segmental pancreas allografts from ACI rats into diabetic Lewis inbred rats confirmed that circadian timing determined the extent of prolongation of graft function [53].

The potential benefit from the circadian timing of cyclosporine was further tested in the dog with a kidney allograft. Treatment was administered IV via an implanted, externally programmable pump (Medtronic Inc., Minneapolis, MN). A circadian sinusoidal schedule of cyclosporine peaking in the middle of the dark span was associated with nearly a doubling in graft survival as compared to a schedule peaking in the middle of the light span [56]. In this experimental model of kidney-allografted dogs, the possibility was then examined that the results obtained with a pump could be exploited for the more practical oral administration of the drug [53].

Kidneys were exchanged between 10 pairs of mongrel dogs, the remaining kidney of each dog being discarded. Quasirandomization was used to assign dogs to one of two treatment groups, receiving single daily doses of 12.5 mg/kg BW cyclosporine orally, for up to 60 days, either at 0830h or 2030h. Dogs in a pair were assigned to different circadian stages, one at 0830h, the other at 2030h. A control group of 6 dogs was kept untreated. Dogs were kept in a regimen of light from 0600 to 1800h alternating with darkness from 1800h to 0600h. At death, rejection was confirmed by laparotomy and graft histology. The chronopharmaokinetics were determined by measuring blood concentrations of cyclosporine around-the-clock (7 samples at 4-hour intervals) in four dogs (two dogs for each treatment time) on the 5th postoperative day. Graft survival was used to assess the chronopharmacodynamics [53].

A statistically significant circadian rhythm was found to characterize cyclosporine blood concentrations from the two dogs treated at 0830h ($P < 0.001$) as well as those from the two dogs treated at 2030h ($P = 0.027$) (Figure 11.11). As anticipated, acrophases at 1542 ± 0041h and at 0322 ± 0113h, respectively, are in near antiphase. From a chronopharmacokinetics point of view, treatment was equally effective at the two timepoints tested, as evidenced by the lack of a statistically significant difference in the areas under the curve (8719 vs. 7740 ng/mL × h, respectively) and in the cyclosporine trough concentrations assessed from 18 dogs (2 dogs were excluded from analysis due to technical failures) (191 ± 60 vs. 141 ± 49 ng/mL, respectively). By contrast, in terms of the chronopharmacodynamics, 8 of the 10 dogs treated at 0830h rejected their graft after 6, 6, 7, 7, 8, 10, 17, and 20 days, whereas only 2 of the

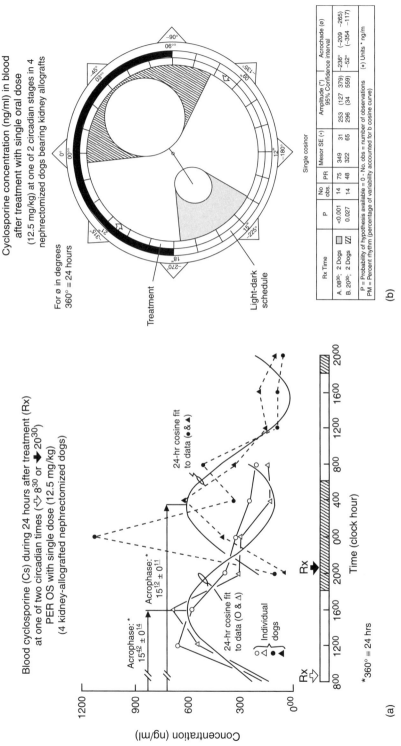

Figure 11.11. Circadian rhythm in cyclosporine blood concentrations from two dogs treated at 0830h (open symbols) and from two dogs treated at 2030h (dark symbols). All dogs were kept in light from 0600h to 1800h daily. Note difference in acrophase (measure of timing of overall high cyclosporine concentrations in blood) in the absence of any difference in chronopharmacologic endpoints, apparent from plot of data as a function of time with best-fitting 24-hour cosine curves (a) and from the polar cosinor display also showing the statistical significance of the circadian rhythms by the rejection of the zero-amplitude (no-rhythm) test (b). Data from M. Cavallini.

8 dogs treated at 2030h rejected their graft after 12 and 15 days ($P < 0.010$ by life table analysis; all 6 control animals acutely rejected their graft within 7 days), See Figure 11.12 [53].

11.5.2 Beyond Circadian Optimization

A circaseptan (about-weekly) periodicity in rejection was found for human kidney transplants in Minnesota, Paris, and Milan [57]. The phase of this circaseptan component was determined by the timing of transplantation rather than by the day of the week when surgery was performed, suggesting that we are dealing with a response rhythm that is amplified after exposure to a single stimulus such as transplantation surgery. The question thus arose as to whether circaseptan rhythms could be exploited to optimize the prolongation of graft function by treatment with an immunosuppressant agent such as cyclosporine [58].

Segmental pancreatic transplantation was performed on Ma Lewis (RT-1^l) recipients with ACI (RT-1^a) donor rats. Animals were kept on staggered regimens of 12 hours of light alternating with 12 hours of darkness. At 7–14 days prior to surgery, all recipients were made diabetic by a single IV injection of 50 mg/kg BW streptozotocin. All rats with a serum glucose over 400 mg% received a segmental pancreas transplant from an ACI rat standardized on the same lighting regimen. Cyclosporine was administered daily, starting on the day of surgery, at one of six different circadian stages, 4 hours apart (either at 2, 6, 10, 14, 18, or 22 hours after light onset, HALO). A given animal was always treated at the same circadian stage each day. One "homeostatic" group (H) received equal daily doses of 3.5 mg/kg cyclosporine. Seven experimental groups (S) received varying daily doses of cyclosporine according to a 7-day sinusoidal pattern, the first largest dose being administered either on the day of surgery or on the second, third, fourth, fifth, sixth, or seventh day after surgery. The average daily dose equaled that of the control group (3.5 mg/kg), with maximal departure of ± 1 mg/kg. Untreated rats and rats receiving the vehicle only served as controls (C).

Serum glucose was measured every 1 or 2 days. The day of graft rejection was defined as the first of at least 3 consecutive days of hyperglycemia (> 200 mg%) and confirmed in most cases by laparotomy and graft histology. The circadian stage-dependent effect of cyclosporine treatment was confirmed in rats of group H, the longest times to rejection occurring at about 20 HALO, in keeping with other studies in rats. But the longest graft function was found to occur for rats receiving varying daily doses of cyclosporine, according to a circaseptan sinusoidal pattern with largest daily doses administered either on the third or fifth day after surgery and at 7-day intervals thereafter [58]. The mean number of days (and standard deviation) elapsed until pancreas rejection was 6.0 ± 1.4 days in the 11 control animals. By comparison, in the 19 rats receiving equal daily doses of cyclosporine, it was 8.8 ± 4.0 days, and in the 49 rats receiving cyclosporine according to a circaseptan schedule, it was 11.5 ± 4.2

days. As shown in Figure 11.13, as compared to the average rejection time of group H, the untreated control rats had a 31% shorter duration of graft function (Student $t = 6.50$, $P < 0.01$), whereas rats in group S had a 30% prolongation of graft function (Student $t = 4.41$, $P < 0.01$) [58]. A 30% increase in treatment efficacy associated with circaseptan optimization is not negligible, for two reasons: first, it can be achieved in addition to benefit from circadian optimization; and second, from a practical viewpoint, chronotherapeutic optimization may be easier to achieve along the scale of the week than along the circadian scale, notably when the best circadian stage happens to fall outside clinic hours and treatment cannot be administered automatically (e.g., via a programmable pump) or by controlled release [59].

Circaseptan optimization was also achieved in studies on the immunomodulation of malignant growth in LOU rats bearing an immunocytoma [60]. The effect of a 7-day pretreatment with the immunomodulator lentinan was compared to that of pretreatment with saline. The growth of the malignant tumor was inhibited and survival time lengthened when lentinan was administered daily during the light (rest) span in doses varying sinusoidally from day to day as a circadian–circaseptan chronotherapy. By contrast, when lentinan was conveniently given during the active span in the usual equal daily doses, tumor growth was accelerated and survival shortened.

For both cyclosporine and lentinan, circannual differences were also documented [58, 60].

11.5.3 Early Detection of Cyclosporine Side Effects in Heart Transplant Patients

Nephrotoxicity represents a frequent and severe complication associated with cyclosporine treatment, reported in heart transplant recipients [61]. Cyclosporine therapy has also been associated with a persistent elevation of blood pressure developing within the first weeks posttransplantation in 60–90% of heart allograft recipients, requiring intensive and combined antihypertensive regimens [61].

Twenty-four-hour ambulatory blood pressure monitoring (ABPM) of 14 patients, 43–61 years of age, 1–33 months after heart transplantation, revealed

---

Figure 11.12. Despite lack of differences in terms of chronopharmacokinetics (Figure 11.11), there is a large difference in pharmacodynamics between treatment at 0830h and 2030h. (a) Intermediate results show that in pairs of dogs with an exchanged kidney, one receiving 12.5 mg/kg cyclosporine at 0830 h and the other at 2030h, the evening dose is consistently associated with a longer time to organ rejection, being over twice as effective as the morning dose in prolonging kidney allograft function. Arrows correspond to functioning graft at time of summary; flat bars correspond to death from rejection. (b) Summary of results at end of study: kidney graft survival in untreated dogs and in dogs receiving oral cyclosporine at 0830h or at 2030h. Dogs were kept in light from 0600h to 1800h daily. Data from M. Cavallini.

Timing oral cyclosporine
Single daily dose

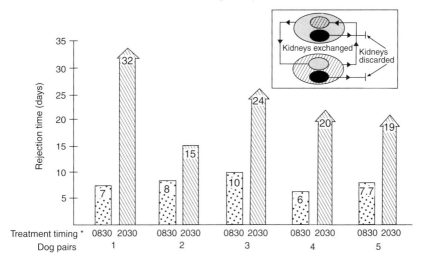

*Timing according to information from study with medtronic pump.

= graft still functioning at time of summary.

= death from rejection.

(a)

Kidney graft survival in mongrel dogs untreated
or treated with oral cyclosporine (Cs; 12.5 mg/kg/day)
at one of two circadian stages[†]

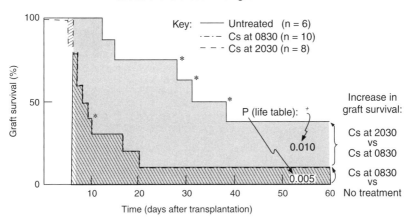

* Died or killed with functioning graft

[†] 08^{30} or 20^{30} (dogs kept in daily light from 06^{00} to 18^{00})

[+] E.T. Lee: statistical methods for survival date analysis. Life-time learning publ. Belmont, Ca., 1980 (552pp.)

(b)

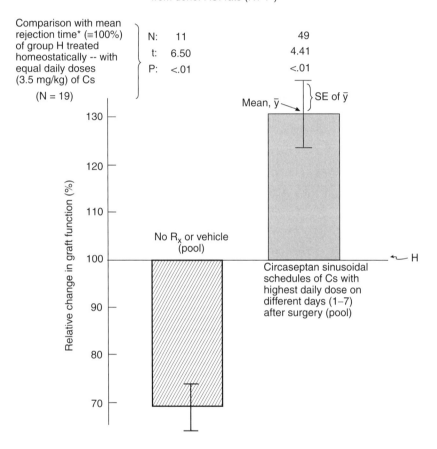

Circaseptan optimization of cyclosporine (Cs)
Transplant-immunotherapy

15-27-week-old diabetic male Ma Lewis (RT-1$^\ell$)
Recipient rats bearing segmental pancreatic allografts
from donor ACI rats (RT-1^a)

Comparison with mean rejection time* ($\equiv$100%) of group H treated homeostatically -- with equal daily doses (3.5 mg/kg) of Cs (N = 19)

N: 11   49
t: 6.50   4.41
P: <.01   <.01

Mean, $\bar{y}$ } SE of $\bar{y}$

Relative change in graft function (%)

130
120
110
100
90
80
70

No R$_x$ or vehicle (pool)

Circaseptan sinusoidal schedules of Cs with highest daily dose on different days (1–7) after surgery (pool)

H

*Time to rejection determined by onset-time of hyperglycemia
(>200 mg% lasting $\geq$ 3 days)

Figure 11.13. Cyclosporine chronotherapy of pancreas-allotransplanted rats suggests further gain in graft function from doses varying from day to day according to a weekly periodicity, beyond the circadian stage dependence of equal daily doses. Data from T Liu.

a nocturnal increase in blood pressure [62]. All patients received standard immunosuppressive therapy. "Hypertension" was diagnosed clinically by the repeated recording of cuff blood pressure readings above 145/95 mm Hg. Antihypertensive treatment, initiated on the basis of isolated readings in the clinic, did not start until after the third month posttransplantation. ABPM revealed nocturnal blood pressure excess already at 2 months after heart transplantation, however. Blood pressure monitoring, as a marker for potential side effects, could prompt the institution of antihypertensive treatment when needed, earlier than on the basis of spotchecks in the clinic. The earlier diagnostic stems both from the fact that abnormality occurred at times when blood pressure is not likely to be checked in the clinic and from the use of time-specified reference values accounting for the usually prominent circadian variation in blood pressure instead of imaginary fixed limits used conventionally [62].

11.6 APPLICATIONS IN CARDIOVASCULAR MEDICINE

11.6.1 Diagnosis of Blood Pressure Disorders

The merit of treating elevated blood pressure is no longer disputed and is widely viewed as a critical way of reducing morbidity and mortality associated with cardiovascular disease [63]. It is also accepted that a diagnosis based on 24-hour ABPM is superior to that based on isolated measurements in the clinic, despite the fact that the latter are taken by trained professionals with an accurate mercury sphygmomanometer under strictly standardized conditions. There are several reasons accounting for the superiority of ABPM over clinic measurements and for the large estimated percentage of misdiagnoses (over 40%) based on single casual readings [64]:

1. The measurements are taken repeatedly, yielding an average value associated with a reduced standard error.
2. They are obtained during usual daily activities rather than at times when the patient's blood pressure may either be spuriously elevated in association with anxiety about the physical examination ("white-coat hypertension") or spuriously lowered in association with the quieter environment away from loads of usual daily life ("masked hypertension").
3. Measurements being obtained around-the-clock, the diagnosis does not depend on when during the day the patient happens to be examined, the current situation ignoring the usually large-amplitude circadian rhythm in blood pressure by neglecting to specify when the measurement is taken and by using fixed rather than time-varying limits for its interpretation; Figure 11.14 [65].
4. Around-the-clock measurements convey not just an average value but patterns of change during both the rest and active span, so that if abnormality is present only during times when the patient is not likely to be examined by a health professional, it will be missed. This was the case of a 78-year-old man treated once a day in the morning with a 24-hour formulation of 10 mg Vasotec (ACE inhibitor) [4]. ABPM revealed

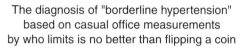

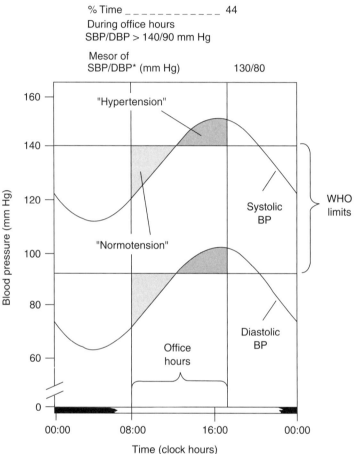

* Circadian amplitude of 20 mm Hg and acrophase of −240° (16h from 00:00).

Figure 11.14. Limitations in dealing with blood pressure (BP) interpreted by fixed limits (and casual measurements or automatic office-hour profiles). Theoretic evidence points to the need to replace fixed thresholds by time-varying reference standards (chronodesms) and to rely on more than one or a few casual BP measurements. Assuming that BP is measured precisely and accurately (without error), ignoring the circadian rhythm in BP results in contradictory diagnoses whether BP is taken in the morning or in the afternoon.

nightly elevated values of diastolic blood pressure during 11 consecutive nights, reaching near 120 mm Hg on the average between midnight and 0300 h, whereas during midday when he saw his treating physician, it was below 90 mm Hg.

Just as there is usually large blood pressure variability from moment to moment, accounted for in part by the circadian variation, there can be large day-to-day, week-to-week, and other variability in the circadian blood pressure pattern as well in some patients, to the point that a decision to treat or not to treat may depend on the day a 24-hour ABPM happened to be obtained [2]. For instance, a 33-year-old untreated man who monitored his blood pressure around the clock for over 30 days was found to have 24-hour average values of systolic blood pressure below 120 mm Hg on some days but above 135 mm Hg on other days, with 77% acceptable values during clinic hours on one day but with all readings above 140/90 mm Hg on another day [1]. The question may be raised as to what constitutes optimal affordable blood pressure monitoring, short of continuous longitudinal records with an inexpensive cuffless device, a goal pursued by the Phoenix Project (www.phoenix. tc-ieee.org), a group of volunteering members of the Institute of Electrical and Electronics Engineers. Table 11.1 lists some advantages and limitations of options available today.

11.6.2 Toward a Chronobiologic Blood Pressure Prevention Clinic

With the possibility to monitor blood pressure automatically around the clock, the conventional question of whether a blood pressure measurement is acceptable or too high (or too low) needs to be replaced by a meaningful interpretation of serial measurements obtained during both the rest and activity spans under usual rather than standardized conditions [66]. Keeping these differences in mind, by 1984 we proposed the use of time-specified reference limits (chronodesms) [67] further qualified by gender and age as replacement for arbitrary time-invariant limits relying on actuarial statistics of morbidity and mortality data from previous generations. By 1984, we also had advocated the use of a set of new endpoints in addition to the actual readings and the circadian rhythm characteristics derived therefrom [68]. The latter are obtained by cosinor, using a two-component model consisting of cosine curves with periods of 24 and 12 hours to account for the usual non sinusoidal circadian waveform of blood pressure and heart rate [69–71]. The new endpoints include the following:

- The percentage time an individual's profile lies above the upper time-specified reference limit during 24 hours (or below the lower limit)
- The extent of excess (or deficit) defined as the area delineated by the reference limit and the individual's profile when it lies outside the reference range
- The timing when most of the excess (or deficit) occurs within 24 hours

These model-independent (nonparametric) endpoints are computer derived by numerical integration. Cosinor-derived parametric and nonparametric

Table 11.1. Advantages and Limitations of Different kinds of Blood Pressure Monitoring

Procedure Number	Procedure	Usage	Advantages	Limitations
1	A few measurements on a few occasions under standardized conditions (rest for 5 min).	Current clinical practice for detecting an elevated blood pressure (BP).	Treatment of thus detected high BP reportedly associated with decline in incidence of heart attacks and strokes.	Does not account for large variability in BP. Potentially associated with misdiagnoses (e.g., "white-coat hypertension," "masked hypertension").
2	24-hour ABPM (ambulatory BP monitoring).	In current practice, reserved for "special cases" (when diagnosis of hypertension is difficult to make).	The 24-hour BP mean has better prognostic value than (1). Allows assessment of BP under usual conditions during both the rest and active daily spans and hence can detect BP abnormality at times when it would usually not be measured. Also allows a rough assessment of the circadian variation.	Does not account for the day-to-day changes in BP and in circadian BP pattern that can be very large in some subjects. Hence it may lead to unwarranted decision to treat or not to treat depending on results on a given day that may or may not be representative. Circadian parameters can only be estimated with a relatively large error margin.

(Continued)

3	48-hour ABPM	Only done in some clinical settings abroad, notably in Japan, reserved for "special cases."	Extending ABPM from 24 to 48 hours is associated with large improvement in estimating circadian characteristics (error term reduced by about 35%). Allows subject to become habituated to monitor.	Still too short to fully account for day-to-day changes in BP characteristics, notably differences often observed between workdays and weekends. Does not allow assessment of any weekly variation in BP that may also contain valuable information in its own right.
4	7-day/24-hour ABPM	Practiced only within BIOCOS.	Yields a more reliable assessment of the circadian characteristics and allows an assessment of the weekly pattern as well. Outcome studies have found associations with results from 7-day record but not with those of first 24 hours.	In some cases, 7-day/24-hour ABPM may not be enough due to large day-to-day changes in BP. When abnormality is detected, a second weeklong profile is advocated. For treated patients, 7-day/24-hour ABPM does not detect any change in patient's response to treatment.

(Continued)

Table 11.1. Continued

Procedure Number	Procedure	Usage	Advantages	Limitations
5	Home monitoring (daily measurement upon awakening and/or at bedtime)	Used in some settings for patients treated for hypertension, notably in Germany and in Japan.	Can detect any change in patient's need for treatment adjustment. Amenable to longitudinal scrutiny, with applications in research.	Does not assess circadian variation or risk associated with abnormalities in BP variability.
6	Home monitoring (daily measurements several times daily, e.g., every 3 hours during waking, with occasional nightly measurement).	Used by some chronobiologists interested in autorhythmometry.	Same advantages as (5) with additional rough assessment of circadian rhythm.	Circadian assessment is often insufficient, notably when nightly values are lacking.
7	Longitudinal ABPM.	Used in some patients in Japan and by a few chronobiologists.	Can detect changes in BP status in a timely fashion. Data also useful for research purposes.	More labor intensive.

endpoints are summarized on a form known as the sphygmochron [1, 2] (www.phoenix.tc-ieee.org/011_Data_Analysis_Methods/Phoenix_Data_Analysis_Methods.htm). In addition to a usually more accurate and more precise estimate of location in the derivation of a MESOR (midline estimating statistic of rhythm) instead of the arithmetic mean, circadian characteristics are also estimated that may reveal abnormalities in their own right.

In 1988, the Mayo Clinic suggested the use of a blood pressure load [72], an index similar to the percentage time elevation, except that it is computed by comparison to fixed limits, rather than chronodesms. Only the latter account for the circadian variation and for differences by gender and age [73]. Clinical issues discussed conventionally by others within the context of ABPM use are the amount of excess, albeit computed versus either fixed limits of 140/90 mm Hg or with respect to daytime and nighttime averages [74]. The use of the hyperbaric index, as the extent of excess has been called, was also advocated by the (U.S.) National High Blood Pressure Education Program Coordinating Committee [75]. As a measure of blood pressure excess, the hyperbaric index helps refine the treatment modality and prognosis that may vary greatly among patients who might have a similar percentage time elevation (or blood pressure load) but different hyperbaric indices, as shown, for instance, in Figure 11.15 [66]. The timing of overall excess is also useful to specify treatment timing.

For a preventive as well as curative medicine, it is critical to map the partly genetically anchored, socioecologically synchronized chronomes (time structures), as their characteristics vary with age, gender, and ethnicity, among others. Chronome maps obtained so far stem from linked cross-sectional (hybrid) studies, in the sense that each individual is sampled around the clock for at least 24 hours, preferably for 7 days or longer. An added longitudinal element along the age scale derived from low-risk, long-lived individuals, validated by outcome, will be indispensable for deriving trustworthy reference standards capable of identifying the presence of a heightened risk in a timely fashion. It will then also become possible to distinguish between rhythm alterations indicative of an elevated risk and naturally occurring changes with age [73]. A website dedicated to this task is being planned by Larry Beaty, a member of the Phoenix Project (www.phoenix.tc-ieee.org/), as a step toward this goal. The merit of such a chronobiologic approach became apparent from a study of pregnant women who were presumably healthy at the start of monitoring, some of them eventually developing complications at a later gestational age [76–78]. Differences on the order of 10 mm Hg were found well within the range of acceptable values between uncomplicated pregnancies and pregnancies that were subsequently complicated by gestational hypertension and/or preeclampsia (Figure 11.16). These MESOR differences detected retrospectively by chronobiological methods could have been acted upon prospectively, already during the first trimester of pregnancy, well before the appearance of any complication, insofar as the systolic and diastolic blood pressure MESORs were below 125/75 mm Hg. This task is a challenge for the future.

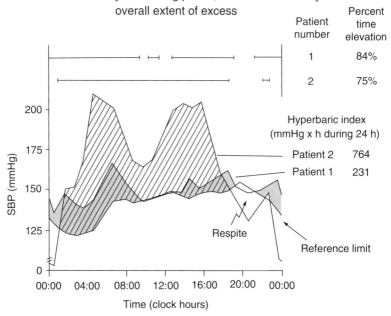

Figure 11.15. The amount of blood pressure excess should be taken into consideration in making decisions regarding treatment since two patients with a similar percentage time elevation (above peer-group chronodesmic limits rather than arbitrary fixed thresholds used to derive blood pressure load) may show drastic differences in extent of excess.

11.6.3 Blood Pressure Variability Disorders

Current guidelines do not specify in the United States the number of measurements to be taken, which in some government-reported studies is less than or equal to 3 [79], whereas the German League Against High Blood Pressure specifies the need for repeated measurements and the Austrian guidelines are even more advanced, specifying a minimum of 30 measurements before a diagnosis is made: hypertension versus normotension if there is more than 26.7% versus less than 23.3% values above fixed limits of 135/85 mm Hg [80]. Indeed, guidelines still focus primarily on the average blood pressure value, with target thresholds of acceptability defined for all adults 18 years or older [81]. The status quo ignores ethnic [82] and gender [83] differences and trends as a function of age both in terms of average value (Figure 11.17), and of the circadian pattern itself (Figure 11.18). Also ignored are results from prospective as well as retrospective studies by others as well as by us indicating that abnormal patterns of blood pressure and/or heart rate are associated with an

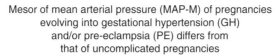

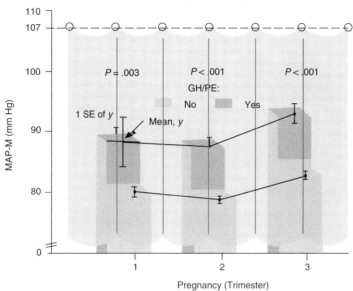

Figure 11.16. Separation on a group basis of the MESOR of mean arterial pressure (MAP) between clinically healthy women at the outset who will develop gestational hypertension and/or preeclampsia ($N = 9$, 21, and 26 in the first, second, and third trimesters, respectively) from those whose pregnancy will remain uncomplicated ($N = 60$, 123, and 88 in the first, second, and third trimesters, respectively). The separation in MAP MESOR between the two groups occurs below a cut off of acceptability at 107 mm Hg. The difference in MAP MESOR exceeds 8 mm Hg on the average between the two groups in all three trimesters. This difference can be detected with statistical significance already during the first trimester of pregnancy, when casual measurements usually fail to recognize a problem (not shown).

increase in vascular disease risk independently of the risk associated with an elevated blood pressure. Risks associated with an excessive pulse pressure [84] and those associated with a decreased heart rate variability [85, 86] have long been recognized and have been confirmed in a 6-year prospective study [87–92] (Table 11.2). An excessive circadian amplitude of blood pressure, a condition known as CHAT (brief for circadian hyperamplitude tension), has also been associated with a large increase in vascular disease risk, notably cerebral ischemic events and nephropathy, even in otherwise MESOR-normotensive patients [1, 2, 87, 91]. An odd timing of the circadian blood pressure rhythm but not of the concomitantly assessed circadian heart rate rhythm, a condition known as ecphasia, sometimes found in patients with non-insulin-dependent diabetes mellitus with autonomic nervous dysfunction [93, 94], has also been

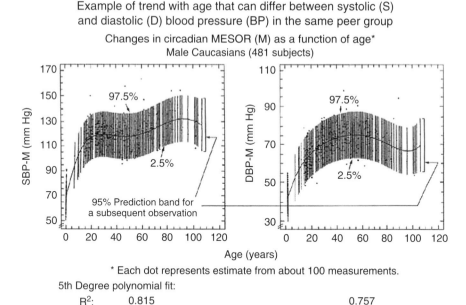

Example of trend with age that can differ between systolic (S)
and diastolic (D) blood pressure (BP) in the same peer group

Changes in circadian MESOR (M) as a function of age*
Male Caucasians (481 subjects)

* Each dot represents estimate from about 100 measurements.

5th Degree polynomial fit:

R^2:	0.815	0.757
P:	< 0.001	< 0.001

Figure 11.17. The diagnosis of blood pressure disorders could be improved by considering differences by gender (not shown here) and changes as a function of age mapped in presumably clinically healthy people, shown for the MESOR of systolic (left) and diastolic (right) blood pressure of healthy Caucasian males. Note that diastolic blood pressure reaches maximal values around 50 years of age but systolic blood pressure increases until about 80 years of age.

associated with a large increase in vascular disease risk [95–97]. Table 11.3 summarizes outcomes of chronobiological screens.

The increased vascular disease risk associated with an excessive blood pressure variability has been corroborated by others, relying on the standard deviation rather than the circadian amplitude [98, 99]. Much literature dealing with risk associated with "nondipping" [100], that is, an insufficient drop in blood pressure by night, another alteration of the circadian pattern, is accounted for in part by ecphasia, a reversal of the circadian blood pressure acrophase [101, 102], rather than by a reduced excursion of the circadian variation in blood pressure, notably in patients with untreated hypertension or in healthy individuals. A comparison of the risk associated with altered circadian characteristics versus a day–night ratio outside acceptable limits indicates the superiority of the chronobiological approach, whether risk is assessed prospectively in terms of actual outcomes [103]—Figure 11.19—or by the left ventricular mass index, used as a surrogate outcome measure available for all study participants [96]—Figure 11.20. Perhaps one reason why the increase in risk associated with an excessive circadian amplitude of blood

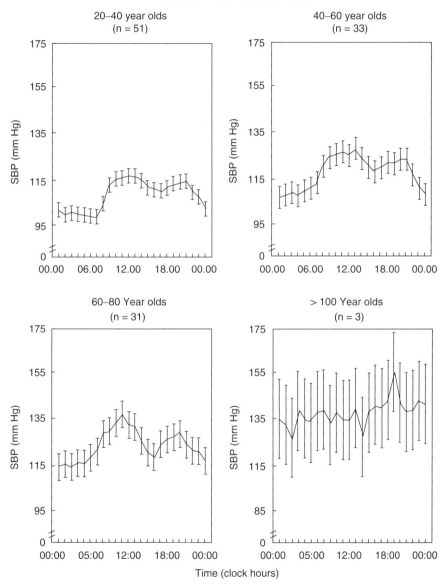

Figure 11.18. Changes in the circadian pattern of systolic blood pressure as a function of age. With increasing age, nightly values tend to increase and the postprandial dip in early afternoon becomes accentuated, at least until 80 years of age. These changes as a function of age seen in presumably clinically healthy people directly affect the day–night ratio. Using fixed values such as 10% and 20% for a classification among nondippers, dippers, and extreme dippers fails to recognize such natural changes with age.

Table 11.2. Relative Risk (RR) and 95% Confidence Interval (CI) of Diastolic Circadian Hyperamplitude Tension (D-CHAT), Decreased Heart Rate Variability (DHRV), and Excessive Pulse Pressure (EPP), Alone or in Combination[a]

Group 1: Reference (N_1) Risk?	Group 2: Test (N_2) Risk?	RR	[95%; CI]
None (214)	D-CHAT (17)	6.294	[2.108; 18.794]
None (214)	DHRV (13)	8.231	[2.847; 23.797]
None (214)	EPP (39)	8.231	[3.600; 18.819]
None (214)	D-CHAT & DHRV (2)	13.375	[2.857; 62.621]
None (214)	D-CHAT & EPP (3)	26.750	[13.554; 52.795]
None (214)	DHRV & EPP (6)	17.833	[7.364; 43.189]
None (214)	D-CHAT & DHRV & EPP (3)	26.750	[13.554; 52.795]
D-CHAT (17)	D-CHAT & DHRV (2)	*2.125*	*[0.417; 10.840]*
D-CHAT (17)	D-CHAT & EPP (3)	4.250	[1.804; 10.013]
D-CHAT (17)	D-CHAT & DHRV & EPP (3)	4.250	[1.804; 10.013]
DHRV (13)	DHRV & D-CHAT (2)	*1.625*	*[0.325; 8.113]*
DHRV (13)	DHRV & EPP (6)	*2.167*	*[0.803; 5.846]*
DHRV (13)	D-CHAT & DHRV & EPP (3)	3.250	[1.438; 7.345]
EPP (39)	EPP & D-CHAT (3)	3.250	[2.030; 5.204]
EPP (39)	EPP & DHRV (6)	2.167	[1.038; 4.523]
EPP (39)	D-CHAT & DHRV & EPP (3)	3.250	[2.030; 5.204]

D-CHAT is defined as circadian amplitude of diastolic blood pressure (BP) above the upper 95% prediction limit of clinically healthy peers matched by gender and age; DHRV is defined as 48-hour standard deviation of heart rate in the lowest 7th percentile of distribution; and EPP is defined as a pulse pressure (MESOR of systolic BP−MESOR of diastolic BP) above 60 mm Hg, where the MESOR is a chronome-adjusted mean value.

[a] Assessed in population of 297 patients, among whom 39 had a morbid event during the following 6 years. RR is computed as ratio of incidence of morbid event in Group 2 versus that of Group 1. A 95% CI not overlapping 1 indicates statistically significant increase in risk in Group 2 versus Group 1.

pressure has not been recognized earlier is that the relationship between risk and blood pressure variability is nonlinear, by contrast to the linear relationship between risk and the MESOR of blood pressure—Figures 11.21 and 11.22 [71, 103]. In most statistical analyses relying on multivariate linear regression, nonlinear associations such as those shown in Figures 11.21 and 11.22 are likely to be missed. Moreover, scholarly papers introducing spectral methods for the study of blood pressure variability [104] or following-up on the same topic include at best variability along the 24-hour scale, while components with periods covering a broad infradian range, including not only circaseptans and circannuals but also transyears and decadal variations, have already been mapped and shown to have congruent counterparts in the near or far environment [105].

11.6.4 Chronotherapy: Experimental Designs

Güllner et al. [106] documented the circadian stage-dependent action of a short-acting anti-hypertensive drug, prazosin, against the background of studies

Table 11.3. Outcomes of Chronobiological Screens of Blood Pressure and Heart Rate[a]

N of Patients (Reference)	N at Follow-up	Sampling	N Measurements: Total (Outcomes)	Finding
10 (1)	10 (up to 5 years)	5/day daily	Up to 9,125 (only partially analyzed)	Among P. Scarpelli's patients, the 4 who died with malignant hypertension had a larger circadian BP amplitude than the 6 who were still alive (SBP: $t = 1.84$; $P = 0.103$; DBP: $t = 2.99$; $P = 0.017$).
63 (2, 3)	21 after 28 years	~q4h for 2 days	756 (252)	9 of 10 Subjects without CHAT are alive while 7 of 11 subjects with CHAT are dead 28 years later ($\chi^2 = 6.390$; $P < 0.01$).
56 (4)	56: Concomitant LVMI	q15 min for 24h	5,376 (5,376)	Classification by Y. Kumagai of patients by LVMI (<100; $100-130$; $>130 \, g/m^2$) reveals elevation of circadian amplitude at LVMI in $100-130$ range whereas MESOR elevation occurs only at LVMI >130.
221 (5, 6)	221 (time of delivery)	q1 h/48 h in each trimester of pregnancy (336 profiles)	16,128 (16,128)	In addition to an 8-mm Hg difference in mean value between women who will or will not develop complications (gestational hypertension, preeclampsia) already observed during the first trimester of pregnancy, the occurrence of complications is also associated with BP profiles characterized by an elevated circadian BP amplitude. In particular, one case (JK) of CHAT where warning was not heeded, was followed 8 weeks later by severe preeclampsia, premature delivery

(Continued)

293

Table 11.3. Continued

N of Patients (Reference)	N at Follow-up	Sampling	N Measurements: Total (Outcomes)	Finding
297 (7–12)	297 after 6 years	q15 min for 48 h	57,024 (57,024)	and 26 months of hospitalization of offspring at a cost of about $1 million. CHAT or a reduced circadian standard deviation of heart rate, or an excessive pulse pressure (>60 mm Hg) are large risk factors (larger than hypertension) for cerebral ischemic events, nephropathy, and coronary artery disease, even when the blood pressure is within acceptable limits.
2039 (13–15)	2039 Concomitant LVMI	Hourly averages for 24 h	48,936 (48,936)	LVMI is increased in patients with CHAT, a reduced circadian standard deviation of heart rate, or an elevated pulse pressure. The relation between LVMI and the circadian endpoints is nonlinear.
23 (16)	12 after 7 years	q15 min for 9 days	19,872 (10,368)	10 of 20 Patients with no consistent BP abnormality are alive and well; 2 of 3 patients with consistent BP abnormality reported an adverse vascular event ($P = 0.015$ by Fisher's exact test).
80 (17, 18)	80: Response to treatment administered 2 h before daily BP peak	q4 h for 24 h before and on treatment	960 (960)	With smaller doses of medications, BP was lowered by R. Zaslavskaya to a larger extent and treatment was accompanied by fewer complications.

(*Continued*)

Treatment: propranolol, clonidine, or α-methyldopa ($P<0.05$ for each effect)

Treating CHAT may prevent adverse vascular events: As compared to placebo, nifedipine (1 mg b.i.d. at 0800 h and 2000 h) increases and benidipine (4 mg/day at 0800 h) decreases the circadian amplitude of blood pressure. The resulting increase versus decrease in the incidence of CHAT on nifedipine versus benidipine may account for the corresponding difference between the number of stroke events of 7.6 versus 3.5 and the total number of cardiovascular events of 20.4 versus 8.8 per 1000 person-years.

vs. control group treated 3 times a day	18 (12 weeks)	q30 min ($\geq$24 h) on 3 regimens	$\geq$2592 ($\geq$2592)	
18 (19)				

Totals:
2,807   2,754   160,769 ($>$141,636)

[a] SBP and DBP, systolic and diastolic blood pressure; HR, heart rate; CHAT, circadian hyper amplitude tension, a condition defined by a circadian amplitude exceeding the upper 95% prediction limit of acceptability (in healthy peers matched by gender and age); LVMI, left ventricular mass index. By comparison with several classical studies, the number of measurements in chronobiological work completed thus far is likely to be larger, and confounding by intersubject variability smaller (Ref. 20).

1. Scarpelli PT, Romano S, Livi R, Scarpelli L, Cornélissen G, Cagnoni M, Halberg F. Instrumentation for human blood pressure rhythm assessment. In: Scheving LE, Halberg F, Ehret CF, eds. *Chronobiotechnology and Chronobiological Engineering.* Dordrecht, The Netherlands: Martinus Nijhoff; 1987: 304–309.

2. Halhuber MJ, Cornélissen G, Bartter FC, Delea CS, Kreze A, Mikulecky M, Müller-Bohn T, Siegelova J, Dusek J, Schwartzkopff O, Halberg F. Circadian urinary glucocorticoid and rhythmic blood pressure coordination. *Scr Med* 2002;75:139–144.

3. Halberg F, Cornélissen G, Katinas G, Hillman D, Schwartzkopff O. Season's appreciations 2000: chronomics complement, among many other fields, genomics and proteomics. *Neuroendocrinol Lett.* 2001;22:53–73.

4. Kumagai Y, Shiga T, Sunaga K, Cornélissen G, Ebihara A, Halberg F. Usefulness of circadian amplitude of blood pressure in predicting hypertensive cardiac involvement. *Chronobiologia.* 1992;19:43–58.

5. Cornélissen G, Halberg F, Bingham C, Kumagai Y. Toward engineering for blood pressure surveillance. *Biomed Instrum Technol.* 1997;31:489–498.

6. Cornélissen G, Rigatuso J, Wang ZR, Wan CM, Maggioni C, Syutkina EV, Schwartzkopff O, Johnson DE, Halberg F. International Womb-to-Tomb Chronome Group. Case report of an acceptable average but overswinging blood pressure in Circadian Hyper-Amplitude-Tension, CHAT. *Neuroendocrinol Lett.* 2003; 24(Suppl 1): 84–91.

7. Otsuka K, Cornélissen G, Halberg F. Predictive value of blood pressure dipping and swinging with regard to vascular disease risk. *Clin Drug Invest.* 1996; 11: 20–31.

8. Otsuka K, Cornélissen G, Halberg F, Oehlert G. Excessive circadian amplitude of blood pressure increases risk of ischemic stroke and nephropathy. *J. Medi Eng Technol* 1997;21:23–30.

9. Otsuka K, Cornélissen G, Halberg F. Circadian rhythmic fractal scaling of heart rate variability in health and coronary artery disease. *Clin Cardiol.* 1997; 20:631–638.

10. Halberg F, Cornélissen G, Halberg J, Fink H Chen C-H, Otsuka K, Watanabe Y, Kumagai Y, Syutkina EV, Kawasaki T, Uezono K, Zhao ZY, Schwartzkopff O. Circadian hyper-amplitude-tension, CHAT: a disease risk syndrome of anti-aging medicine. *J Anti-Aging Med.* 1998;1:239–259.

11. Cornélissen G, Otsuka K, Chen C-H, Kumagai Y, Watanabe Y, Halberg F, Siegelova J, Dusek J. Nonlinear relation of the circadian blood pressure amplitude to cardiovascular disease risk. *Scr Med.* 2000; 73:85–94.

12. Cornélissen G, Otsuka K, Bakken EE, Halberg F, Siegelova J, Fiser B. CHAT (circadian hyper-amplitude-tension) and CSDD-HR (circadian standard deviation deficit of heart rate): separate, synergistic vascular disease risks? *Scr Med.* 2002;75:87–94.

13. Chen CH, Cornélissen G, Halberg F, Fiser B. Left ventricular mass index as 'outcome' related to circadian blood pressure characteristics. *Scr Med.* 1998; 71:183–189.

14. Chen C-H, Cornélissen G, Siegelova J, Halberg F. Does overswinging provide an early warning of cardiovascular disease risk when non-dipping may fail? A meta-analysis of 2039 cases. *Scr Med* 2001; 74:75–80.

15. Cornélissen G, Chen C-H, Siegelova J, Halberg F. Vascular disease risk syndromes affecting both MESOR-normotensives and MESOR-hypertensives: a meta-analysis of 2039 cases. *Scr Med* 2001; 74:81–86

16. Schaffer E, Cornélissen G, Rhodus N, Halhuber M, Watanabe Y, Halberg F. Outcomes of chronobiologically normotensive dental patients: a 7-year follow-up. *JADA* 2001;132:891–899.

17. Zaslavskaya RM. *Chronodiagnosis and Chronotherapy of Cardiovascular Diseases.* 2nd ed. Translation into English from Russian. Moscow: Medicina, 1993.

18. Cornélissen G, Zaslavskaya RM, Kumagai Y, Romanov Y, Halberg F. Chronopharmacologic issues in space. *J Clin Pharmacol.* 1994;34:543–551.

19. Shinagawa M, Kubo Y, Otsuka K, Ohkawa S, Cornélissen G, Halberg F. Impact of circadian amplitude and chronotherapy: relevance to prevention and treatment of stroke. *Biomed Pharmacother.* 2001;55 (Suppl 1):125–132.

20. Halberg F, Cornélissen G, Halberg E, Halberg J, Delmore P, Shinoda M, Bakken E. Chronobiology of human blood pressure. Medtronic Continuing Medical Education Seminars, 1988, 4th ed.

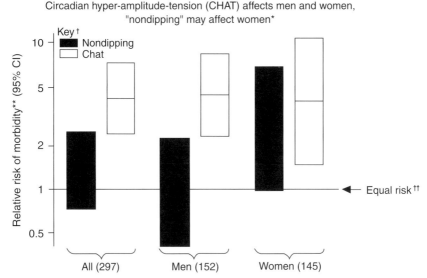

Figure 11.19. The relative risk (RR) of morbidity occurring within 6 years of 297 patients in Tokyo, Japan, associated with an excessive circadian amplitude of diastolic blood pressure (diastolic CHAT) is statistically significant for both men and women, as well as overall, as evidenced by the 95% confidence intervals of RR values not overlapping one (representing equal risk). By contrast, the relative risk associated with "nondipping" (day–night ratio less than 10%) is only marginally elevated, and only so for women and not for men. Data from K. Otsuka.

testing the timing of hydrochlorothiazide [107]. A follow-up approach, successful on a population basis, relied on just two groups, consisting of comparing the merits of treatment administered at the presumed optimal circadian stage, accounting for the pharmacokinetics of the chosen antihypertensive agent and for the individual's own blood pressure profile obtained prior to the start of treatment, with those of traditional treatment. As shown in Figure 11.23, in studies by Zaslavskaya, treating 1.5–2 hours prior to the time of largest blood pressure excess with propranolol, clonidine, or α-methyldopa was associated with a hypotensive effect of greater extent, achieved with a lesser dose, as compared to treatment with equal doses three times a day [108, 109]. Not shown in Figure 11.23 are additional benefits from chronotherapy, namely, an earlier response to treatment and fewer side effects such as overdosages and treatment-related complications.

Another approach attempting to determine an optimal circadian stage of treatment administration consists of following the Phase 0 design [9–11]. As shown elsewhere in this volume, this approach was successful in finding

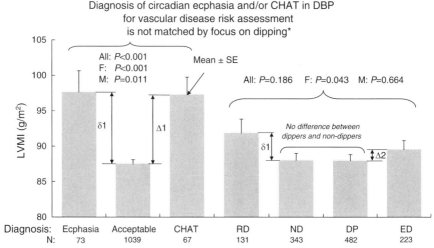

Figure 11.20. The left ventricular mass index (LVMI), used as a surrogate outcome measure, was available from all 1179 participants. It is compared overall and separately for men (M) and women (F) by one-way analysis of variance (ANOVA) among patients classified in terms of circadian characteristics assessed by cosinor (3 columns on left) or in terms of the day–night ratio (DNR) of diastolic blood pressure ("dipping," 4 columns on right). LVMI values are greatly elevated when diastolic ecphasia or CHAT is diagnosed, corresponding to circadian patterns of diastolic blood pressure abnormal in terms of timing or extent of predictable change within a day. This is not the case when patients are classified as reverse dippers (DNR < 0%), nondippers (0% < DNR < 10%), or extreme dippers (DNR > 20%). Ambulatory blood pressure monitoring may serve the broader derivation of normative values in health for circadian parameters. Data from C.H. Chen.

that low-dose aspirin is effective as an anticlotting agent when administered after awakening, but not when taken 12 hours later [110]. In the same six subjects, low-dose aspirin was found to be more effective as a hypotensive agent when given in the middle of the activity span [111], a result corroborated independently on a larger sample [112]. This is illustrated in Figures 11.24 and 11.25. Blood pressure was measured around the clock for a total of 16 days by 6 clinically healthy young women. During the first 7 days, aspirin was taken once a day, the timing of its administration differing among the 6 subjects: one took it upon awakening, four others either 3, 6, 9, or 12 hours after awakening, and the last one at bedtime. During the next 2 days, treatment was interrupted (washout), and for the last 7 days, a placebo was administered daily at the same time aspirin was taken during the first week. Each blood pressure profile was analyzed by a cumulative sum (CUSUM) control chart to determine whether

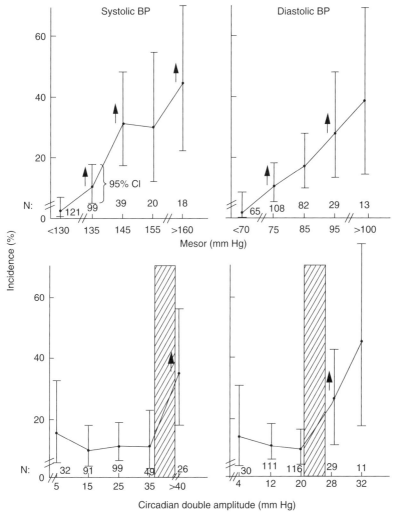

Threshold (hatched; bottom) must be exceeded before
the circadian double amplitude (2A) of Blood Pressure
(BP) indicates a disease risk syndrome; the BP-2A relates
nonlinearly to vascular disease incidence,
the 24-hour mean (MESOR; Top) does so nearly linearly*

* Statistically significant ($P < 0.05$) increase (↟) found between some consecutive MESORs (top) but
only at the transition to the highest (or second highest) 2A from the preceding one(s) (bottom);
▨ threshold, N = number of subjects per group; incidence of coronary artery disease, ischemic
stroke, nephropathy and/or retinopathy, within 6 years of a 48-hour ambulatory profile of BP in
297 patients in Tokyo, Japan. Data of K. Otsuka.

Figure 11.21. The circadian double amplitude (2A) of blood pressure must exceed a
threshold (hatched; bottom) before cardiovascular disease risk increases. The circadian
blood pressure amplitude relates nonlinearly to vascular disease incidence. By contrast,
the blood pressure MESOR relates linearly to the incidence of morbid events (top). Data
from K. Otsuka.

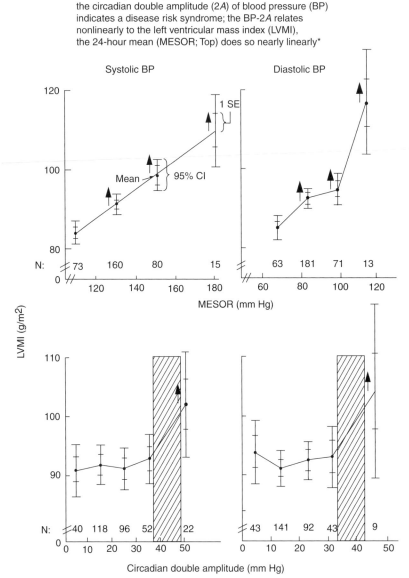

Threshold (Hatched; Bottom) must be exceeded before
the circadian double amplitude (2A) of blood pressure (BP)
indicates a disease risk syndrome; the BP-2A relates
nonlinearly to the left ventricular mass index (LVMI),
the 24-hour mean (MESOR; Top) does so nearly linearly*

* Statistically significant ($P < 0.01$ corrected for multiple testing) increase (↟) found between
consecutive MESORs (top) but only at the transition to the highest 2A from the preceding
one(s) (bottom); ⧄ threshold; N = number of subjects per group; 328 untreated men and
women, 30–88 years of age, in Taiwan, each providing a 24-hour ambulatory profile.
Data of C-H. Chen et al.

Figure 11.22. The circadian double amplitude (2A) of blood pressure must exceed a
threshold (hatched; bottom) before cardiovascular disease risk increases. The circadian
blood pressure amplitude relates nonlinearly to the left ventricular mass index (LVMI),
used as a surrogate outcome measure. By contrast, the blood pressure MESOR relates
linearly to LVMI (top). Data from C. H. Chen.

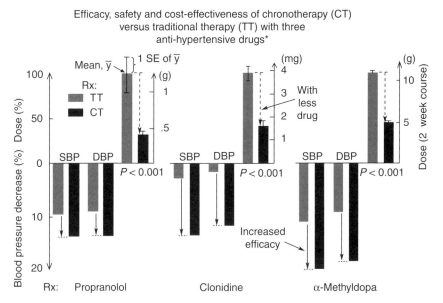

Figure 11.23. As compared to treatment with equal doses 3 times a day, treating 1.5–2 hours prior to the time of largest blood pressure excess with propranolol, clonidine, or α-methyldopa is associated with a hypotensive effect of greater extent from smaller doses of the drug. Not shown is the finding that the effect occurs sooner and leads to fewer overdosages and to fewer complications. Data from R. Zaslavskaya.

aspirin was associated with a statistically significant change in blood pressure [19]. A CUSUM consists of two lines, one indicating an increase in mean, the other a decrease in mean. As long as the two curves remain within a given decision interval, any change in blood pressure remains "in control" (no statistically significant change). But once one of the two curves breaks outside the decision interval, it indicates a statistically significant increase (if the positive CUSUM curve breaks above the upper limit of the decision interval) or decrease (if the negative CUSUM curve breaks below the lower limit of the decision interval) in blood pressure.

Figure 11.24 indicates an increase in blood pressure after switching from aspirin to placebo 6 or 9 hours after awakening, but not at other circadian stages. When the response is assigned to the circadian stage of treatment administration, pooling results from all 6 subjects, the circadian stage dependence of the effect becomes apparent (Figure 11.25), as subjects were randomly assigned to a circadian stage of treatment. Parenthetically, it has been reported that aspirin, albeit at a higher dosage, may be better tolerated in the evening [113], yet this report has been later disputed [114, 115]. The different optimal circadian stage of aspirin administration, after awakening for its anticlotting

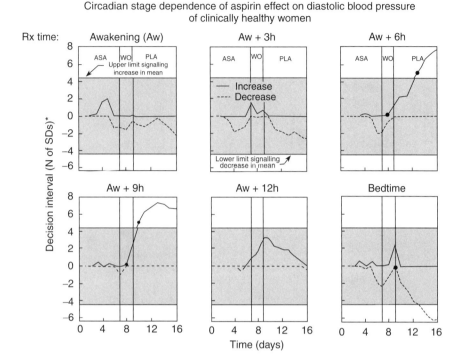

Circadian stage dependence of aspirin effect on diastolic blood pressure of clinically healthy women

ASA = Aspirin stage (100 mg/day for 1 week); PLA = Placebo; WO = Wash-out.
* Standard deviation from CUSUM: If there is displacement of 1 SD, it would be diagnosed by a slope of (1-0.5=) 0.5 SD.

Figure 11.24. In an N-of-6 pilot study, 6 clinically healthy women took low-dose aspirin (100 mg per day) for 1 week, and after a 2-day wash-out were switched to another week of placebo. Each woman was treated at a different circadian stage, either upon awakening, 3, 6, 9, 12 hours after awakening, or at bedtime. The treatment time was kept the same for a given subject. Blood pressure was measured around the clock throughout the study. Changes in the MESOR of blood pressure were assessed by means of a self-starting cumulative sum control chart. While the series of daily MESORs of diastolic blood pressure is proceeding "in control" (i.e., before the switch from aspirin to placebo), the cumulative sum (CUSUM) comprises two line graphs that generally stay within the limits of the "decision interval" (shaded area). The two curves signal increase and decrease in mean (in this case daily diastolic blood pressure MESORs), respectively. When one curve breaks out of the (shaded) decision interval boundary, it provides the rigorous validation of the change (increase or decrease) in DBP MESOR. The time at which the MESOR changed is estimated by tracking the line segment leading to the breakout back to the last occasion on which it lay on the horizontal axis. An increase in DBP MESOR is observed only when aspirin was replaced by placebo 6 or 9 hours after awakening, and treatment at bedtime has the opposite effect. Treatment at other times was not associated with any statistically significant change in diastolic blood pressure. Data from P. Prikryl.

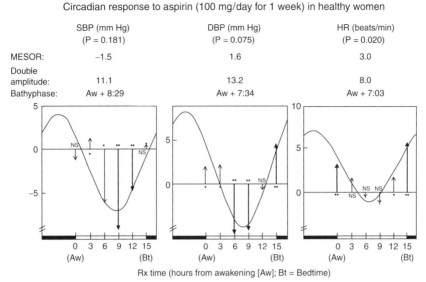

Circadian response to aspirin (100 mg/day for 1 week) in healthy women

Figure 11.25. Because women in Figure 11.24 were randomly assigned to one of six different treatment times, the response to treatment can be allocated to the timing of its administration. The least squares fit of a 24-hour cosine curve then tests whether the response to treatment was circadian stage dependent. For diastolic blood pressure, the circadian stage dependence of low-dose aspirin treatment reaches borderline statistical significance ($P = 0.075$), the largest effect being observed for aspirin taken in the afternoon, in keeping with independent results on a larger population. Data from P. Prikryl.

properties, midactivity span for its hypotensive effect, or possibly, still to be clarified, before bedtime to reduce its side effects, are a reminder of the need to triangulate among different effects, with consideration for the given patient's condition and susceptibility.

A similar protocol was followed to determine the optimal circadian stage of administration of Micardis (Telmisartan) [116], except that in this study patients served as their own longitudinal control, the time of treatment administration being changed at intervals.

One problem related to this design when it is applied longitudinally rather than in a group is the choice of an interval during which treatment is taken at a given time. In the Micardis study, the time of treatment administration was rotated by 3 hours every day. This may be too rapid, the first treatment time tending to be associated with a larger response, as it also corresponds to the patient's first response to the drug. One way to circumvent this problem is to repeat the rotation around all test times several times. Another consists of starting with different treatment times for different patients and of assessing effects on a group basis rather than for the individual patient. Considering a longer interval before changing the treatment time also presents some problem as it lengthens the duration of study, during which trends related to infradian components such as the circannual rhythm may complicate the interpretation of the results that can then no longer be attributed primarily to the response to treatment. Changing treatment times at intervals of 1 to 2 weeks seems preferable, and has been done for an antihypertensive agent [105] and for a nutriceutical with an effect on blood pressure [117].

11.6.5 Chronotherapy: Restoration of an Acceptable Blood Pressure Pattern

Much emphasis is placed today on lowering an elevated blood pressure, but not much attention is given to restoring an altered circadian variation in blood pressure (and/or heart rate). There is evidence, however, that the reduction of an excessive circadian amplitude of blood pressure to eliminate CHAT is associated with a reduction in adverse cardiovascular outcomes. Large clinical Asian trials [118, 119] indicated that treatment with benidipine in the morning was more beneficial than treatment twice a day (in the morning and evening) with nifedipine. A crossover randomized study comparing both treatments on patients followed by ABPM indicated that treatment with nifedipine was associated with a slight increase in the circadian amplitude of blood pressure. By contrast, benidipine treatment was associated with a reduction of the circadian amplitude of blood pressure (Figure 11.26), and hence with a reduction in the incidence of CHAT [120]. Of further interest is the observation that even though nifedipine lowered the average value of blood pressure more than benidipine, the latter halved undesirable events, in keeping with its reducing the circadian amplitude of blood pressure.

That the timing of treatment administration was relevant rather than the choice of the antihypertensive agent was further demonstrated in N-of-1 studies, that repeatedly showed the presence of a larger circadian amplitude of blood pressure when the same dose of the same drug was taken in the evening as compared to the morning [120]. This is illustrated, for instance, in

Figure 11.26. (a) A crossover study investigates the effect of two different treatments on the circadian pattern of blood pressure. Whereas nifedipine (taken twice a day, in the morning and in the evening, Rx1) is associated with a slightly more pronounced decrease in the MESOR of systolic blood pressure as compared to benidipine (taken once a day upon awakening, Rx2), it is also associated with a numerical increase rather than with a decrease in the circadian amplitude of systolic blood pressure. For patients with a circadian blood pressure amplitude close to the upper limit of acceptability, taking Rx1 or Rx2 may make the difference between iatrogenic CHAT or reducing the amplitude well within the range of acceptable values. Data from K. Otsuka. (b) Rx2 was found in large Asian clinical trials to be associated with better outcomes than Rx1. Reducing the incidence of CHAT may be the reason accounting for the difference (almost by a factor of 2) in outcomes, whether strokes or all cardiovascular events are considered.

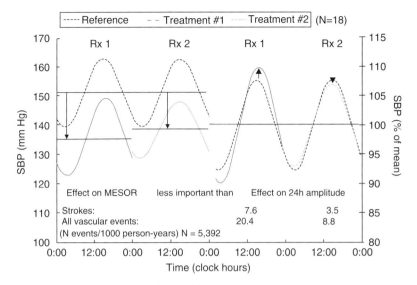

Does treating CHAT reduce morbidity?
(18 Patients in double blind placebo controlled study)
(M Shinagawa et al. Biomed pharmacother 2002; 55: 125–132)

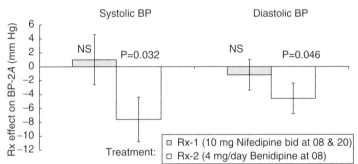

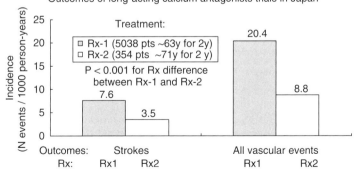

CHAT: Circadian hyper-amplitude-tension, condition defined by
circadian double amplitude (2A) of blood pressure (BP) above 95% prediction limit
of healthy peers matched by gender and age.
Outcomes of 2-year calcium antagonist trials on 5392 patients.
Over 50% reduction of strokes (left) and of all severe vascular events (right)
by treatment (Rx) that reduces (Rx2, white bars) vs. one that does not reduce
(Rx1, black bars) BP-2A. Rx1 vs Rx2 comparison: P < 0.001.

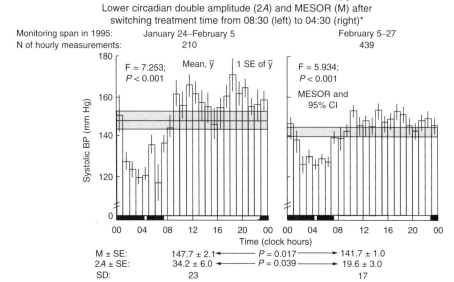

Individualized blood pressure (BP) chronotherapy
Lower circadian double amplitude (2A) and MESOR (M) after
switching treatment time from 08:30 (left) to 04:30 (right)*

Monitoring span in 1995: January 24–February 5 February 5–27
N of hourly measurements: 210 439

M ± SE:	147.7 ± 2.1 ◄——— P = 0.017 ———► 141.7 ± 1.0
2A ± SE:	34.2 ± 6.0 ◄——— P = 0.039 ———► 19.6 ± 3.0
SD:	23	17

* 240 mg Diltiazem HCl taken daily by 75-year-old man (FH) after getting up (left) or during an interruption of sleep (right).

Figure 11.27. Techniques are available to test on an individualized basis the efficacy of treatment. One such method consists of testing the equality of rhythm parameters before and after the start of treatment. In the case of this 75-year-old man, the same dose (240 mg) of the same drug (Diltiazem HCl) was taken either upon awakening (left) or during an interruption of sleep (right). The change in timing of medication was associated with both a further decrease in the MESOR of systolic blood pressure and with a decrease in the circadian amplitude of this variable. Timing treatment (chrono-therapy) can hence be useful to treat CHAT as well as MESOR-hypertension.

Figure 11.27. Not only is the MESOR of systolic blood pressure lowered more when the same dose (240 mg) of the same drug (Diltiazem HCl) is taken around 0430h than around 0830h, treatment at 0430h is also associated with a statistically significant decrease in the circadian amplitude of blood pressure [4], as ascertained by parameter tests, another approach applicable to assessing the response to treatment for the individual patient.

Clinical studies have also shown that not all antihypertensive agents act similarly on the circadian amplitude of blood pressure. For instance, long-acting carteolol is capable of lowering the circadian amplitude of blood pressure in most subjects, but captopril Retard is not (Figure 11.28) [121]. This differential effect of different antihypertensive agents in their action on the circadian amplitude of blood pressure was already noted in 1991 [122].

11.6.6 Treating an Elevated Risk: Primary Prevention

Blood pressure variability disorders such as CHAT can occur in otherwise MESOR-normotensive individuals who may not need antihypertensive

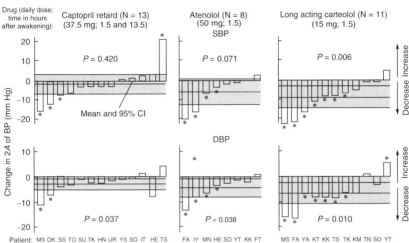

Figure 11.28. Whereas anti-hypertensive drugs are administered to decrease an elevated blood pressure mean, their effect on the circadian pattern of blood pressure, often ignored, can be very different from one drug to another. For instance, on the average, long-acting carteolol but not captopril can reduce the circadian amplitude of blood pressure of most patients participating in the study. This difference should be taken into consideration when CHAT is diagnosed. Data from Y. Watanabe.

medication. Even in MESOR-normotension, CHAT is associated with a large increase in vascular disease risk, however [1, 2]. The diagnosis of CHAT should thus prompt the institution of primary prevention before there is target organ damage.

When there is no need for a pharmacologic intervention, several options are available for the treatment of CHAT. One consists of using relaxation techniques such as autogenic training [121, 123, 124]. Another promising avenue of research relates to the use of ubiquinone (CoQ10), a powerful antioxidant and an integral component of the mitochondrial respiratory chain for energy production [125]. It is found in all tissues and organs of the body, with highest concentrations in the heart. Blood and tissue concentrations of CoQ10 are reportedly reduced with advancing age and in the presence of cardiovascular disease [126]. A recent meta-analysis of 12 clinical trials (362 patients) assessing the efficacy of CoQ10 in reducing an elevated blood pressure concluded that this nutriceutical has the potential of lowering systolic blood pressure by up to 17 mm Hg and diastolic blood pressure by up to 10 mm Hg without marked side effects [127].

In an *N*-of-1 study, a clinically healthy woman, 55 years of age, monitored her blood pressure around the clock for several months prior to the start of CoQ10 softgels supplementation (Tishcon Corporation) in daily doses of 100 mg. During the first week, CoQ10 was taken upon awakening, during weeks 2–5, it was taken 3.5, 7, 10.5, and 14 hours after awakening, and during week 6, it was taken 17.5 hours after awakening (corresponding to bedtime). The last 6 weeks prior to the start of treatment were used as reference. A circadian rhythm was invariably demonstrated for systolic and diastolic blood pressure during each of these 12 weeks ($P<0.001$). As compared to the reference span, CoQ10 was associated with a reduction of the circadian amplitude of both systolic ($P<0.001$) and diastolic ($P<0.001$) blood pressure, the effect being circadian stage-dependent (SBP: $P=0.043$; DBP: $P=0.012$). The largest reduction in circadian amplitude was associated with CoQ10 supplementation in the evening (around 14 hours after awakening) [117]. Notably in the absence of MESOR-hypertension, CoQ10 supplementation may be preferred to antihypertensive medication for the treatment of CHAT.

11.6.7 Chronotheranostics

Rhythms need to be assessed individually. The most opportune time to administer treatment may differ drastically from one patient to another. A patient diagnosed with CHAT is likely to have blood pressure excess primarily in the afternoon, whereas a "nondipper," or rather a patient with ecphasia, is likely to have blood pressure excess primarily by night, even when their blood pressure MESOR, percentage time elevation, and hyperbaric indices are similar. Model fitting to fractionated indices of excess, that is, hyperbaric indices computed not for the entire 24-hour span but for consecutive intervals of 1 to 3 hours, can determine the time of highest excess [66], an approach underlying the results illustrated in Figure 11.23 [108, 109].

Individualization of treatment includes the consideration of a given drug's effects on the variability of blood pressure and heart rate, in addition to its blood pressure lowering effect. Any differential effects of antihypertensive agents should be targeted to the patient's chronodiagnosis. Figure 11.29 summarizes results from a study comparing the effect of lercanidipine and felodipine on Chinese patients with primary hypertension [128]. Both drugs lower the blood pressure MESOR and reduce the pulse pressure, but only lercanidipine increases the standard deviation of heart rate, while felodipine but not lercanidipine may decrease the circadian amplitude of blood pressure. Lercanidipine may thus be the preferred treatment for patients with a decreased heart rate variability, whereas felodipine may be the preferred treatment for patients with CHAT [2].

For the treatment of risk elevation (prehabilitation) [129], drugs available to restore acceptable patterns of blood pressure and heart rate, thereby eliminating variability disorders, should be chosen as a function of the chronodiagnosis specifying the kind of abnormality encountered. As a first step, Figure 11.29 shows the kinds of questions to be raised and how they may be answered with specific molecules (as no more than illustrative examples). The individualized

Toward multiply-individualized chronotherapy*
Different calcium channel blockers can have different effects on blood pressure (BP)
and heart rate (HR) deviations associated with elevated vascular disease risk

	For a specific requirement, we ask of each drug:	
NO	1. Does it reduce the circadian amplitude of BP ?	YES
YES	2. Does it increase the circadian HR variability (CHRV) ?	NO
YES	3. Does it reduce pulse pressure (PP) ?	YES
YES	4. Does it reduce the BP MESOR ?	YES

*Individualized by 1. kind of chronome alteration detected by a chronodiagnosis that recognizes risk elevation as well as disease (against a gender- and age-qualified standard), 2. kind of drug, i.a., with respect to the desired effect on variabilities of BP and/or HR, and 3. multiple considerations also of timing. For instance, decisions regarding drug choice can be based on a chronodiagnosis using felodipine in the presence of CHAT (circadian hyper-amplitude-tension) (1), with MESOR-hypertension (2) and/or an elevated PP, but not with a decreased CHRV; or using lercanidipine in the presence of a deficit in CHRV, with MESOR-hypertension and/or an elevated PP, but not with CHAT. In each case, individualization is further desirable in relation to the timing of any BP or HR alteration, including the timing of blood pressure excess (1,2). Evidence thus far for the above drugs is available only in MESOR-hypertension. In MESOR-normotension, non-drug, approaches are indicated first, and the action in MESOR-normotension remains to be explored.

1. Halberg. F. Cornélissen G. Schack B. Self-experimentation on chronomes, time structures, chronomics for health surveillance and science: also transdisciplinary civic duty? Behavioral and Brain Sciences, http://www.bbsonline.org/Preprints/Roberts/Commentators/Halberg.html

2. Cornélissen G, Delmore P, Halberg F. Healthwatch 3. Why 7-day blood pressure monitoring: What everyone should know about blood pressure. Minneapolis: Halberg Chronobiology Center, University of Minnesota; 2003. 31 pp.

Figure 11.29. Differential effects of lercanidipine and felodipine on the variabilities of blood pressure and heart rate may be used for the individualization of treatment in the light of a chronodiagnosis established on the basis of around-the-clock monitoring of blood pressure and heart rate, analyzed chronobiologically, with results interpreted in the light of time-specified reference values of gender- and age-matched healthy peers. Data from B. Tomlinson and B. Fok.

therapy of risk elevation will eventually have to become an as-one-goes bootstrap operation. It is facilitated by the longitudinal monitoring of blood pressure and heart rate as marker variables useful both for the chronodiagnosis and as a guide for chronotherapy also aimed at restoring altered time structures [97, 105]. A dividend from longitudinal monitoring for self surveillance is the continued checking of the patient's response to treatment, so that any needed adjustment is immediately identified and acted upon, notably since blood pressure disorders are mostly asymptomatic. The aim is to prevent silent incipient target organ damage, such as an elevation of the left ventricular mass index, which was shown to be associated with an increase in the circadian amplitude of blood pressure possibly leading to CHAT, before there is a clear elevation of the blood pressure MESOR [130] (Figure 11.30). In keeping with this result are studies showing the higher prevalence of CHAT among patients with borderline hypertension by comparison with MESOR-hypertensive or MESOR-normotensive individuals [131].

With accumulating databases documenting the great day-to-day variability in blood pressure not just in isolated cases but in most individuals who have

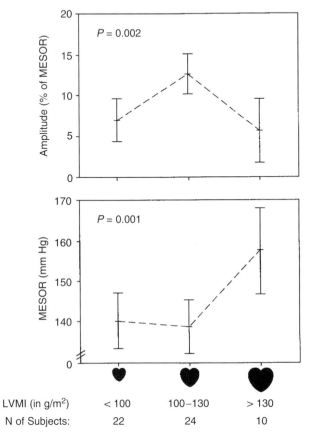

Elevation of circadian amplitude of systolic blood
pressure (SBP) associated with larger left ventricular
mass index (LVMI) when there is no increase in overall
rhythm-adjusted mean (MESOR)

Figure 11.30. When 56 untreated subjects newly diagnosed conventionally as hypertensive are classified in terms of their left ventricular mass index (LVMI), differences are observed in terms of the MESOR and circadian amplitude of blood pressure automatically measured around-the-clock every 15 minutes for 24 hours with an ambulatory monitor. Results shown here for systolic blood pressure are similar for mean arterial and diastolic blood pressure. A transient elevation of the circadian blood pressure amplitude is observed for subjects with intermediate LVMI values, while an elevated blood pressure MESOR is only observed for subjects with the highest LVMI values. Corroborating this finding are results from subsequent studies indicating that CHAT was more frequently observed among patients with borderline hypertension than among MESOR-hypertensive patients or among MESOR-normotensive subjects. Data from Y. Kumagai.

monitored for months, years, and even decades, the wisdom of current treatment modalities that most of the time "fly blind" [132] may also come under new scrutiny. Since blood pressure is so highly variable, should the treatment remain the same every day, in keeping with emphasis now placed on the development of 24-hour formulations? Or should the pharmaceutical industry turn to biosensors that would enable them to close the loop? An implanted blood pressure sensor linked to a drug delivery device capable of programmed patterned delivery of fast-acting antihypertensive medication by means of telemetry relaying the information from the sensor to the pump may be within reach, at least for high-risk patients already requiring the use of an implanted device such as a pacemaker or a defibrillator.

11.7 CONCLUSION

The idea of adjusting the treatment to individual needs emerged a few years ago from advances in molecular biology [133]. The profile of metabolites present in urine before drugs are administered may also help identify whether a patient is a good candidate for a drug. Based on studies in the experimental laboratory, Clayton et al. [134] report that predose metabolic profiles can predict how an individual might respond to a particular drug, a technique dubbed "pharmaco-metabonomics." Unlike pharmacogenomics [135], pharmacometabonomics in-cludes environmental as well as genetic factors. It has also been suggested that the use of biomarkers for personalized medicine can help reduce drug risks [136], Others have pointed to the danger of relying on averages that can hide individual differences in clinical trials [137]. As an example, these authors cite results from the ATLANTIS B trial that looked at the outcome of stroke patients treated 3 – 5 hours after the onset of symptoms. Whereas collective results showed no difference between t-PA treatment or placebo, benefit from t-PA was found among the one-third of patients who had the least risk of hemorrhage.

Notwithstanding the merits of such recent advances, one critical element remains missing from the aforementioned approaches, namely, the ubiquitous, broad time structures that have repeatedly been shown to make the difference between life and death in the experimental laboratory [8] or between the success or failure of a given treatment in the clinic [23], The transition from conven-tional treatment, if not from theranostics, to chronotheranostics is facilitated by the development of several technologies for monitoring health status, screening not only for disease conditions but also for risk elevation, for timely treatment scheduled according to bodily rhythms, and for the continued surveillance of the patient's response to treatment:

- Availability of portable, personal, long-term ambulatory monitors of biological variables, such as blood pressure, heart rate, the ECG and EEG, gastric acidity, core temperature and motor activity
- Availability of database systems to acquire and analyze volumes of data

- Availability of statistical procedures to analyze and model the data to devise dosage time patterns optimized for each individual patient
- Availability of portable, programmed devices to administer treatment (e.g., pacemakers, defibrillators, drug pumps)
- A chronobiologic understanding of the health effects of photic and nonphotic cycles

All these technologies could lead to marker rhythms-guided chronotherapy adjusted for the chronodiagnosis of each individual patient.

Table 11.4. Beginnings of Chronopharmacology and Chronotherapy

Year	Description	Author(s)
1952, 1953	2800-fold increase in sensitivity of a corticosteroid assay by accounting for circadian stage	Halberg (1, 2)
1955	Circadian susceptibility rhythm to noise	Halberg, Bittner, Gully, Albrecht, Brackney (3)
1955	Circadian susceptibility rhythm to an endotoxin	Halberg, Spink, Albrecht, and Gully (4)
1958	Detection of (growth) hormone effect on mitoses depends on circadian stage	Litman, Halberg, Ellis, and Bittner (5)
1959	Effect of ethanol depends on circadian stage	Haus, Hanton, and Halberg (6)
1959	Circadian susceptibility rhythm to a drug (ouabain)	Halberg and Stephens (7)
1960	LD_{50} to whole body X-ray irradiation depends on circadian stage	Halberg (8, discussion)
1961	Circadian susceptibility rhythm to Librium	Marte and Halberg (9)
1963	Circadian susceptibility rhythm to acetylcholine	Jones, Haus, and Halberg (10)
1964	Circadian susceptibility rhythm to fluothane	Matthews, Marte, and Halberg (11)
1969	Circadian susceptibility rhythm to penicillin	Reinberg Zagula-Mally, Ghata, and Halberg (12)
1970, 1972	Circadian susceptibility rhythm to arabinosyl cytosine	Cardoso Scheving, and Halberg (13), Haus et al. (14)
1973	Chronotherapy with hydrochlorothiazide and adriamycin	Halberg et al. (15)
1973	Marker rhythmometry introduced for hydrochlorothiazide chronotherapy	Levine Thampson, Shiotsuka, Krzanowski and Halberg (16)

(Continued)

Table 11.4. Continued

Year	Description	Author(s)
1974	Formulation of rules of chronopharmacology and chronotherapy	Halberg (17)
1977	Doubling of 2-year survival by timing radiotherapy	Halberg (18)
1979	Ara-C chronotherapy-related cancer cures	Halberg, Nelson, Cornélissen, Haus, Scheving, and Good (19)

1. Halberg F. Some correlations between chemical structure and maximal eosinopenia in adrenalectomized and hypophysectomized mice. *J Pharmacol Exp Ther*. 1952;106:135–149.

2. Halberg F. Some physiological and clinical aspects of 24-hour periodicity. *Lancet*. 1953;73: 20–32.

3. Halberg F, Bittner JJ, Gully RJ, Albrecht PG, Brackney EL. 24-hour periodicity and audiogenic convulsions in I mice of various ages. *Proc Soc Exp Biol* (NY). 1955;88:169–173.

4. Halberg F, Spink WW, Albrecht PG, Gully RJ. Resistance of mice to brucella somatic antigen, 24-hour periodicity and the adrenals. *J Clin Endocrinol*. 1955;15:887.

5. Litman T, Halberg F, Ellis S, Bittner JJ. Pituitary growth hormone and mitoses in immature mouse liver. *Endocrinology*. 1958; 62:361–364.

6. Haus E, Hanton EM, Halberg F. 24-hour susceptibility rhythm to ethanol in fully fed, starved and thirsted mice and the lighting regimen. *Physiologist*. 1959;2:54.

7. Halberg F, Stephens AN. Susceptibility to ouabain and physiologic circadian periodicity. *Proc Minn Acad Sci*. 1959;27:139–143.

8. Halberg F. Temporal coordination of physiologic function. *Cold Spring Harb Symp Quant Biol*. 1960;25:289–310. Discussion on LD_{50} p 310.

9. Marte E, Halberg F. Circadian susceptibility rhythm of mice to librium. *Fed Proc*. 1961;20:305.

10. Jones F, Haus E, Halberg F. Murine circadian susceptibility-resistance cycle to acetylcholine. *Proc Minn Acad Sci*. 1963;31:61–62.

11. Matthews JH, Marte E, Halberg F. A circadian susceptibility-resistance cycle to fluothane in male B_1 mice. *Can Anaesthetists' Soc J*. 1964;11:280–290.

12. Reinberg A, Zagula-Mally ZW, Ghata J, Halberg F. Circadian reactivity rhythm of human skin to house dust, penicillin and histamine. *J Allergy*. 1969;44:292–306.

13. Cardoso SS, Scheving LE, Halberg F. Mortality of mice as influenced by the hour of the day of drug (ara-C) administration. *Pharmacologist*. 1970;12:302.

14. Haus E, Halberg F, Scheving L, Pauly JE, Cardoso S, Kühl JFW, Sothern R, Shiotsuka RN, Hwang DS. Increased tolerance of leukemic mice to arabinosyl cytosine given on schedule adjusted to circadian system. *Science*. 1972;177:80–82.

15. Halberg F, Haus E, Cardoso SS, Scheving LE, Kühl JFW, Shiotsuka R, Rosene G, Pauly JE, Runge W, Spalding JF, Lee JK, Good RA. Toward a chronotherapy of neoplasia: tolerance of treatment depends upon host rhythms. *Experientia (Basel)*. 1973;29: 909–934.

16. Levine H, Thompson D, Shiotsuka R, Krzanowski M, Halberg F. Autorhythmometrically determined blood pressure ranges and rhythm of 12 presumably healthy men during an 18-day span. *Int J Chronobiol*. 1973; 1: 337–338.

17. Halberg F. Protection by timing treatment according to bodily rhythms: an analogy to protection by scrubbing before surgery. *Chronobiologia*. 1974;1 (Suppl. 1):27–68.

18. Halberg F. Biological as well as physical parameters relate to radiology. Guest Lecture, Proceedings of the 30th Annual Congress Radiology, January 1977, Post-Graduate Institute of Medical Education and Research, Chandigarh, India.

19. Halberg F, Nelson W, Cornélissen G, Haus E, Scheving LE, Good RA. On methods for testing and achieving cancer chronotherapy. *Cancer Treatment Rep*. 1979;63:1428–1430.

Some milestones in the development of chronopharmacology and chronotherapy are listed in Table 11.4. Already in 1952, it became apparent that the use of timing in a bioassay accounting for rhythms allowed a 2800-fold increase in sensitivity [138], a finding pertinent to drug development. Also, over half a century ago, a small electrical device, cobbled together with spare parts according to a diagram for an electronic metronome borrowed from a popular magazine, kept an infant heart patient alive, by pacing the basic rhythm of the heart. This chronotheranostic ("chrono" since it restored a rhythm) intervention (Bakken, 1999; [139–141] led to current implantable devices, useful in disease. The challenge of the next generation of devices is not only to close the loop between diagnosis and treatment, but to do so by prophylactic intervention in the presence of a heightened risk, before the onset of overt disease.

ACKNOWLEDGMENT

Support: US Public Health Service (GM-13981; FH), University of Minnesota Supercomputing Institute (GC, FH).

REFERENCES

1. Halberg F, Cornélissen G, Halberg J, Fink H, Chen CH, Otsuka K, Watanabe Y, Kumagai Y, Syutkina EV, Kawasaki T, Uezono K, Zhao ZY, Schwartzkopff O. Circadian hyper-amplitude-tension, CHAT: a disease risk syndrome of anti-aging medicine. *J Anti-Aging Med*. 1998; 1: 239–259.
2. Cornélissen G, Halberg F, Bakken EE, Singh RB, Otsuka K, Tomlinson B, Delcourt A, Toussaint G, Bathina S, Schwartzkopff O, Wang ZR, Tarquini R, Perfetto F, Pantaleoni GC, Jozsa R, Delmore PA, Nolley E. 100 or 30 years after Janeway or Bartter, Healthwatch helps avoid "flying blind." *Biomed Pharmacother*. 2004; 58(suppl 1): S69–S86.
3. Halberg F, Cornélissen G, Wang ZR, Wan C, Ulmer W, Katinas G, Singh Ranjana, Singh RK, Singh Rajesh, Gupta BD, Singh RB, Kumar A, Kanabrocki E, Sothern RB, Rao G, Bhatt MLBD, Srivastava M, Rai G, Singh S, Pati AK, Nath P, Halberg F, Halberg J, Schwartzkopff O, Bakken E, Shastri VK. Chronomics: circadian and circaseptan timing of radiotherapy, drugs, calories, perhaps nutriceuticals and beyond. *J Exp Ther Oncol*. 2003; 3: 223–260.
4. Halberg F, Cornélissen G, International Womb-to-Tomb Chronome Initiative Group. Resolution from a meeting of the International Society for Research on Civilization Diseases and the Environment (New SIRMCE Confederation), Brussels, Belgium, March 17–18, 1995. *Fairy Tale or reality*? Medtronic Chronobiology Seminar #8, April 1995, 12 pp. text, 18 figures. Available at http://www.msi.umn.edu/~halberg/.
5. Halberg F. When to treat. *Hæmatologica (Pavia)*. 1975; 60: 1–30.
6. Carandente A, Halberg F. Drug industry and chronobiology: achievements and prospects. *Ann NY Acad Sci*. 1991; 618: 484–489.

7. Halberg F. Protection by timing treatment according to bodily rhythms: an analogy to protection by scrubbing before surgery. *Chronobiologia.* 1974; 1(suppl 1): 27–68.

8. Ertel RJ, Halberg F, Ungar F. Circadian system phase-dependent toxicity and other effects of methopyrapone (SU-4885) in mice. *J Pharmacol Exp Ther.* 1964; 146: 395–399.

9. Bingham C, Cornélissen G, Halberg F. Power of Phase 0 chronobiologic trials at different signal-to-noise ratios and sample sizes. *Chronobiologia.* 1993; 20: 179–190.

10. Cornélissen G, Bingham C, Wilson D, Halberg F. Illustrating power of cost-effective "Phase 0" chronobiologic trials in endocrinology, psychiatry and oncology. In: Cornélissen G, Halberg E, Bakken E, Delmore P, Halberg F, eds. *Toward Phase Zero Preclinical and Clinical Trials: Chronobiologic Designs and Illustrative Applications.* University of Minnesota Medtronic Chronobiology Seminar Series #6, September 1992, pp 138–181.

11. Halberg F, Bingham C, Cornélissen G. Clinical trials: the larger the better? *Chronobiologia.* 1993; 20: 193–212.

12. Zaslavskaya RM. *Chronodiagnosis and Chronotherapy of Cardiovascular Diseases,* 2nd ed. Translation into English from Russian. Moscow: Medicina; 1993.

13. Halberg F, Halberg J, Halberg E, Halberg F. Chronobiology, radiobiology and steps toward the timing of cancer radiotherapy. In: Kaiser H, ed. *Cancer Growth and Progression,* vol 9, chap 19. Dordrecht: Kluwer Academic Publishers; 1989: 227–253.

14. Peto R, Pike MC, Armitage P, Breslow NE, Cox DR, Howard SV, Mantel N, McPherson K, Peto J, Smith PG. Design and analysis of randomized clinical trials requiring prolonged observation of each patient. I. Introduction and design. *Brit J Cancer.* 1976; 34: 585–612.

15. Peto R, Pike MC, Armitage P, Breslow NE, Cox DR, Howard SV, Mantel N, McPherson K, Peto J, Smith PG. Design and analysis of randomized clinical trials requiring prolonged observation of each patient. II. Analysis and examples. *Br J Cancer.* 1977; 35: 1–39.

16. Fedorov VV, Khabarov V. Duality of optimal designs for model discrimination and parameter estimation. *Biometrika.* 1986; 73: 183–190.

17. Kitsos CP, Titterington DM, Torsney B. An optimal design problem in rhythmometry. *Biometrics.* 1988; 44: 657–671.

18. Bingham C, Arbogast B, Cornélissen Guillaume G, Lee JK, Halberg F. Inferential statistical methods for estimating and comparing cosinor parameters. *Chronobiologia.* 1982; 9: 397–439.

19. Hawkins DM. Self-starting cusum charts for location and scale. *Statistician.* 1987; 36: 299–315.

20. Cornélissen G, Halberg F, Hawkins D, Otsuka K, Henke W. Individual assessment of antihypertensive response by self-starting cumulative sums. *J Med Eng Technol.* 1997; 21: 111–120.

21. Johnson EA, Haus E, Halberg F, Wadsworth GL. Graphic monitoring of seizure incidence changes in epileptic patients. *Minn Med.* 1959; 42: 1250–1257.

22. Halberg F. Temporal coordination of physiologic function. *Cold Spring Harb Symp Quant Biol.* 1960; 25: 289–310.

23. Halberg F. Biological as well as physical parameters relate to radiology. Guest Lecture, Proceedings of the 30th Annual Congress Radiology, January 1977, Post-Graduate Institute of Medical Education and Research, Chandigarh, India.

24. Halberg F, Prem K, Halberg F, Norman C, Cornélissen G. Cancer chronomics I: origins of timed cancer treatment: early marker rhythm-guided individualized chronochemotherapy. *J Exp Ther Oncol.* 2006; 6: 55–61.

25. Haus E, Fernandes G, Kühl JFW, Yunis EJ, Lee JK, Halberg F. Murine circadian susceptibility rhythm to cyclophosphamide. *Chronobiologia.* 1974; 1: 270–277.

26. Halberg F, Halberg E, Haus E, Walker R, Fujii S, Berg H, Takagi M, Cornélissen G. Markers for the diagnosis and prevention of malignancy. *Bioquimia.* 1994; 19: 41–42.

27. Halberg F, Cornélissen G, Bingham C, Fujii S, Halberg E. From experimental units to unique experiments: chronobiologic pilots complement large trials. *In vivo.* 1992; 6: 403–428.

28. Cornélissen G, Halberg F. *Introduction to Chronobiology.* Medtronic Chronobiology Seminar #7, April 1994. (Library of Congress Catalog Card #94-060580). Available at http://www.msi.umn.edu/~halberg.

29. Cornélissen G, Halberg F, Walker R, Zaslavskaya RM, Fine RL, Haus E. Chronobiologic aspects of urinary gonadotropin peptide (UGP). *In Vivo.* 1995; 9: 359–362.

30. Xu FJ, Yu YH, Bast RC Jr, Cornélissen G, Fujii S, Takagi M, O'Brien T, Halberg F. Toward salivary–urinary chronosensitivity testing: chronomes of OVX1, M-CSF and CA130. *In Vivo.* 1995; 9: 407–412.

31. Halberg E, Long HJ III, Cornélissen G, Blank MA, Elg S, Touitou Y, Bakken E, Delmore P, Haus E, Sackett-Lundeen L, Prem K, Halberg F. Toward a chronotherapy of ovarian cancer with taxol: Part II: Test pilot study on CA125. *Chronobiologia.* 1992; 19: 17–42.

32. Cornélissen G, Halberg F, Halberg E, Bingham C, Haus E, Bast RC Jr, Fujii S, Long HJ III, Halberg F, Tamura K. Toward a chronotherapy of ovarian cancer. Part III: Salivary CA125 for chronochemotherapy by efficacy. *Chronobiologia.* 1992; 19: 131–149.

33. Halberg E, Cornélissen G, Haus E, Fine RL, Walker R, Von Hoff D, Halberg F, Halberg J, Halberg F. Amplification [on comments by Berry DA. Power of chronobiologic pilots: a statistician's opinion. *Chronobiologia.* 1993; 20: 213–214]. *Chronobiologia.* 1993; 20: 214–218.

34. Klevecz RR, Shymko RM, Blumenfeld D, Braly PS. Circadian gating of S-phase in human ovarian cancer. *Caner Res.* 1987; 47: 6267–6271.

35. Elg S, Halberg E, Ramakrishnan R, Cornélissen G, Haus E, Nicolau G, Carson L, Twiggs L, Long HJ III, Halberg F. Marker rhythmometry with macrophage colony stimulating factor (M-CSF). *Chronobiologia.* 1991; 18: 141–152.

36. Carenza L, Villani C, Rulli G, Labi FL, Prosperi Port R. Ovarian cancer: relationship between in vitro chromosensitivity and clinical response. *Gynecol Oncol.* 1990; 36: 13–18.

37. Fine RL, Cornélissen G, Haus E, Bast RC Jr, Walker R, Berg H, Jatoi A, Dahl J, Sturner ML, Nelson R, Cardarelli I, Mikhail L, Hunter D, Halberg J, Halberg F, Von Hoff DD, Halberg F, Halberg E. Erna-test: chemosensitivity assays and

marker rhythmometry target cancer treatment in time and kind. 16th World Congress of Anatomic and Clinical Pathology, Acapulco, Mexico, October 5–9, 1993.

38. Levi F, Zidani R, Brienza S, Dogliotti L, Perpoint B, Rotarski M, Letourneau Y, Llory JF, Chollet P, Le Rol A, Focan C. A multicenter evaluation of intensified, ambulatory, chronomodulated chemotherapy with oxaliplatin, 5-fluorouracil, and leucovorin as initial treatment of patients with metastatic colorectal carcinoma. International Organization for Cancer Chronotherapy. *Cancer.* 1999; 85: 2532–2540.

39. Halberg F, Gupta BD, Haus E, Halberg E, Deka AC, Nelson W, Sothern RB, Cornélissen G, Lee JK, Lakatua DJ, Scheving LE, Burns ER. Steps toward a cancer chronopolytherapy. In: *Proceedings of the XIV International Congress of Therapeutics.* Montpellier, France: L'Expansion Scientifique Française; 1977: 151–196.

40. Halberg F, Haus E, Cardoso SS, Scheving LE, Kühl JFW, Shiotsuka R, Rosene G, Pauly JE, Runge W, Spalding JF, Lee JK, Good RA. Toward a chronotherapy of neoplasia: tolerance of treatment depends upon host rhythms. *Experientia (Basel).* 1973; 29: 909–934.

41. Hrushesky WJM. The clinical application of chronobiology to oncology. *Am J Anat.* 1983; 168: 519–542.

42. Hrushesky WJM. Automatic chronotherapy: an integral part of the future of medicine. In: Hekkens WTJM, Kerkhof GA, Rietveld WJ, eds. *Trends in Chronobiology.* Oxford, UK: Pergamon Press; 1988: 281–293.

43. Cornélissen G, Halberg F. *The chronobiologic pilot study with special reference to cancer research: Is chronobiology or, rather, its neglect wasteful?* In: Kaiser H, ed. *Cancer Growth and Progression,* vol 9. chap 9. Dordrecht: Kluwer Academic Publishers; 1989: 103–133.

44. Kennedy BJ. A lady and chronobiology. *Chronobiologia.* 1993; 20: 139–144.

45. Blank MA, Gushchin VA, Halberg F, Portela A, Cornélissen G. X-irradiation chronosensitivity and circadian rhythmic proliferation in healthy and sarcoma-carrying rats' bone marrow. *In Vivo.* 1995; 9: 395–400.

46. Halberg F, Cornélissen G, Schwartzkopff O, Katinas GS, Chibisov SM, Khalitskaya EV, Mitsutake G, Otsuka K, Scheving LA, Bakken EE. Chronometaanalysis: magnetic storm associated with a reduction in circadian amplitude of rhythm in corneal cell division. In: *International Conference on the Frontiers of Biomedical Science: Chronobiology,* Chengdu, China, September 24–26, 2006, pp 40–42.

47. Blank MA, Blank OA, Duke VA. The hemodepressive effect of irradiation in humans. *Dokl Biol Sci.* 2003; 393: 424–426.

48. Blank MA, Blank OA, Gershanovich ML. Influence of geomagnetic activity on mustophoran hematotoxicity. *Dokl Biol Sci.* 2005; 404: 835–838.

49. Takahashi R, Halberg F, Walker C, eds. *Toward Chronopharmacology.* New York: Pergamon Press; 1982 .

50. Di Santo A, Chodos D, Halberg F. Chronobioavailability of three erythromycin test preparations assessed by each of four indices: time to peak, peak, nadir and area. *Chronobiologia.* 1975; 2(suppl 1): 17.

51. Morris PJ. Cyclosporin A overview. *Transplantation.* 1981; 32: 349–354.

52. Ferguson RM, Rynasiewicz JJ, Sutherland DER, Simmons RS, Najarian JS. Cyclosporin A in renal transplantation. A prospective randomized trial. *Surgery*. 1982; 92: 175–182.

53. Cavallini M, Halberg F, Sutherland DER, Cornélissen G, Heil J, Najarian JS. Optimization by timing of oral cyclosporine to prevent acute kidney allograft rejection in dogs. *Transplantation*. 1986; 41: 654–657.

54. Magnus G, Cavallini M, Halberg F, Cornélissen G, Sutherland D, Hrushesky W, Najarian JS. Circadian toxicology of cyclosporine. *Toxicol Appl Pharmacol*. 1985; 77: 181–185.

55. Cavallini M, Magnus G, Halberg F, Liu T, Field MY, Sibley R, Najarian JS, Sutherland DER. Benefit from circadian timing of cyclosporine revealed by delay of rejection of murine heart allograft. *Transplant Proc*. 1983; 15(4, suppl 1): 2960–2966.

56. Cavallini M, Halberg F, Cornélissen G, Enrichens F, Margarit C. Organ transplantation and broader chronotherapy with implantable pump and computer programs for marker rhythm assessment. *J Control Release*. 1986; 3: 3–13.

57. DeVecchi A, Carandente F, Fryd DS, Halberg F, Sutherland DE, Howard RJ, Simmons RL, Najarian JS. Circaseptan (about 7-day) rhythm in human kidney allograft rejection in different geographic locations. In: Reinberg A, Halberg F, eds. *Chronopharmacology, Proceedings of the Satellite Symposium of the 7th International Congress on Pharmacology*, Paris 1978. New York: Pergamon Press; 1979: 193–202.

58. Liu T, Cavallini M, Halberg F, Cornélissen G, Field J, Sutherland DER. More on the need for circadian, circaseptan and circannual optimization of cyclosporine therapy. *Experientia*. 1986; 42: 20–22.

59. Cornélissen G, Gubin D, Halberg F, Milano G, Halberg F. Chronomedical aspects of oncology and geriatrics (review). *In Vivo*. 1999; 13: 77–82.

60. Halberg E, Halberg F. Chronobiologic study design in everyday life, clinic and laboratory. *Chronobiologia*. 1980; 7: 95–120.

61. Rottembourg J, Mattei MF, Cabrol A, Leger P, Aupetit B, Beaufils H, Gluckman JC, Pavie A, Gandjbakhch I, Cabrol C. Renal function and blood pressure in heart transplant recipients treated with cyclosporine. *J Heart Transplant*. 1985; 4: 404–408.

62. McDonald K, Sanchez de la Peña S, Cavallini M, Olivari MT, Cohn JN, Halberg F. Chronobiologic blood pressure and heart rate assessment of patients with heart transplants. *Prog Clin Biol Res*. 1990; 341B: 471–480.

63. Lenfant C. Reflections on hypertension control rates: a message from the director of the National Heart, Lung, and Blood Institute. *Arch Intern Med*. 2002; 162: 131–132.

64. Veerman DP, de Blok K, Elemarre BJ, van Montfrans GA. Office, nurse, basal and ambulatory blood pressure as predictors of hypertensive target organ damage in male and female patients. *J Hum Hypertens*. 1996; 10: 9–15.

65. Cornélissen G, Halberg F. Impeachment of casual blood pressure measurements and the fixed limits for their interpretation and chronobiologic recommendations. *Ann NY Acad Sci*. 1996; 783: 24–46.

66. Cornélissen G, Otsuka K, Halberg F. Blood pressure and heart rate chronome mapping: a complement to the human genome initiative. In: Otsuka K, Cornélissen G, Halberg F, eds. *Chronocardiology and Chronomedicine: Humans in Time and Cosmos*. Tokyo: Life Science Publishing; 1993: 16–48.

67. Nelson W, Cornélissen G, Hinkley D, Bingham C, Halberg F. Construction of rhythm-specified reference intervals and regions, with emphasis on "hybrid" data, illustrated for plasma cortisol. *Chronobiologia*. 1983; 10: 179–193.

68. Halberg F, Drayer JIM, Cornélissen G, Weber MA. Cardiovascular reference data base for recognizing circadian mesor- and amplitude-hypertension in apparently healthy men. *Chronobiologia*. 1984; 11: 275–298.

69. Halberg F. Chronobiology. *Annu Rev Physiol*. 1969; 31: 675–725.

70. Halberg F. Chronobiology: methodological problems. *Acta Med Rom*. 1980; 18: 399–440.

71. Cornélissen G, Halberg F. Chronomedicine In: Armitage P, Colton T, eds. *Encyclopedia of Biostatistics*, 2nd ed. Chichester, UK: John Wiley & Sons Ltd; 2005: 796–812.

72. Zachariah PK, Sheps SG, Ilstrup DM, Long CR, Bailey KR, Wiltgen CM, Carlson CA. Blood pressure load — a better determinant of hypertension. *Mayo Clinic Proc*. 1988; 63: 1085–1091.

73. Cornélissen G, Haus E, Halberg F. *Chronobiologic blood pressure assessment from womb to tomb*. In: Touitou Y, Haus E, eds. *Biological Rhythms in Clinical and Laboratory Medicine*. Berlin: Springer-Verlag; 1992: 428–452.

74. White WB. Analysis of ambulatory blood pressure data in antihypertensive drug trials. *J Hypertens*. 1991; 9(suppl 1): S27–S32.

75. National High Blood Pressure Education Program Coordinating Committee Working Group Report on Ambulatory Blood Pressure Monitoring. *Arch Intern Med*. 1990; 150: 2270–2280.

76. Cornélissen G, Halberg F, Bingham C, Kumagai Y. Toward engineering for blood pressure surveillance. *Biomed Instrum Technol*. 1997; 31: 489–498.

77. Cornélissen G, Halberg F, Bingham C, Kumagai Y. More on software chronobio-engineering for blood pressure surveillance. *Biomed Instrum Technol*. 1997; 31: 511–513.

78. Cornélissen G, Siegelova J, Halberg F. Blood pressure and heart rate dynamics during pregnancy and early extra-uterine life: methodology for a chrononeo-natology. In: Halberg F, Kenner T, Fiser B, eds. *Proceedings, Symposium: The Importance of Chronobiology in Diagnosing and Therapy of Internal Diseases*. Faculty of Medicine, Masaryk University, Brno, Czech Republic, January 10–13, 2002. Brno: Masaryk University; 2002: 58–96.

79. Kshirsagar AV, Carpenter M, Bang H, Wyatt SB, Colindres RE. Blood pressure usually considered normal is associated with an elevated risk of cardiovascular disease. *Am J Med*. 2006; 119: 133–141.

80. Magometschnigg D. Definition und Klassifikation der Hypertonie. *J Hyperton*. 2004; 8: 12–13. Deutsche Hochdruckliga e.V. (DHL) und Deutsche Hypertonie-gesellschaft (DHL/DHG). Leitlinien zur Hypertonie. Available at http://www.paritaet.org/RR-Liga/Hypertonie-Leitlinien05.pdf.

81. Hagen P, ed. Mayo Clinic Guide to Self-Care: Answers for Everyday Health Problems. Rochester, MN: Mayo Clinic; 2003: 180–181.

82. Taylor AL, Lindenfeld J, Ziesche S, Walsh MN, Mitchell JE, Adams K, Tam SW, Ofili E, Sabolinski ML, Worcel M, Cohn JN, A-HeFT Investigators. Outcomes by gender in the African-American Heart Failure Trial. *J Am Coll Cardiol.* 2006; 48: 2263–2267.

83. Hayes SN, Taler SJ. Hypertension in women: current understanding of gender differences. *Mayo Clin Proc.* 1998; 73: 157–165.

84. Celis H, Fagard RH, Staessen JA, Thijs L. Systolic Hypertension in Europe Trial Investigators. Risk and benefit of treatment of isolated hypertension in the elderly: evidence from the Systolic Hypertension in Europe Trial. *Curr Opin Cardiol.* 2001; 16: 342–348.

85. Kleiger RE, Miller JP, Bigger JT, Moss AJ. Multicenter Post-Infarction Research Group. Decreased heart rate variability and its association with increased mortality after acute myocardial infarction. *Am J Cardiol.* 1987; 59: 256–262.

86. Tsuji H, Venditti FJ, Manders ES, Evans JC, Larson MG, Feldman CL, Levy D. Reduced heart rate variability and mortality risk in an elderly cohort: the Framingham Heart Study. *Circulation.* 1994; 90: 878–883.

87. Otsuka K, Cornélissen G, Halberg F. Predictive value of blood pressure dipping and swinging with regard to vascular disease risk. *Clin Drug Investi.* 1996; 11: 20–31.

88. Otsuka K, Cornélissen G, Halberg F. Circadian rhythmic fractal scaling of heart rate variability in health and coronary artery disease. *Clin Cardiol.* 1997; 20: 631–638.

89. Otsuka K, Cornélissen G, Halberg F. Age, gender and fractal scaling in heart rate variability. *Clin Sci.* 1997; 93: 299–308.

90. Otsuka K, Cornélissen G, Halberg F. Heart rate variability measures and the autonomic nervous function. *Diagn Treatment.* 1997; 85: 1500–1506.

91. Otsuka K, Cornélissen G, Halberg F, Oehlert G. Excessive circadian amplitude of blood pressure increases risk of ischemic stroke and nephropathy. *J Med Eng Technol.* 1997; 21: 23–30.

92. Baevsky RM, Petrov VM, Cornélissen G, Halberg F, Orth-Gomér K, Åkerstedt T, Otsuka K, Breus T, Siegelova J, Dusek J, Fiser B. Meta-analyzed heart rate variability, exposure to geomagnetic storms, and the risk of ischemic heart disease. *Scr Med.* 1997; 70: 199–204.

93. Nakano S, Fukuda M, Hotta F, Ito T, Ishii T, Kitazawa M, Nishizawa M, Kigoshi T, Uchida K. Reversed circadian blood pressure rhythm is associated with occurrence of both fatal and nonfatal vascular events in NIDDM subjects. *Diabetes.* 1998; 47: 1501–1506.

94. Sanchez de la Pena S, Gonzalez C, Cornélissen G, Halberg F. Blood pressure (BP), heart rate (HR) and non-insulin-dependent diabetes mellitus (NIDDM) chrono-biology. Abstract S8-06, 3rd International Congress on Cardiovascular Disease, Taipei, Taiwan, November 26–28, 2004. *Int J Cardiol.* 2004; 97(suppl 2): S14.

95. Cornélissen G, Chen CH, Halberg F. Predictive value of blood pressure variability: merits of circadian parameters versus dipping patterns. *N Engl J Med.* 2006; 355: 850.

96. Cornélissen G, Halberg F, Otsuka K, Singh RB, Chen CH. Chronobiology predicts actual and proxy outcomes when dipping fails. *Hypertension*. 2007; 49: 237–239.

97. Halberg F, Cornélissen G, Halberg J, Schwartzkopff O. Pre-hypertensive and other variabilities also await treatment. *Am J Med*. 2007; 120: e19–e20.

98. Mancia G, Frattola A, Parati G, Santucciu C, Ulian L. Blood pressure variability and organ damage. *J Cardiovasc Pharmacol*. 1994; 24(suppl A): S6–S11.

99. Parati G, Di Rienzo M, Ulian L, Santucciu C, Girard A, Elghozi JL, Mancia G. Clinical relevance of blood pressure variability. *J Hypertens*. 1998; 16: S25–S33.

100. Verdecchia P, Schillaci G, Guerrieri M, Gatteschi C, Benemio G, Boldrini F, Porcellati C. Circadian blood pressure changes and left ventricular hypertrophy in essential hypertension. *Circulation*. 1990; 81: 528–536.

101. Chen CH, Cornélissen G, Siegelova J, Halberg F. Does overswinging provide an early warning of cardiovascular disease risk when non-dipping may fail? A meta-analysis of 2039 cases. *Scr Med*. 2001; 74: 75–80.

102. Cornélissen G, Chen CH, Siegelova J, Halberg F. Vascular disease risk syndromes affecting both MESOR-normotensives and MESOR-hypertensives: a meta-analysis of 2039 cases. *Scr Med*. 2001; 74: 81–86.

103. Cornélissen G, Otsuka K, Chen CH, Kumagai Y, Watanabe Y, Halberg F, Siegelova J, Dusek J. Nonlinear relation of the circadian blood pressure amplitude to cardiovascular disease risk. *Scr Med*. 2000; 73: 85–94.

104. Parati G, Saul JP, Di Rienzo M, Mancia G. Spectral analysis of blood pressure and heart rate variability in evaluating cardiovascular regulation. *Hypertension*. 1995; 25: 1276–1286.

105. Halberg F, Cornélissen G, Katinas G, Tvildiani L, Gigolashvili M, Janashia K, Toba T, Revilla M, Regal P, Sothern RB, Wendt HW, Wang ZR, Zeman M, Jozsa R, Singh RB, Mitsutake G, Chibisov SM, Lee J, Holley D, Holte JE, Sonkowsky RP, Schwartzkopff O, Delmore P, Otsuka K, Bakken EE, Czaplicki J, International BIOCOS Group. Chronobiology's progress: Part II, chronomics for an immediately applicable biomedicine. *J Appl Biomed*. 2006; 4: 73–86. Available at http://www.zsf.jcu.cz/vyzkum/jab/4_2/halberg2.pdf.

106. Güllner HG, Bartter FC, Halberg F. Timing antihypertensive medication. *Lancet*. 1979; Sept 8: 527.

107. Levine H, Halberg F. Clinical aspects of blood pressure autorhythmometry. In: Scheving LE, Halberg F, Pauly JE, eds. *Chronobiology, Proceedings of the International Society for the Study of Biological Rhythms*, Little Rock, Arkansas. Tokyo: Igaku Shoin Ltd; 1974 406–414.

108. Zaslavskaya RM, Varshitsky MG, Teibloom MM. *Effectiveness of chronotherapy of hypertensive patients with hypotensive drugs*. In: Tarquini B, ed. *Social Diseases and Chronobiology*. Bologna: Esculapio; 1987: 373–380.

109. Cornélissen G, Zaslavskaya RM, Kumagai Y, Romanov Y, Halberg F. Chrono-pharmacologic issues in space. *J Clin Pharmacol*. 1994; 34: 543–551.

110. Cornélissen G, Halberg F, Prikryl P, Dankova E, Siegelova J, Dusek J. International Womb-to-Tomb Chronome Study Group. Prophylactic aspirin treatment: the merits of timing. *JAMA*. 1991; 266: 3128–3129.

111. Siegelova J, Cornélissen G, Dusek J, Prikryl P, Fiser B, Dankova E, Tocci A, Ferrazzani S, Hermida R, Bingham C, Hawkins D, Halberg F. Aspirin and the blood pressure and heart rate of healthy women. *Policlinico (Chrono)*. 1995; 1(2): 43–49.

112. Hermida RC, Fernández JR, Ayala DE, Iglesias M, Halberg F. Time-dependent effects of ASA administration on blood pressure in healthy subjects. *Chronobiologia*. 1994; 21: 201–213.

113. Moore JG, Goo RH. Day and night aspirin-induced gastric mucosal damage and protection by ranitidine in man. *Chronobiology Int*. 1987; 4: 111–116.

114. Nold G, Drossard W, Lehmann K, Lemmer B. Daily variation of acute gastric mucosal injury after high- and low-dose acetylsalicylic acid. *Biol Rhythm Res*. 1995; 26: 428.

115. Nold G, Drossard W, Lehmann K, Lemmer B. Gastric mucosal lesions after morning versus evening application of 75 mg or 1000 mg acetylsalicylic acid (ASA). *Naunyn-Schmiedeberg's Arch Pharmacol*. 1995; 351: R17.

116. Prikryl P, Cornélissen G, Neubauer J, Prikryl P Jr, Karpisek Z, Watanabe Y, Otsuka K, Halberg F. Chronobiologically explored effects of telmisartan. *Clin Exp Hypertens*. 2005; 2 & 3: 119–128.

117. Cornélissen G, Halberg F, Schwartzkopff O, Gvozdjakova A, Siegelova J, Fiser B, Dusek J, Mifkova L, Chopra RK, Singh RB. Coenzyme-Q10 effect on blood pressure variability assessed with a chronobiological study design. In: *Noninvasive Methods in Cardiology*, Brno, Czech Republic, September 14, 2005. Brno: Masaryk University; 2005: 10.

118. Gong L, Zhang W, Zhu Y, Zhu J, Kong D, Page V, Ghadirian P, LeLorier J, Hamet P. Shangai trial of nifedipine in the elderly (STONE). *J Hypertens*. 1996; 14: 1237–1245.

119. Liu L, Wang JG, Gong L, Liu G, Staessen JA, for the Systolic Hypertension in China (Sys-China) Collaborative Group. Comparison of active treatment and placebo for older Chinese patients with isolated systolic hypertension. *J Hypertens*. 1998; 16: 1823–1829.

120. Shinagawa M, Kubo Y, Otsuka K, Ohkawa S, Cornélissen G, Halberg F. Impact of circadian amplitude and chronotherapy: relevance to prevention and treatment of stroke. *Biomed Pharmacother*. 2001; 55(suppl 1): 125–132.

121. Watanabe Y, Cornélissen G, Watanabe M, Watanabe F, Otsuka K, Ohkawa S- I, Kikuchi T, Halberg F. Effects of autogenic training and antihypertensive agents on circadian and circaseptan variation of blood pressure. *Clin Exp Hypertens*. 2003; 25: 405–412.

122. Tamura K, Kohno I, Saito Yuzo, Wakasugi K, Achiwa S, Imanishi Y, Cugini P, Halberg F. Antihypertensive individualized therapeutic strategy. *Difesa Sociale*. 1991; 6: 109–124.

123. Watanabe Y, Cornélissen G, Halberg F, Saito Y, Fukuda K, Otsuka K, Kikuchi T. Chronobiometric assessment of autogenic training effects upon blood pressure and heart rate. *Perceptual Motor Skills*. 1996; 83: 1395–1410.

124. Watanabe Y, Cornélissen G, Halberg F, Saito Y, Fukuda K, Revilla M, Rodriguez C, Hawkins D, Otsuka K, Kikuchi T. Method and need for continued assessment

of autogenic training effect upon blood pressure: case report. *New Trends Exp Clin Psychiatry.* 1996; 12: 45–50.

125. Overvad K, Diamant B, Holm L, Holmer G, Mortensen SA, Stender S. Coenzyme Q10 in health and disease. *Eur J Clin Nutr.* 1999; 53: 764–770.

126. Langsjoen PH, Langsjoen AM. Overview of the use of CoQ10 in cardiovascular disease. *Biofactors.* 1999; 9: 273–284.

127. Rosenfeldt FL, Haas SJ, Krum H, Hadj A, Ng K, Leong JY, Watts GF. Coenzyme Q10 in the treatment of hypertension: a meta-analysis of the clinical trials. *J Hum Hypertens.* 2007; 21: 297–306.

128. Fok BSP, Cornélissen G, Halberg F, Chu TTW, Thomas GN, Tomlinson B. Different effects of lercanidipine and felodipine on circadian blood pressure and heart rate among hypertensive patients. Abstract 15, HK College of Cardiology, 12th Annual Science Congress. *J Hong Kong Coll Cardiol.* 2004; 12: 33.

129. Cornélissen G, Halberg F, Schwartzkopff O, Delmore P, Katinas G, Hunter D, Tarquini B, Tarquini R, Perfetto F, Watanabe Y, Otsuka K. Chronomes, time structures, for chronobioengineering for "a full life". *Biomed Instrum Technol.* 1999; 33: 152–187.

130. Kumagai Y, Shiga T, Sunaga K, Cornélissen G, Ebihara A, Halberg F. Usefulness of circadian amplitude of blood pressure in predicting hypertensive cardiac involvement. *Chronobiologia.* 1992; 19: 43–58.

131. Watanabe Y, Cornélissen G, Halberg F, Bingham C, Siegelova J, Otsuka K, Kikuchi T. Incidence pattern and treatment of a clinical entity, overswinging or circadian hyperamplitudetension (CHAT). *Scr Medica.* 1997; 70: 245–261.

132. Fossel M. Editorial. *J Anti-Aging Med.* 1998; 1: 239.

133. Picard FJ, Bergeron MG. Rapid molecular theranostics in infectious diseases. *Drug Discov Today.* 2002; 7: 1092–1101.

134. Clayton TA, Lindon JC, Cloarec O, Antti H, Charuel C, Hanton G, Provost JP, Le Net JL, Baker D, Walley RJ, Everett JR, Nicholson JK. Pharmaco-metabonomic phenotyping and personalized drug treatment. *Nature.* 2006; 440: 1073–1077.

135. Shastry BS. Pharmacogenetics and the concept of individualized medicine. *Pharmacogenomics J.* 2006; 6: 16–21.

136. Mukhtar M. Evolution of biomarkers: drug discovery to personalized medicine. *Drug Discov Today.* 2005; 10: 1216–1218.

137. Kent D, Hayward R. When averages hide individual differences in clinical trials. *Am Scientist.* 2007; 95: 60–68.

138. Halberg F. Some correlations between chemical structure and maximal eosinopenia in adrenalectomized and hypophysectomized mice. *J Pharmacol Exp Ther.* 1952; 106: 135–149.

139. Bakken EE. *One Man's Full Life.* Minneapolis, MN: Medtronic Inc; 1999.

140. Bakken EE, Heruth K. Temporal control of drugs. *Ann NY Acad Sci.* 1991; 618: 484–489.

141. Halberg F, Cornélissen G, Otsuka K, Katinas G, Schwartzkopff O. Essays on chronomics spawned by transdisciplinary chronobiology: witness in time: Earl Elmer Bakken. *Neuroendocrinol Lett.* 2001; 22: 359–384.

INDEX

Chronopharmaceutics: Science and Technology for Biological Rhythm-Guided Therapy and Prevention of Diseases, edited by Bi-Botti C. Youan
Copyright © 2009 John Wiley & Sons, Inc.